Venus Envy

Venus Envy

A HISTORY OF

COSMETIC SURGERY

ELIZABETH HAIKEN

THE JOHNS HOPKINS UNIVERSITY PRESS

Baltimore and London

The Johns Hopkins University Press
2715 North Charles Street
Baltimore, Maryland 21218-4319
The Johns Hopkins Press Ltd., London

Library of Congress Cataloging-in-Publication Data will be found
at the end of this book.
A catalog record for this book is available from the British Library.

ISBN 0-8018-5763-5

Contents

Acknowledgments

I have accrued a number of debts while writing this book and am grateful for the chance to acknowledge them publicly.

First, I owe a great deal to my original dissertation committee at the University of California at Berkeley: Paula Fass, Günter Risse, and Todd Gitlin. I thank Paula Fass especially, who from the day she agreed to supervise my senior honors thesis always encouraged me to ask the hard questions, and provided a model of how to do that in her own work. I was fortunate to go through graduate school with a talented, committed, and supportive group of scholars who became friends; for their encouragement, constructive criticism, and blind faith I will be everlastingly grateful to Jesse Berrett, Karen Bradley, Julia Rechter, Tina Stevens, and Jessica Weiss. The Group in the History of Medicine and Culture provided sustenance and challenge; special thanks to Tom Laqueur and David Barnes. For financial support, I thank the Woodrow Wilson National Fellowship Foundation for a Mellon Fellowship in the Humanities, the Graduate Division of the University of California, Berkeley, for a Humanities Research Grant, and the American Association for the History of Medicine for the Richard Shryock medal (1993).

In 1994–95, I had the privilege of holding a postdoctoral fellowship in the History of Health Sciences at the University of California, San Francisco. I thank Günter Risse and Jack Pressman, whose leadership makes the department such a supportive place to work, and the group with whom I shared that year: Bob Bartz, Sally Hughes, JoAnn Lopez, Elizabeth Murray, Deirdre O'Reilly, Nancy Rockafellar, Francis Schiller, Victoria Sweet, Colin Talley, and Michael Thaler.

To my colleagues at the University of Tennessee, who made my first years of full-time teaching enjoyable and reminded me to take time for my own work, I owe a great debt; I am especially grateful to Russell Buhite, to Bruce Wheeler for his unflagging enthusiasm and support, and to Kim Harrison and Penny Hamilton for their unstinting aid. A History Department Enrichment Fund Mini-Grant and a grant from the University of Tennessee, Knoxville, Exhibit, Performance, and Publication Expense (EPPE) Fund aided greatly during the final stages of manuscript preparation.

I am grateful to Dr. Robert Goldwyn for encouraging me to make use of the National Archives of Plastic Surgery, and to curatorial assistant Madeleine Mullin, who helped me do so. I thank Richard Hollinger (who has by now moved on) for the aid he provided during my stay at the Jerome Pierce Webster Library of Plastic Surgery, and Paul Yohannes and Bob Vietrogoski, who helped me wrap things up. For additional research help, I thank Chris Orr of the *San Francisco Chronicle,* Kristine Krueger of the National Film Information Service at the Academy of Motion Picture Arts and Sciences, Michael Shulman of Archive Photos, Nancy Whitten Zinn at the University of California, San Francisco, and the periodical room staffs at the Oakland, California, and Knoxville, Tennessee, public libraries. I am especially grateful to JoLynn Milardovich and the staff of Interlibrary Borrowing Services at the University of California, Berkeley, who with patience and humor demonstrated that successful research is collaborative in the best sense of the word.

Various people read the manuscript, in whole or in part, at different stages, and others listened as I thought through my ideas aloud. Careful and considered readings by Eric Arnesen, Beth Bailey, Jesse Berrett, Cynthia Blair, Hans Pols, Susan Reverby, Jessica Weiss, and particularly Charles Rosenberg, whose patience and commitment to younger scholars is unequaled, made this a far better book than it would otherwise have been. A special thanks to the growing community of feminist scholars— many of them approaching that "certain age"—who have shared with me their humor and their misgivings.

At the Johns Hopkins University Press, I am grateful to M. J. Devaney for her inventive and ingenious talent at hunting down illustrations and to Fred DeKuyper for his sage advice. My best luck was to find an editor whose vision of the book matched mine; to kindred spirit Jacqueline Wehmueller, my heartfelt gratitude. Thanks too to my agent, Beth Vesel, and to Peter Strupp of Princeton Editorial Associates.

For their continued friendship and support, I thank Mark Bradley, Susan Etlinger, Susan Glosser, Lisa and Peter Levi, Amy Segal, Elise Sheffield, Susan Southall, Jane Stahlhut, Melissa Weese-Goodill, and Audrey Wu.

To my far-flung family—Jean McEwen, Matt, Melanie, Sally, and Claire Haiken, Sallie Weissinger, Eric, Melia, Linnea, and Karen Shurig, the Singletons, the Hardings, Fred and Harriet Aibel, and the Content clan—I can only say I could never have done this without you.

Finally, thanks to my grandmother, Marjorie Rickard McEwen, the first woman I ever knew who had a Ph.D., and to Steve, who thinks her faith in me was justified.

Venus Envy

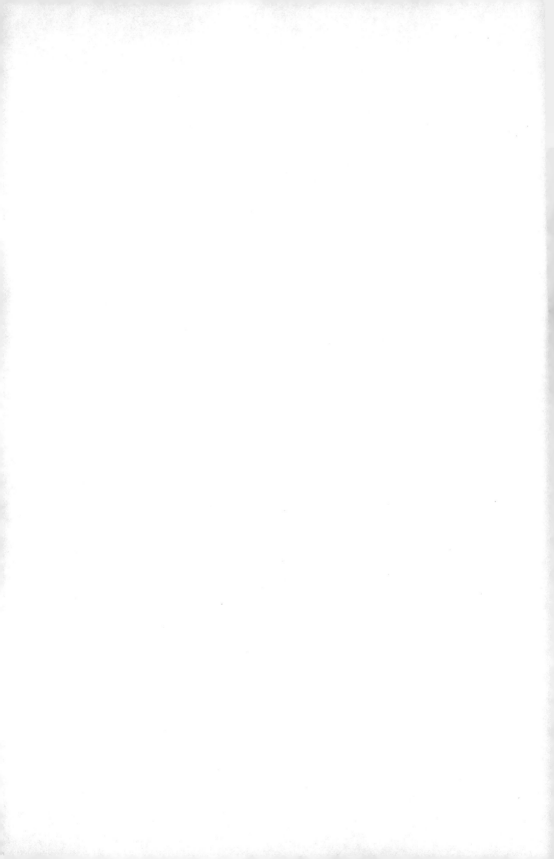

Present at the Re-Creation

In 1923, Americans clamored for an explanation of why Fanny Brice, beloved vaudeville actress, successful comedienne, and star of Florenz Ziegfeld's new Follies, had bobbed her nose. Forty years later, in similar circumstances, Americans asked a very different question. When Barbra Streisand emerged on the national scene—ironically, her first significant role was as Brice in the musical *Funny Girl*—Americans wanted to know why she had not.

That Brice's nose job was performed as a publicity stunt in a hotel room by a traveling quack both reflected and confirmed what most Americans thought about plastic surgery in 1923, just as the "why on earth not" question Streisand repeatedly parried reflected the reality of the early 1960s, by which time the nose job—safe, sterile, predictable, even routine—was simply one of the many wonders of postwar medicine. The inversion of the original question, then, signifies a sea change in American medical and cultural attitudes toward cosmetic surgery and encapsulates the subject of this book.

At the turn of the century, cosmetic surgery appeared to contradict both the traditional American injunction against vanity and the Hippocratic injunction against doing harm. Those surgeons who considered themselves "reputable" (and, as such, undertook to organize the emergent specialty of plastic surgery) believed that by placing healthy patients at risk, cosmetic surgery contradicted the fundamental tenets of the medical profession; "beauty surgery" was the province of quacks

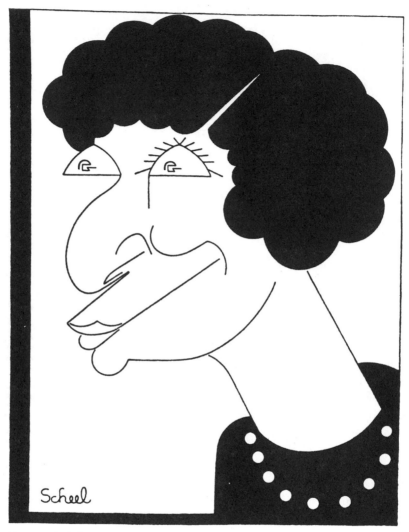

Fanny Brice's face seemed to invite caricature at the beginning of the century...

and charlatans. Like their physicians, most Americans condemned cosmetic surgery. Big noses, small breasts, and wrinkles of all sizes, they believed, were simply facts of life, and the dignity with which one bore them testified to the strength of one's character.

Americans might have been more comfortable with the idea of cosmetic surgery had they viewed it simply as a newfangled form of the

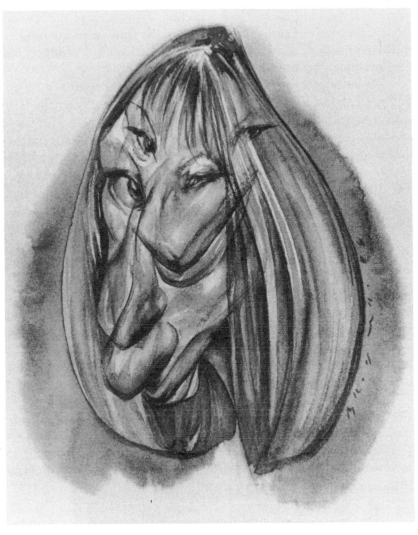

... as does Barbra Streisand's at the end.

vaunted American tendency toward self-improvement, but they did not. Perfectibility, as originally conceived, was defined in religious (or at least spiritual) terms. The physical culture movement of the late nineteenth and early twentieth centuries did encourage Americans to pursue physical perfection, but its adherents, too, framed this project in terms that, if not specifically religious, were at least imbued with spiritual and moral meaning. Steeped in this tradition, most turn-of-the-century Americans regarded cosmetic surgery with the same suspicion modern fitness enthusiasts display toward new pharmaceutical products like fenfluramine-phentermine (fen/phen) and Redux.

Over the course of this century, these conflicts ceased to pose significant barriers to the profession's growth. *Plastic surgery* (the term encompasses both reconstructive and cosmetic surgery) is now one of the largest and fastest-growing medical specialties in the United States. Its clientele increases yearly in both size and diversity, and the entire body—male as well as female—is now within its purview. According to the American Society of Plastic and Reconstructive Surgeons, Inc., between 1982 and 1992 the number of people who approve of plastic surgery increased by 50 percent, while the number who disapprove decreased by 66 percent.[1]

Cosmetic (or aesthetic) surgery, broadly defined as surgery undertaken solely for reasons of appearance, accounts for an increasing proportion of this growth. Aging faces, flat breasts, and small penises, which as facts of life were considered undeserving of medical attention, have been progressively redefined as problems worthy of medical concern and more recently as pathologies or deformities requiring medical solutions.

How, when, and why did so many Americans, over the course of the century, broaden their definition of self-improvement to encompass the pursuit of physical perfection through surgery? And what were the mechanisms by which surgeons, who in the early twentieth century eschewed cosmetic surgery as beneath the dignity of their profession, came to embrace it and to stress its benefits?

Because its development was powered as much by consumer dream and desire as by perceived medical necessity, plastic surgery constitutes a peculiar historical puzzle. But because plastic surgeons proudly proclaim themselves practitioners of both an ancient art and an ancient medical practice, the history of medicine provides one of the essential contexts. Modern surgeons trace their history to India, where, as early as 600 B.C., the Hindu surgeon Sushruta described a method of reconstructing a nose from a patient's cheek: "A careful physician having taken a plant leaf of the size of the nose of that person, and having cut adjoining cheek according to that measurement, and having scarified the nose tip should attach it to the nose tip and quickly join it with perfect sutures." The technique known as the Indian (or forehead) reconstruction rhinoplasty was performed as early as A.D. 1000 (although the first written account of this operation was not published until 1794). Plastic surgeons also claim kinship with Gasparo Tagliacozzi of Bologna, Italy, often credited as the "father of modern plastic surgery." Sometime prior to 1586, inspired by "the great need for plastic operations during the sixteenth century due to the frequent duels, street brawls, and other clashes of armed men," Tagliacozzi pioneered the Italian method of nasal reconstruction, in which a flap from the upper arm is gradually transferred to the nose.[2]

The small group of self-defined "reputable surgeons" who would eventually found and organize the specialty of plastic surgery in the United States agreed that because few surgeons on either side of the Atlantic followed the path Tagliacozzi had forged, not until World War I was plastic surgery "reborn," as an art and a profession; even then, they said, it was a medical response to the medical emergency of modern warfare. The language they used to describe their work evokes the classical context in which they preferred to place themselves; the term *plastic surgery* derives from the Greek *plastikos,* to shape or mold. They chose the term *plastic surgeon* to distinguish themselves from the practitioners they called "beauty doctors" and claimed the inclusive term *plastic surgery* to differentiate their work from what they variously called "featural," "beauty," "cosmetic," or "aesthetic" surgery.[3]

Yet in proclaiming World War I the wellspring of their specialty, these surgeons were claiming a particular version of their history: as Chapter One suggests, interest in "beauty surgery" predated the war. And, while it is clear that those who considered themselves "reputable" took care to distinguish themselves from those they called "beauty doctors," as we see in Chapter Two it is also clear that this latter group, however despised by their more restrained colleagues, did much to shape the specialty.

Medicine remains an important context because plastic surgeons are physicians. Early in the century, plastic surgeons (like most would-be specialists) forged their own paths through medical school, individually sought out apprenticeships with experienced physicians here or in Europe, and struggled to make a place for themselves in medical practice. After World War I, again like many of their colleagues, plastic surgeons organized professional societies, negotiated the boundaries of their specialty, and then—once the specialty was established—attempted to control its image and parameters. Today they attend medical school, complete internships and residencies, work in medical offices, surgical suites, and hospitals, and define their work in medical terms. Like other physicians, they see patients who come to them seeking help and who judge their worth according to their ability to effect cure. And in many ways their specialty has evolved much the same way as has medicine in general. As the World Health Organization now defines health as "complete physical, mental, and social well-being, and not merely the absence of disease or infirmity," so plastic surgeons have come to see their work as facilitating patients' total mental and physical health rather than merely removing a distressing flaw.[4]

The history of medicine, then, provides a natural context for the history of plastic surgery, but it is by no means the only (nor, perhaps, even the most important) context. Its explanatory power is limited because much of plastic surgery—in particular, that part we generally call cosmetic surgery—diverges from other medical practices in fundamental ways. The patients upon whom surgeons perform cosmetic surgery are physically healthy. The diseases for which these patients seek cures—aging, ugliness, poor self-esteem—are many, but they share the characteristic of being difficult to diagnose in the precise terms medicine normally employs. In medical terms, the etiology (causes), nosology (classification), and symptomology (effects) of these diseases are individualized: they are defined by the patient before they are diagnosed by the surgeon, and they are impossible to quantify.

A more significant difference, however, is plastic surgery's unique historical status. Human Growth Hormone and Prozac offer comparatively recent examples of cases in which popularity and public enthusiasm have driven medical developments and shaped the response to them, but plastic surgery was the first, and it is the longest-lived. Largely in response to market demand, plastic surgeons moved to incorporate cosmetic surgical techniques and concerns into their specialty and by doing so created an entirely new range of optional medical treatments that were available for purchase. Equally important is that in doing so they both ratified and reified the medicalized and psychologized culture of twentieth-century America. Plastic surgeons have been influenced by the process of medicalization, "whereby the language and ideology of scientific medicine come to predominate in explanations of human behavior"; that they have equally contributed to it is evidenced by the words practitioners and patients use to describe the conditions for which they seek remedy: ugliness, like many other qualities, has been pathologized. But in this tangled web, the psychological thread is even more significant.[5]

Early in the twentieth century, the interrelated processes of industrialization, urbanization, and immigration and migration transformed the United States from a predominantly rural culture, in which identity was firmly grounded in family and locale, to a predominantly urban culture, in which identity derives from "personality" or self-presentation. The ethos of acquisitive individualism that emerged from this brave new world encouraged Americans to rethink their attitudes toward cosmetic surgery. Today the stigma of narcissism that once attached to cosmetic surgery has largely vanished, leaving in its place the comfortable aura of American pragmatism, with a whiff of an optimistic commitment to self-improvement thrown in.[6]

Chapter Three thus argues that, as both explanation and justification for their move toward cosmetic surgery, surgeons drew from two related developments. Inspired by this new culture, they began to discuss and emphasize as an article of faith the social and economic importance of external appearance, as determined by clear normative standards. A more important shift was that the psychological lens through which Americans were beginning to examine themselves gave cosmetic surgery a new look. The inferiority complex, in particular, offered a compelling explanation and justification for the practice of cosmetic surgery, and it forms the basis for the broader concept of "self-esteem" that is more often used today. Seen through this lens, the decision to alter one's face or body surgically, once taken as a sign of weakness, often becomes a sign of strength—a pragmatic, psychologically healthy response to the (admittedly stringent) requirements of the modern world.

Because it took shape in the public realm, plastic surgery represents a revealing and ambiguous case in the negotiation of professional authority. As in other medical specialties, education, training, and credentials constitute one set of variables that create the plastic surgeon's professional authority. In the case of cosmetic surgery, however, authority derives as much from the patient (and, more broadly, from the realm of the consumer culture the patient both inhabits and embodies) as from the surgeon.

Consider this illustrative case. Miss Cecily Clemons, a twenty-two-year-old secretary at the Singer Sewing Machine Company, wrote to the College of Physicians and Surgeons at Columbia Presbyterian Medical Center in Manhattan on January 11, 1934: "Dear Sirs: I am considering having my nose reconstructed and want information." Do such operations work? Can you recommend a doctor? she asked. Letters of this type (they were not rare) were routinely routed to Jerome Pierce Webster, head of the Division of Plastic Surgery. On January 19, Webster advised Clemons that it was difficult to answer questions without seeing the patient and that, if she wished, she might call for an appointment. Instead, Clemons wrote again on January 27, explaining that it was "simply a matter of appearance. If you do this please let me know," so that she might make an appointment. Webster replied that some conditions could be improved by surgery, while others could not. It was impossible to tell until he saw her, he stressed, but he promised that he would be frank. On March 10, 1934, Clemons and Webster met. Webster's notes on the appointment read, "Very slightly wide. Not large. Strongly advised against having any operation." On June 7 of that year, Clemons penned her final communication to Webster. She was in receipt of his bill, she confirmed, but would not pay it. "When I made the appointment, your secretary said there was no charge for a mere inquiry. As no charge was mentioned in advance and you said you would not handle my sort of case your bill is entirely out of line and I do not feel obliged to send a remittance." In this exchange, Webster exercised his professional authority in refusing her case, but Clemons clearly called the shots in determining the nature, and the price, of their interaction.[7]

In 1934, at twenty-two, Cecily Clemons was a more sophisticated medical consumer than many Americans today, and in fact her age is the only aspect of this transaction that should surprise us. Americans, after all, have long suspected that, in the marketplace of consumer culture, beauty is a commodity whose worth may be quantified. Economists Daniel Hamermesh and Jeff Biddle provided support for this view in 1993, when they concluded that attractive people make more money. Good looks increase one's hourly income by approximately 5 percent, while the lack of looks decreases it by about 7 percent, these researchers found. And while attractive people do tend to congregate in certain occupations, this did not account for the difference. "It's not just a matter of good-looking people going to work in Hollywood and bad-looking people digging ditches," Hamermesh told the *San Francisco Chronicle*. "Even within any given occupation, good-looking people make more."[8]

Yet there is something about the coolness of Clemons's negotiation that does jar us, just as there is something about the conclusions these researchers so dispassionately draw that rankles. For Americans, in fact, have been peculiarly reluctant to acknowledge the "undemocratic fact that beautiful women and handsome men are liked better than homely ones." Like nineteenth-century author Calvin Colton, we prefer to believe that "Ours is a country, where men start from an humble origin. . . . No exclusive privileges of birth, no entailment of estates, no civil or political disqualifications, stand in their path; but one has as good a chance as another, according to his talents, prudence, and personal exertions." Americans have begun to acknowledge the extent to which gender, race, and class have limited opportunities for success, but our culture continues to hold dear a vision of itself as a place in which the length of one's arms and the strength of one's proverbial bootstraps are all that determine one's possibilities. For every American who smiles in grim recognition at the revelation of yet another glass ceiling, another frowns in disbelief.[9]

Yet the idea that beautiful people have a leg up on success is not exactly news. The finding that appearance may determine income could not have come as a surprise to America's women, whose beauty expenditures scandalized commentators as early as the 1920s and who now spend more than $20 billion annually on cosmetics alone and many billions more on diets, clothes, hair care, and surgery. Despite the personal and professional gains women have made in recent years, appearance remains key to women's sense of self-worth. As Mary Lou Weisman observed wryly in her 1984 essay "The Feminist and the Face-Lift," "I do not think . . . that too many men worry that their wives will leave them for a younger, smooth-skinned man." In terms of numbers, the more than fifty athletes who surprised a researcher by saying they would be willing to take a "magic pill" guaranteeing both an Olympic gold medal and death within a year are nothing compared to the 33,000 women who confided to researchers "that they would rather lose ten to fifteen pounds than achieve any other goal."[10]

Women, in fact, have driven, as well as supported, the growth of cosmetic surgery. Granted, women have not always acted freely in the arena of beauty. Consumer culture, in America, has acquired a power that at times approaches coercion, and a variety of other imperatives— such as the post–World War II expansion of the specialty of plastic surgery—have acted in concert with this power. But as Chapter Four suggests, women were more than hapless victims in the story of cosmetic surgery's evolution. They dogged surgeons for solutions to problems they identified. They wrote letters to newspapers, to magazines, to the American Board of Plastic Surgery, and even to their senators, asking for information and help. They researched and published articles about plastic surgery, and they passed information on in informal ways as well—on the job, on the golf course, in the beauty parlor, at the PTA, and sometimes even at home. And, most important, they put their money on the table. Perhaps one of the deepest ironies in this story is that, as a direct result of the economic gains women made in the post–World War II years, by the 1970s and 1980s more women than ever before could afford to buy the things they wanted, and among the goods they bought were smoother faces, bigger breasts, and thinner thighs.

Equally haunting is the indication that, by recognizing "ugliness," diagnosing inferiority complexes, and prescribing surgery, plastic surgeons reproduced and replicated a definition of beauty that clearly derived from and relied on Caucasian, even Anglo-Saxon, traditions and standards. Plastic surgeons claim consistently that the standards of beauty on which they rely are individual rather than normative. Yet as they organized, they chose as their symbol the Venus de Milo, a classic icon of white, western beauty.

It is easy to react with disdain to explanations like that of Hilda Novak, a gentile who told Jerome Webster in 1939 that, while she had always disliked her nose, the "last straw" had come when someone assumed that she was Jewish; such comments, above all, reveal the depth and breadth of American prejudices. But consider the words of surgeon Jacques Maliniak, who at almost the same time proclaimed that "the great masters of art have agreed upon certain criteria—or canons, as they are called—based upon the measurements of models that represent the ideal in form and proportion." Listen, too, to surgeon Henry Junius Schireson, who in 1938 wrote that "composite measurements" made from the beautiful noses of Sunday supplement and magazine cover girls "indicate that the American ideal now is an angle of 28.5 degrees—thus giving the nose a saucy tilt one degree higher than that of the Venus de Milo." Comments like Novak's speak to questions of power, or lack of it, and access to it. The specific attributes Americans seek to alter have changed, as new techniques have expanded the remediable area from noses to faces, through breasts and buttocks, to upper arms and lower legs, but their reasons for seeking surgery have remained remarkably consistent. What most claim to want, and what they believe cosmetic surgery will give them, is the privilege of "civil inattention," which "makes it possible to move unhindered in public places and to conduct one's affairs without fear of personal intrusion." They may feel misgivings about acquiescing to a cultural system that so strongly emphasizes external appearance, but, as practical Americans, they hedge their bets.[11]

Yet there is an irony here too, in that the economic success that has made it possible for more Americans to entertain the idea of cosmetic surgery has not engendered the confidence that leads to self-acceptance. Chapter Five thus traces the way plastic surgeons and their patients have conceptualized and negotiated issues of ethnicity and race and places this process in the larger context of the American project of creating race. Framed as individualism, the project of recreating the self through surgery has led instead to conformity. Only when taken to an extreme, as in the hauntingly fragile face of Michael Jackson, does this trend give us pause.

The rhetoric that has been used to market cosmetic surgery underscores not only how "raced" but how fundamentally gendered is the relationship between supply (provider) and demand (consumer). St. Luke's Hospital in San Francisco made this point in 1992 with a newsletter devoted almost entirely to selling its services in cosmetic surgery. "Denise," a married mother of five and the satisfied recipient of a tummy tuck and a breast lift and enlargement, enthused, "I'm very pleased with what was done. I feel much younger now and much more confident about my body. And I feel that I now have a better relationship with my husband." She continued, "Most cosmetic procedures are not covered by insurance plans, but I was able to work out a package price. . . . There's no way that I would have had the surgery if they hadn't given me such a great deal." The philosophy behind this effort—"Give the customer what she wants at a price she can afford"—has become more common in medicine as practitioners have been forced to take their patients,' or their patients' insurers,' cost-consciousness into account. In "marketing medicine," however, plastic surgeons were pioneers, and until recently their target audience was largely female.[12]

Statistics for cosmetic surgery are notoriously incomplete, but it is clear that until around 1970 women accounted for more than 90—some say 95—percent of patients (and by all available estimates, still account for more than 80%). Female surgeons are even fewer in number than male patients. In the United States, Alma Dei Morani and Kathryn Lyle Stephenson practiced in the middle of the century, and both achieved some prominence in the profession; in recent years more women have chosen to specialize in plastic surgery, but their numbers remain strikingly few. The moniker *Dr. Pygmalion,* which mid-century surgeon Maxwell Maltz chose as the title for his autobiography, thus has a haunting resonance, and it seems appropriate that in Chapter Six, when we turn to the history of sculpting the female form through breast surgery, we return to the subject of gender.[13]

Cosmetic surgery lies at the nexus of medicine and consumer culture. It was the combination of medical knowledge, leisure, and money that made possible its entrance on the American stage in the early years of this century, and it was the confluence of technological prowess, cultural confidence, and postwar abundance that fueled the boom after World War II. As New York plastic surgeon Gustave Aufricht put it in his 1957 article on the "Philosophy of Cosmetic Surgery," everyone recognizes the importance of and awards priority to necessary surgery like reconstruction after cancer, but, fortunately, "life's demands are not always of an emergency matter, of life or death, bread or starvation . . . among other achievements of science for better living, surgery also offers its contribution beyond the absolute necessities."[14]

Thus, while Americans were intrigued by what they read about plastic surgery as an innovative branch of medicine, it was consumer culture that taught them to stop worrying and love the nose job. American journalists' focus on the reconstructive side of plastic surgery ended on Armistice Day. In the 1920s, Americans learned instead about Fanny Brice's nose job and the alleged face-lifts of the Dowager Duchess of Rutland and her daughter, Lady Diana Manners. Those who read the *New York Mirror* could vote to elect the city's homeliest girl, who received free plastic surgery and an opera audition.

The public's fascination with the topic only grew in subsequent decades. In 1935, Americans flocked to theaters to see Bela Lugosi's *The Raven,* in which a sadistic surgeon creates a monster by making a disfigured man even uglier. They came back in 1941 to watch Joan Crawford in *A Woman's Face,* playing a woman whose soul carries a scar larger than the one on her face. They returned again in 1945 to ponder the meaning of beauty during *The Enchanted Cottage,* which starred Robert Young and Dorothy McGuire as an ugly couple who, with the help of a

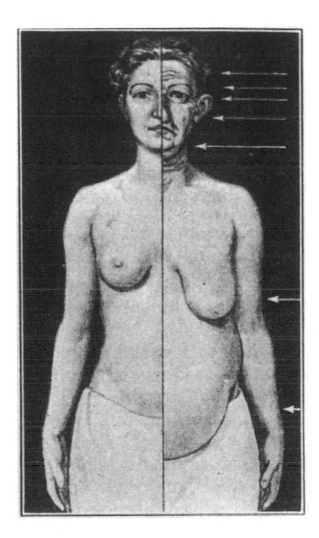

New York plastic surgeon Jacob Sarnoff drew this vision of total transformation—entitled "diagrammatic illustration of common deformities amenable to plastic surgery"—in 1936.

blind friend, come to see that it is enough that their love makes them beautiful to each other. And of course, in 1947, thousands watched breathlessly as Lauren Bacall carefully unveiled Humphrey Bogart's new face in *Dark Passage.* That same year, *Look* readers learned that Milton Berle was so thrilled with his own nose job he had begun to give them as gifts to friends and associates—a practice that had earned him the nickname "Santa Schnozo." By the 1950s, cosmetic surgery was a staple topic of the ever-increasing number of women's magazines, as well as of newspapers across the country, and it would become a staple topic for

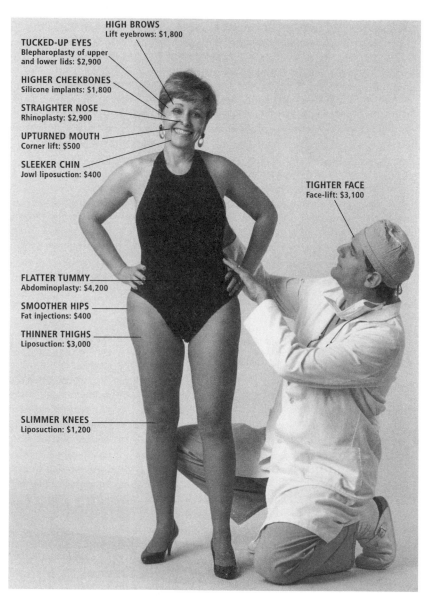

HIGH BROWS
Lift eyebrows: $1,800

TUCKED-UP EYES
Blepharoplasty of upper
and lower lids: $2,900

HIGHER CHEEKBONES
Silicone implants: $1,800

STRAIGHTER NOSE
Rhinoplasty: $2,900

UPTURNED MOUTH
Corner lift: $500

SLEEKER CHIN
Jowl liposuction: $400

TIGHTER FACE
Face-lift: $3,100

FLATTER TUMMY
Abdominoplasty: $4,200

SMOOTHER HIPS
Fat injections: $400

THINNER THIGHS
Liposuction: $3,000

SLIMMER KNEES
Liposuction: $1,200

Plastic surgeon Henry Austin and his wife Carol demonstrate what a complete transformation cost in 1988.

the new medium of television: witness the *Oprah Winfrey Show* on April 29, 1992, "Plastic Surgeons Create Their Perfect Wives."[15]

In one sense, the widespread adoption of the surgical solution reveals a frightening vision of Americans as conformists, bent on achieving a commodified, advertising-driven standard of perfection. Throughout the twentieth century, the public discourse on plastic surgery has not only acknowledged but decried this trend. Every new scandal, every revelation of wrongdoing on the part of a surgeon or a company, elicits cries of outrage and sadness. Every announcement that yet another part of the body, or another category of citizens, has come under the scalpel's purview generates a round of soul-searching: have we come to this? In 1991, the Dow Corning Wright trials generated an extraordinary outcry that was only partially appeased by the decision of the Food and Drug Administration to restrict the availability of silicone breast implants and, two years later, by the largest damage award in consumer history. Yet the specific historical mechanisms that might enable us to understand not just where we have come but how—and by whose guidance—have remained largely unexamined.

They have remained unexamined, I think, because the surgical solution has allowed us to hold on to an idealized self-image: we may dream of kinder, gentler worlds, but we are realists, pragmatists at heart, and above all individualists, bent on creating and recreating ourselves in the most modern of all possible ways. This is the view, presumably, that in 1988 led the editors of *Ms.* to select Cher as "an authentic feminist hero." Given the complexity of the modern world, it is not surprising that individuals conclude that it is easier to change the self: the problem, in other words, clearly lies with the world, but the easiest solution, just as clearly, lies with the patient. But in our readiness to define the problem as too complex to tackle, we have encouraged the belief that the only practical solution is the individual one. Our increasing tendency to individualize social problems of inequality suggests just how fundamentally we have lost faith in the possibility that commitment and collective action can transform the society in which we live.[16]

When I was little—even though, like most small children, I was cute—my favorite fairy tale was the Ugly Duckling. Over and over again, I empathized with that poor pathetic little creature, and I shared its triumph when it became beautiful and flew away. As an adolescent, I was convinced I was hideous. Chubby, gawky, sporting both braces and glasses, I spent my time reading and dreaming about being someone else; when my grandmother took me to see the musical *A Chorus Line,* the phrase "different is nice but it sure isn't pretty; pretty is what it's about" is the one I came out singing. When I came across the feminist version of Duckling—in which a fairy godmother gives a teenaged princess a magic mirror with the power to alter her every feature and attribute and the princess, after experimenting with a wide variety of transformations, decides that she likes herself best the way she is—I rolled my eyes in disbelief. Anyone dumb enough to fall for that trick, I thought, deserved to stay ugly.

But I was blessed with a father who kept a photo of me, in profile, on his desk because he said it showed strength, and a mother who told me that, while I would never be pretty, I would be elegant and interesting, which was much better. I did not of course believe them then, but, like the fairy godmother in the tale I dismissed, they were right. And while I am reluctant to judge those who seek surgery, today I tell my nieces the modern version rather than the original.

CHAPTER ONE

Plastic Surgery Before and After

Two seemingly unrelated events occurred in the late summer of 1921. On August 8, Dr. Henry Sage Dunning of New York and Drs. Truman W. Brophy and Frederick B. Moorehead of Chicago met at the Chicago Athletic Club to organize the first association in North America of specialists in what would come to be called plastic surgery. Less than a month later, eight contestants participated in the first Miss America pageant, which was held in Atlantic City, New Jersey, on September 5, in a calculated attempt to extend the summer season past Labor Day.

Most plastic surgeons would see the timing of these two inaugural events as a coincidence and an irrelevant one at that. In their view, the history of plastic surgery is the history of medical and surgical practices and techniques; while antecedents can be traced across centuries, surgeons generally agree that the specialty in its modern form dates from World War I. This interpretation suggests that reconstructive surgery predates cosmetic surgery in both a valuative and a chronological sense. During the war, surgeons say, Americans heard and read about new surgical miracles that were seemingly invented daily, as surgeons attempted to treat the unprecedented numbers of facial injuries with which the war presented them. Not until after the war, according to surgeon Max Thorek, did plastic surgery begin to make its way into the American cultural consciousness, as Americans began to realize that these techniques might have potential in civilian life. "No stranger aftermath" developed after the war, Thorek recalled, "than the sudden hope, surging through feminine—and sometimes masculine—hearts, that where nature had been niggardly in her gifts of pulchritude, the knife of the surgeon could remedy the lack. If soldiers whose faces had been torn away by bursting shell on the battlefield could come back into an almost normal life with new faces created by the wizardry of the new science of plastic surgery, why couldn't women whose faces had been ravaged by nothing more explosive than the hand of the years find again the firm clear contours of youth?"[1]

An emphasis on World War I also paints plastic surgery as purely, or at least primarily, a medical phenomenon. The "renaissance" in plastic surgery, surgeons say, was due in part to the significant advances in surgical technique made during the war and in part to the interest and participation that the war inspired among established, reputable surgeons, including Sir Harold Delf Gillies and Sir Arbuthnot Lane of England and Varaztad Kazanjian, Vilray Blair, John Staige Davis, and Jerome Pierce Webster of the United States. The society that would become the American Association of Plastic Surgeons (AAPS) was founded in 1921 as a direct result of the war. What linked these men together, despite their diverse training, was their common interest and their experience in reconstructive surgery during World War I. Almost all of the original members had worked in the various medical establishments that had been founded to address the needs of facially mutilated soldiers; some, such as Vilray Blair, had played pivotal roles.[2]

For many of the "first generation" of American plastic surgeons, World War I was indeed a turning point; for these, interest in reconstructive surgery did predate (and in some cases exclude) an interest in cosmetic surgery. But if some surgeons made the intellectual leap from recreating male faces to creating female faces only after the war's end, others, along with an indeterminable number of prospective patients, had already crossed this chasm. Late-nineteenth- and early-twentieth-century medical literature suggests that the impetus toward plastic surgery had been building among doctors and the public well before the First World War; many of the issues that would shape the field had already been raised. Plastic surgery cannot be viewed solely in a medical context because it is more than a medical practice; in the public mind, at least, it was and is inextricably intertwined with the cultural practice of self-presentation. The specialty's early development, then, must be viewed in a cultural, as well as medical, context—specifically, that of the American culture of beauty. During the decades bridging the turn

of the century, American culture was transformed from "Protestant Victorianism to a secular consumer culture," and American ideas about beauty changed accordingly. Although Victorian culture had held that beauty derived solely from internal qualities of character and health, by 1921 most Americans (and particularly American women) had come to understand physical beauty as an external, independent—and thus alterable—quality, the pursuit of which demanded a significant amount of time, attention, and money.[3]

Thus, the year 1921 is not so much a watershed as a useful point at which to stop and review the converging currents of American medicine and American culture. In 1921, plastic surgery was neither a recognized medical specialty nor a cultural phenomenon. The first association meeting, like the first Miss America pageant, was small. Twenty men were selected as founding members (one of whom died shortly thereafter); only nine were present at the first formal meeting, held in October 1921 in conjunction with the Clinical Congress of the American College of Surgeons. Founding members had received their training in a number of areas and were listed in the *Year Book of the American College of Surgeons* under various headings, including oral surgery, laryngology, rhinology-laryngology, rhino-oto-laryngology, and surgery. And, in 1921, plastic surgery had not yet had a significant impact on American culture. Although some Americans were aware that correction of congenital and acquired deformities such as cleft lips and palates and saddle noses might be attempted, the "nose job" as we know it was comparatively uncommon, face-lifts were brand new, and body surgery for cosmetic purposes was unknown, although some dreamt of it.[4]

But however coincidental, the proximity in timing of the meeting and the pageant suggests a new perspective through which to view the history of plastic surgery. When placed in the broader context of American culture in general and of the American culture of beauty in particular, plastic surgery in 1921 appears to have had the makings of a cultural, as well as a medical, phenomenon.

Beauty and Surgery at the Turn of the Century

Late-nineteenth- and early-twentieth-century medical literature reveals that physicians were not only beginning to experiment with some of the operations that would supply the modern plastic surgeon's arsenal but also to discuss many of the concerns that would shape the profession well

into the twentieth century. Two stories in particular—one of a medical practice and one of a medical practitioner—offer a window onto the world of plastic surgery in these years. The practice of injecting paraffin and the career of Charles C. Miller have been largely relegated to footnotes in medical histories, but they illuminate some of the ways in which cultural beliefs and medical practices influence each other. Specifically, they suggest that physicians, as they began to explore ways to correct physical flaws, shared with other Americans prevailing cultural concerns about beauty, aging, gender, and economic status.

Surgeons in Europe and the United States began to experiment with nasal operations in the late nineteenth century. Rochester, New York, surgeon John Orlando Roe published the first reports of intranasal rhinoplasty (in which incisions are hidden inside the nose) in 1887 and 1891. Dr. John B. Roberts, in 1892, assured his colleagues that "nearly all undesirable distortions of the nose can be improved or entirely corrected by cosmetic operation . . . the Roman nose, the Jewish nose, and the nose with an angular prominence on its dorsum can, in many instances, be satisfactorily modified." Dr. J. P. Clark presented a "case operated on for exaggerated Roman Nose" at the Massachusetts General Hospital in 1901.[5]

Although Drs. Roe, Roberts, and Clark were concerned with reducing large noses, most early nasal operations were undertaken to build up the condition, much more common then than now, called "saddle-nose." A saddle-nose can be inherited or caused by trauma, an abscess, or infection, but scrofula, lupus, and especially syphilis were the more common causes. The Wassermann test, which provided the first reliable means of identifying syphilis, was invented in 1906, and arsenical compounds such as Salvarsan (immortalized as *Dr. Ehrlich's Magic Bullet* by Edward G. Robinson in the Warner Bros. 1940 feature film) were used with some success to treat it after 1909, but the Wassermann was not foolproof and the arsenicals were far from perfect. As William Osler advised Johns Hopkins University medical students in these years, "Know syphilis in all its manifestations and relations, and all other things clinical will be added unto you." Not until penicillin was found to be effective against syphilis in 1943 was a simple and predictable cure found.[6]

Surgeons who attempted to correct depressed noses were aware that they were responding to a cultural, as well as a medical, problem. Syphilis was popularly viewed as the scourge of the American landscape, and Americans knew that one of the most common results of untreated syphilis

was a depressed nose. As New York surgeon Joseph Safian observed in a 1926 radio address, "Many persons with a saddle nose . . . are suspected of having inherited disease and are greatly handicapped, both in their social and business relations." Dr. James T. Campbell of Chicago also noted the stigma such a nose might evoke: "The unfortunates with depressed noses are subject to remarks and stares of the thoughtless and the ignorant. . . . By shaping their features like those of normal men, we will earn their lasting gratitude."[7]

The "saddle-nose deformity," as it was called, was particularly difficult to treat because adding substance to the human body is harder than subtracting it. Some surgeons had recorded attempts to build up noses using internal prostheses or bone and cartilage grafts, but these techniques were challenging, time-consuming, and often unsuccessful. Grafts sometimes failed to take, and the human body, they found, had an unfortunate tendency to reject foreign substances such as ivory, often years later. Paraffin, in contrast, seemed ideal. It was relatively easy to inject, it did not require any troublesome incisions, and, at least initially, it appeared to remain inert once introduced into the body.

Apparently simultaneously, J. Leonard Corning, a New York City neurologist, and Viennese physician Robert Gersuny began to experiment with paraffin in the late nineteenth century, and news of this apparently ideal substance began to spread through the medical community. In September 1903, Leadville, Colorado, physician F. Gregory Connell noted cautiously that although the surgical use of paraffin was still "more or less" experimental, its potential was rapidly increasing: "prosthetic operations, undertaken solely for cosmetic effect," he forecast confidently, "should be absolutely harmless." Apparently successful in treating saddle-noses, paraffin quickly came to be seen, by some practitioners, as an instant panacea for soft-tissue defects: it was used to fill out facial wrinkles, in one case to create a testicle, and was rumored to have been injected into breasts.[8]

Paraffin, however, proved not to be the miracle cure originally described. Physicians soon began to observe that it had an unfortunate tendency to migrate, particularly if patients spent time in the sun. More seriously, many recipients began to develop paraffinomas, or "wax cancers." Removing paraffin proved to be much more difficult than injecting it; the process often left the patient severely scarred. These findings worried doctors, but they were loath to abandon a practice that had seemed to hold such promise; instead, they experimented with different mixtures of substances and different methods and temperatures of injection. Gersuny, for example, had used, at different times, paraffin and Vaseline, Vaseline alone, or Vaseline with olive oil. Dr. J. Carlyle DeVries of Chicago described the use of unadulterated paraffin as "almost medieval in its brutality" and advised also against mixing paraffin with either goose grease or white oak bark, recommending instead "a mixture of white vaseline, white wax, a shade of glycerin and a shade of paraffin," all of which was to be boiled with carbolic acid "to render it antiseptic."[9]

By 1920, these recipes had also proved problematic, and most reputable physicians had abandoned the practice of injecting paraffin, adulterated or not. Dr. Seymour Oppenheimer of New York, who that year chronicled paraffin's rise and fall, tried to draw some lessons from the episode. He attributed paraffin's meteoric rise in popularity to the belief, common among even "skilled and well-recognized surgeons and rhinologists," that "the operation was practically without pain, caused no scars . . . and corrected nasal deformities that could not well be overcome otherwise." The more significant problem, however, was the widespread awareness and fear of the moral implications of such deformities that drove public demand and made patients particularly vulnerable: "The charlatans, the advertising 'beauty doctor' and others of that ilk were quick to see the possibilities in a financial sense in its appeal to the popular imagination, and seized upon the method with avidity, and with this added to their armentarium reaped, and still reap, a harvest from the willing victims among the laity." He called on his colleagues to participate in an educational campaign to inform the public that paraffin injections, while "dangerous even in the hands of the well-equipped surgeon," were "doubly more dangerous . . . at the hands of the ignorant, unscrupulous and uneducated 'beauty doctor.'"[10]

As plastic surgeon Robert M. Goldwyn has observed, "What emerges [from the story of paraffin] is the too-familiar sequence of the introduction of a treatment, its avid acceptance without sufficient testing, and its disastrous sequelae for many patients." From a medical viewpoint, this is an accurate description of the episode: the practice of injecting paraffin is simply one of many footnotes to medical history, albeit one that foreshadowed the later experience with silicone and may yet prove analogous to the more recent case of collagen.

But the medical literature related to paraffin also suggests that, well before the First World War, surgeons were beginning to identify and discuss issues we tend to assume are of more recent vintage, including the social value of beauty and the social cost of ugliness, and the clear financial potential of surgery with a cosmetic goal. Moreover, surgeons' desire to differentiate themselves, as responsible, reputable members of the medical profession, from the so-called quacks on the profession's fringes, and their commitment to educating the public about this difference, suggest that they were watching with interest not only their colleagues' moves toward specialization but also the impressive growth of the American beauty business.[11]

In the late nineteenth and early twentieth centuries, according to historian Lois Banner, "natural" standards of beauty vied with artificial ones. Both feminist and progressive thought advocated natural beauty, and beauty literature influenced by these schools of thought was highly moralistic: the development of character, combined with living right, eating right, and even thinking right, were the means by which women might achieve true beauty. But inventiveness and advancing technologies, revealed in new cosmetics and hair care techniques and publicized through equally new marketing and advertising strategies, combined with the cultural imperative of consumption for pleasure to undermine Victorian strictures against the artificial enhancement of beauty. With the advent of consumer culture after the turn of the century, in short, outward appearance, achieved solely by external means made available by the growth of commercial beauty culture, easily superseded inner character in the quest for beauty.[12]

On the economic level, the new consumer beauty culture appeared to advance American democratic principles by offering advantageous career opportunities, with more autonomy and higher salaries than most other fields open to women. As *Woman Beautiful* magazine reported, by 1907 America had 36,000 female hairdressers (compared to 18,000 in 1900 and only 9,000 in 1890); 25,000 manicurists and 30,000 specialists in face massage and skin culture were also women. But the democratic implications of the beauty business extended beyond the economic level. By making the same tools available to all women and by enabling all women, regardless of the vagaries of birth, to achieve beauty, Americans believed, the new beauty culture stemmed from and fostered democratic impulses. Contemporary observers placed the beauty culture squarely within America's democratic tradition of self-improvement. According to *Woman Beautiful,* "the cult of the beauty specialist is the cult of decent respect for oneself, of optimistic belief in one's heritage of beauty and a desire to come into one's own." Writer Elinor Glyn similarly commended the beauty parlor for improving American life by engendering "a greater feeling of self-respect and hope amongst all classes." It was, she noted, "difficult to exaggerate the importance of the influence of the 'Beauty Parlor' on American life."[13]

Although many Americans believed that the beauty business offered women equality, it clearly offered them equality only with one another, not with men. The discussion of aging in these years offers an interesting perspective on just how "democratic" America's beauty culture was. In contrast to nineteenth-century standards, which more or less classified women over thirty-five as elderly, the early twentieth century was, some claimed, a "Renaissance of the Middle Aged." The extent of the change, however, was limited. As Lois Banner argues, it was not that the "normal physical attributes of old age—white hair, wrinkles, sagging muscles" came to be seen as beautiful or accepted as the natural result of women's life experiences. Rather, "the cultural prohibitions against older women's attempting to look youthful were dropped," and older women were encouraged to join their younger sisters in the democratic arena of beauty. Some saw this as a liberating development for older women, but others believed its effects were mixed. Women were given to understand that they must avoid mental and physical exertion to avoid the appearance of aging—that conserving unwrinkled skin was more important than anything else they might achieve—and older women were not only allowed, but expected, to spend time and effort maintaining their looks.[14]

Whether or not the expanded opportunities the consumer beauty culture offered compensated women for the new demands on their time and energy is debatable. There can, however, be no doubt that the market women identified and created was large and growing, and that men, as well as women, took advantage of it. The women who shaped the new beauty culture were undoubtedly influenced by the many irregular physicians who set up "colleges" and "schools" in this era and who claimed to represent a new specialization within the medical profession. According to muckraking journalists, many beauty salons, as well as dermatologists and "featural specialists," offered paraffin injections, as well as the option of face peeling or skinning. Both the business of beauty and the profession of medicine were in the process of formation in these years, and practitioners borrowed widely from one another as they attempted to carve out satisfying and lucrative practices.[15]

Dr. Charles C. Miller of Chicago was one such pioneer. One plastic surgeon has called him "the father of modern cosmetic surgery," while others have called him "an unabashed quack." But despite his dubious reputation, Miller's story deserves more than a footnote. In his many articles and books, Miller articulated the overwhelming contemporary concern with beauty and anticipated many of the themes that continue to shape the specialty, including the social and market value of beauty and the effect aging had on women's social, economic, and mental status. Even more prophetic was his vision of the part cosmetic surgery would play in the modern world.[16]

A brief review of Miller's career is sufficient to explain why plastic surgeons have been reluctant to include him in their genealogy. Born in 1880 in New Albany, Indiana, Miller graduated from the Hospital College of Medicine in Louisville, Kentucky, in 1899. He set up practice in Chicago and taught clinical surgery at a small medical college. In 1906 he began to publish articles on "featural surgery," a seemingly endless series of which appeared in county, state, and some national medical journals. In 1907 alone he published more than twenty articles, as well as a textbook entitled *Cosmetic Surgery: The Correction of Featural Imperfections.* Between 1908 and 1923, Miller published little, perhaps because of legal problems resulting from his acknowledged ownership of three "quack" drugstores in the Chicago area, which the *Chicago Daily Tribune* targeted in its Progressive era campaign against narcotic misuse. The charge of selling drugs without a prescription was dropped in 1914 when the *Tribune* reporter failed to appear in court.[17]

Miller reappeared in 1915 as editor of a lay publication entitled *Medicine and Health.* He opened a new office in Chicago's fashionable New North Side, to which his tireless recruiting reportedly drew flocks of patients. His 1907 textbook was reissued in 1924, and in 1927 he began publishing his own journal, *Dr. Charles Conrad Miller's Review of Plastic and Esthetic Surgery,* copies of which seem not to have survived. In addition to reducing humped noses and bulbous nasal tips, building up small noses, and lifting faces, Miller described operations to correct crow's feet, eyelid, forehead, and nasolabial wrinkles, thick and thin lips, large, small, and protruding ears, and excessively small or large mouths, as well as an original method for creating dimples. In his more adventurous articles, Miller advocated "subcutaneous dissection" of certain facial nerves and muscles to prevent formation of the "expression lines" to which he believed women were particularly prone. The later

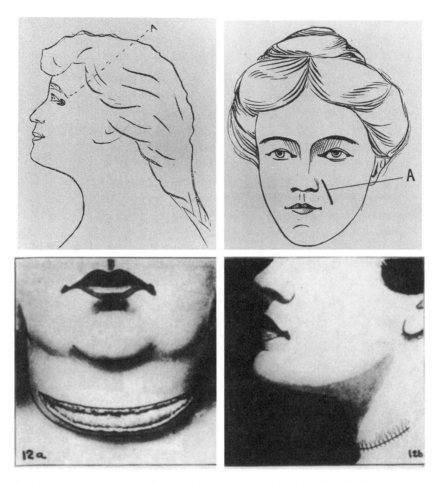

Excising crow's feet, preventing wrinkles, and correcting a double chin, from Charles C. Miller's *Cosmetic Surgery: The Correction of Featural Imperfections* (1907 and 1924).

years of his career are shrouded in obscurity, although the 1924 edition of his text suggests that he abandoncd his pathbreaking "featural" work in favor of a return to general surgery. After his first wife's suicide in 1930, Miller married again and fathered three children. He died of a heart attack in 1950.[18]

Like those who used paraffin to correct congenital and acquired deformities, Miller acknowledged the power of social forces and images, but he was explicit about his interest in what would come to be known as cosmetic surgery. The "defects" to which he directed his attention were primarily those of luck and age, and he optimistically proclaimed his belief that others would come to share his conviction that these were as deserving of attention as any others. In the "prefatory remarks" to his textbook, he recalled, "Four or five years ago ethical practitioners laughed or grew hostile when I mentioned my interest in elective surgery of the face for the correction of featural imperfections which were not actual deformities. Two years ago medical publishers refused to consider a manuscript upon the subject. Today . . . it is established beyond a doubt that featural surgery is destined to take its place as a recognized specialty."[19]

For those who remained in doubt, Miller offered a compelling argument, which anticipated his colleagues' thinking, if it did not directly shape it. Escalating coverage in the lay press, he asserted, was exacerbating Americans' preoccupation with physical beauty and increasing public demand for surgery. "For years," he warned in 1907, "the newspapers and magazines have been devoting many pages to 'Beauty Chats,' 'Beauty Hints,' etc., and the people have gradually developed a desire for knowledge of those means which will enable them to appear to the best advantage. 'The Beauty Page' . . . continually hints at the possibilities of surgery." This coverage was dangerous not just because it sparked dreams of beauty but because those same publications carried scores of advertisements for unqualified practitioners. "Unscrupulous charlatans" and "advertisers of indifferent ability" were, according to Miller, "reaping a harvest of dollars" and leaving in their wake "mutilations and disfigurements, which mean the lifelong distress of their unhappy victims."[20]

For this, Miller blamed neither the charlatans nor the gullible patients, but the physicians who did not take seriously their patients' needs. "Physicians cannot longer disregard the effect of the 'Beauty Columns,'" Miller insisted. "Every practitioner who laughs at the paticnt who questions him regarding an operation for improving the appearance of the face takes the chance of seeing that patient return from the advertiser disfigured for life." Although he voiced some sympathy for those physicians whose refusal to perform cosmetic operations reflected their personal convictions, Miller believed that it was too late to turn the tide of public interest: "the demand for featural surgeons is too great on the part of the public."[21]

Finally, Miller argued, doctors should perform cosmetic surgery because it offered a challenging and fulfilling practice. "Operations for improving the appearance cannot be botched," he asserted proudly. "The operator must be skillful and fully capable in this field more than in any other." He wished to encourage reputable physicians to participate in part because "it promises to be, before many years, a most profitable and satisfactory specialty"—satisfactory not just for the financial potential it offered but also because it contributed to "the future happiness and peace of mind of the patient," who was, predictably, almost invariably envisioned as female.[22]

Assessing Miller's contribution to plastic surgery is difficult, in part because his published work is hyperbolic; he was obsessed with the importance of feminine beauty and sought to portray himself as women's sole ally in the quest for beauty. While his articles and books were lavishly illustrated, they included few photographs; it is thus difficult to deduce whether or not he actually performed all of the operations he described (and, if he did, what kind of long-term results he achieved). Finally, as one surgeon has noted, although the title "father of cosmetic surgery . . . implies a generative role, . . . Miller . . . remained always a solitary figure, working in the eddies outside the mainstream of plastic surgery. He left no school of followers. Few of the next generation of plastic surgeons (even those in Chicago) have ever heard of him."[23]

Miller may indeed have been a quack with no "generative" legacy; certainly, in later years, plastic surgeons who rediscovered or reinvented the surgical practices Miller advocated, and the arguments he used to justify them, believed themselves original. To say that he practiced "outside the mainstream of plastic surgery," however, does not tell us much, especially as it was during these years that those in the mainstream of plastic surgery (if there was one) were enthusiastically injecting paraffin and other substances into patients. Miller's defense of cosmetic surgery—which began by identifying public demand as a driving force, moved on to paint cosmetic surgery as a form of public protection, and closed with a reference to "peace of mind"—anticipated the reasoning of the first official generation of plastic surgeons, who began to organize the specialty after the First World War. It is perhaps the greatest irony of Miller's story that he is remembered only as one of the quacks he so prolifically condemned.[24]

The First World War and the First Generation

With the advent of World War I, those who would later be hailed as plastic surgery's "first generation" entered the field. The war drew general surgeons, dentists and dental surgeons, otolaryngologists, and others into the practice of plastic surgery, but Miller was not among them. Perhaps he was preoccupied with his legal affairs, or perhaps his experience with cosmetic surgery was regarded as irrelevant to the pathbreaking maxillofacial surgery that war injuries required. Reflecting the concerns of soldiers and surgeons alike, almost everything the American public heard about plastic surgery during the war years concerned reconstructive rather than cosmetic efforts.

World War I resulted in staggering numbers of casualties, and facial wounds were immediately recognized as "both a surgical and a social problem." Injuries to the mouth and jaws were not unknown prior to the war. Surgery for malignant disease sometimes resulted in bone or soft-tissue loss, as did fights, falls, and carriage and elevator accidents, but in general, as one surgeon recalled, "prior to 1915, the treatment of maxillofacial injuries was not one of the major preoccupations of surgery." This changed, suddenly and dramatically, with the advent of World War I, and the change was evident early on. Trench warfare meant that heads and necks were particularly vulnerable. The provision of steel helmets saved many lives but contributed to facial injury, as fragments of helmets (and of the projectiles that shattered on them) often hit the soldiers' unprotected faces. Pilots and passengers in the new and dangerous airplanes often suffered serious facial injuries during crashes. According to one surgeon, war injuries resulted in a greater loss of bony framework than did the civilian injuries with which surgeons were familiar, and the situation was further complicated by the fact that several days might elapse before a wounded soldier arrived at a base hospital. Facial injuries and resulting deformities received great attention not just because they were visible and often horrifying, but because these particular types of injuries were among the most numerous.[25]

At the beginning of the war, the British Army had no dental corps and only fifteen dentists. After meeting with Sir William Osler in London early in 1915, Ambassador Robert Bacon suggested to James Lowell, then president of Harvard, that the university participate in sponsoring a medical aid unit. Harvard, Columbia, and Johns Hopkins subsequently joined in sponsoring the first Harvard Unit, consisting of about thirty-five physicians and surgeons, three dentists, and seventy-five nurses, all of whom were commissioned as officers in the Royal Army Medical Corps. Among those for whom the founding of the first Harvard Unit was a career turning point was Varaztad Kazanjian, then a dentist with two years of medical school, who was appointed chief dental officer. The unit's members left New York on June 26, 1915, and after spending two weeks in London observing their colleagues' work, sailed for France on July 17.[26]

The American doctors were immediately confronted with facial wounds so horrifying that, as Kazanjian later recalled, "no one knew what to do with them." Kazanjian's skill and inventiveness at wiring small fragments of jaws together, devising splints to hold the jaws of patients who had no remaining teeth, and constructing internal facial splints of vulcanized rubber, which would essentially prevent the patient's face from contracting until more extensive bone grafting could be attempted in the States, earned him the name "the miracle man of the Western Front." Under his direction, the hospital where the Harvard Unit operated became the British Army's first Maxillofacial Treatment Center in France. Although the general policy was to return wounded soldiers to England within three weeks, Kazanjian was authorized to keep those who wished to remain for further treatment, and many did: "The severely wounded and disfigured men," he later recalled, "were loath to be seen by members of their families." The *New York Times* proudly reported, "the skill of American dentistry holds undisputed first place, and is particularly highly esteemed in France."[27]

Perhaps the most famous wartime establishment for facial surgery was Queen's Hospital at Sidcup in Kent. Early in 1916 the Royal Army Medical Corps had established the Cambridge Military Hospital under Sir Arbuthnot Lane. Lane convinced the queen to sponsor the new establishment when existing facilities proved inadequate for the large number of casualties generated by the battle of the Somme. To direct Sidcup, Lane chose Harold Delf Gillies, a young otolaryngologist from New Zealand, who had been inspired by French surgeon Hippolyte Morestin's work at Val-de-Grâce military hospital near Paris and had subsequently become Lane's assistant. He was supported by American, British, and Commonwealth doctors and surgeons.[28]

The experimental approach characteristic of both the American and British medical services resulted in new developments in many areas. One was anesthesia. Surgeons and patients alike detested ether and chloroform, initially the only available anesthetics. Surgeons found them unsatisfactory because they needed to be reapplied during long operations, which meant that the anesthetist had to touch the patient and, in the process, contaminate the surgical field. Patients hated them because they were unpleasant: one surgeon recalled that "the sight of a man in a white coat hovering near with a chloroform bottle and gauze pad in one hand and a tongue forceps in the other terrified a generation of soldiers." At Sidcup, anesthetists worked with Gillies to develop new techniques. The tubed pedicle was equally important. Devised independently by Vladimir Petrovich Filatov, an ophthalmic surgeon in Odessa, Russia, in 1916 and by Gillies at Sidcup in 1917, the tubed pedicle enabled surgeons to transfer skin in stages from one location to another while maintaining the blood supply, which helped to ensure that grafts would take. Some soldiers may have been dubious about participating in such experiments, but in general they were grateful for surgeons' efforts. One surgeon recalled that the plastic surgical service's "effect on morale throughout the Army was widespread and entirely beneficial. For the first time the Army knew something was being done to return men to civilian life whatever their facial disfigurements."[29]

Although surgeons emphasized that function was their primary goal, they were committed to restoring patients' appearance. Facial disfigurements were particularly debilitating because they were visible; they could not be covered up by clothes or gloves. As Lane observed, "It's the poor devils without noses and jaws, the unfortunates of the trenches who come back without the faces of men that form the most depressing part of the work." Their families may love them and their country may honor them, he noted, but "the race is only human, and people who look as some of these creatures look haven't much of a chance." Surgeons' commitment to improving their patients' appearance reflected patients' concerns. As one surgeon recalled: "We know from a considerable experience the patient wants to be left as nearly normal in appearance as possible. He will undergo untold hardships to be restored to the normal. This rule has no exceptions. . . . What is the use of life if he is not in a condition to seek and to earn a livelihood, is the view that the patient who wishes to support himself takes."[30]

This last point is significant, because for soldiers (all of whom were male) wartime surgery was driven by the goal of economic independence—the ability to secure a job and support self and perhaps family. Early in 1916, Mrs. William K. Vanderbilt excitedly told readers of the *New York Times* about her visit to the American Ambulance Hospital in France. She acknowledged that many of the men looked "frightful" when they came in, but assured readers that the condition was temporary as the "big thing" at the hospital was "re-making": "The Ambulance takes these torn, mutilated beings, without any faces, who would otherwise be unbearably repulsive and almost certainly economically dependent, and makes them over. It turns them into normal men again, so that they can live normal lives, as individuals, and be of service to their country as well." Mrs. Vanderbilt emphasized that such surgical work carried economic significance on a national as well as an individual level: it would allow them to reenter society, whereas without it they would remain public wards. Miss Eve Hammond of San Francisco, who spent five years in Europe working with the facially wounded under the auspices of the Red Cross, concurred with Mrs. Vanderbilt's enthusiasm: "The things that can be done to make it worth while for [a wounded soldier] to go on living . . . were surprising to us, to whom they were an everyday matter, and to the uninitiated they were a revelation."[31]

Doctors, too, hailed the new miracles. In 1918, Major George A. Stewart of the Rockefeller Institute's War Demonstration Hospital told *New York Times* readers that medicine and surgery had advanced a half century in four years. Sir James Mackenzie of the British Medical Mission agreed: "There is no other branch of surgery in which such wonderful progress has been made since the beginning of the war, nor any class of wounded who call more for our sympathies and help." The following year, Dr. William Seaman Bainbridge of the Navy medical corps told *Current Opinion* readers that the surgical work being done was "little short of miraculous . . . one of the greatest triumphs ever achieved by the beneficent art of surgery."[32]

Cosmetic surgery for men would not become significant, in terms of numbers of patients or amount of attention paid to it, until much later in the century. But the equation of manhood with economic independence had become standard in nineteenth-century definitions of masculinity, and, during the war, surgeons and the American public accepted the idea that a man's appearance was crucial to his economic status. True, during these years it was wartime exigency that fostered acceptance of this principle; true too that the repair of serious disfigurement is quite different, in some ways, from the cosmetic improvement of perceived flaws. Yet once the idea that appearance has a market value for men, as well as for women, had been given voice, it would not be easily ignored.

Surgeons and patients made unprecedented progress, but in many cases their best efforts fell short of the challenges the trenches posed. Both the British and the French medical services employed artists to construct full or partial facial masks for those whom surgery could not help further. Only a comparatively small number of soldiers fell into this category, but the poignant experiences of those who made the masks and those who wore them point to some of the limits of plastic surgery in these years. Using photographs of the men taken before the war, Captain Derwent Wood, an artist attached to Britain's Third London General Hospital, created portrait masks "cast and galvanized in silvered copper" and painted in oil. "My work begins when the work of the surgeon is completed," he explained. "When the surgeon has done all he can to restore function, to heal wounds, to support fleshy tissues by bone grafting, to cover areas by skin grafting, I endeavor by means of the skill I happen to possess as a sculptor to make a man's face as near as possible to what it looked like before he was wounded." American socialite and sculptress Anna Coleman Ladd undertook similar work under the auspices of the American Red Cross in France. With her assistants, she eventually produced ninety-seven masks. An American magazine noted that Frenchmen especially appreciated the mustaches and whiskers of fine copper wire, which were sturdy enough to be "pulled and twirled." Leon Dufourmentel, a French otolaryngologist turned surgeon, acknowledged that Ladd's prostheses were invaluable in those cases that could not be repaired surgically, and all surgeons acknowledged that many of those whom surgery did help would bear severe scars for the rest of their lives. Years later, Ernest Hemingway described "les gueules cassées," who still bore visible signs of their war experience: "There were other people too who lived in the quarter and came to the Lilas, and some of them wore Croix de Guerre ribbons in their lapels and others also had the yellow and green of the Médaille Militaire, and I watched how well they were overcoming the handicap of the loss of limbs, and saw the quality of their artificial eyes and the degree of skill with which their

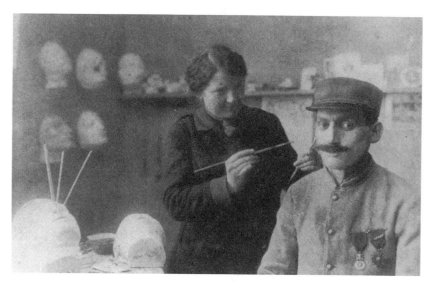

Anna Coleman Ladd puts the finishing touches on a mask.

faces had been reconstructed. There was always an almost iridescent shiny cast about the considerably reconstructed face, rather like that of a well packed ski run, and we respected these clients more than we did the *savants* or the professors."[33]

The First Generation at Home

Although French, British, and American surgeons worked together during the war, plastic surgery grew after the war only in the United States. Gillies was knighted, but while this increased plastic surgery's prestige throughout the British empire, it did not generate significant interest. At Sidcup, he trained "practically no one from Britain"; instead, he trained the American surgeons who came over to study with him. Richard Battle, in 1936 a young British general surgeon considering specialization in plastic surgery, later recalled being told, "Really I do not think you have a chance, my boy. There are four plastic surgeons in the country and I can't think there can be room for more." In France, Leon Dufourmentel was remembered as the only surgeon practicing plastic surgery after the war.[34]

American surgeons, in contrast, returned from the war eager to build the specialty (and by the beginning of World War II would claim about sixty practicing plastic surgeons—more than ten times as many as Britain, and almost twice as many as the rest of the world combined). Kazanjian, who returned to Harvard in 1919 to finish medical school, later recalled that although previously plastic surgery had never been "looked upon too favorably by the medical profession at large," the war "created an interest and demand for reconstructive surgery." Vilray Blair returned from Sidcup to found the plastic surgery department at Washington University School of Medicine and Barnes Hospital in St. Louis, the first separate plastic surgical service in the country; many who had been inspired by his wartime work, including Jerome Webster, made the trek south to study with him. At the Johns Hopkins University, John Staige Davis became the first titled professor of plastic surgery in the United States, following the publication in 1919 of his textbook *Plastic Surgery*, which Frank McDowell, an eminent plastic surgeon, later called "perhaps the first respected book with that title in the English language."[35]

Surgeons realized that the success of the reconstructive work they had undertaken during the war years enabled them to make a claim, however tenuous, for medical legitimacy. Like that of their colleagues in other arenas of medicine who found in their wartime experience a basis for professionalization and organization, the plastic surgical literature of the late teens and early twenties suggests a new self-consciousness, a sense of a profession with a shared past and common aims and goals for the future, that was seldom evident in prewar medical literature. New York surgeon Gustav Tieck, for example, reported in 1920 that he had corrected the noses of more than a thousand patients over the past twelve years. He had hesitated to report his work previously, he stated, because he had wanted to be "absolutely certain of my ground," and he was: "I believe that I have placed this branch of surgery on a definite scientific basis." Seymour Oppenheimer, describing his and others' success in plastic surgery during the war, noted that he was addressing his colleagues "to bring to your notice the advancement of this branch of surgery within the last few years, and to suggest that it be more often employed in civilian practice than has been the custom heretofore."[36]

Wartime reconstructive surgery had enabled surgeons to gain experience and confidence, but the war had also shown them the limits of their knowledge and skill. Physicians and surgeons who wished to practice plastic surgery when they returned home were thus aware that they were in a transitional position. Unlike the well-established field of general or abdominal surgery, plastic surgery was still in its infancy, and while reconstructive surgery had achieved some status, cosmetic surgery was still regarded with suspicion. As Seymour Oppenheimer observed, "Plastic and cosmetic surgery in general has signally failed to keep apace of the tremendous advance which has been made in other domains of surgery, and furthermore, cosmetic surgical endeavors seem to have fallen into more or less disrepute until the advent of the war when reconstruction became the by-word."[37]

The closing days of the "war to end all wars" seemed to signal the likely contraction of reconstructive surgery. At the same time, however, surgeons saw that cosmetic surgery offered great potential for growth. Oppenheimer, for example, noted that although "the world war, with its pressing demands for the practice of reconstructive surgery . . . has not alone brought cosmetic rhinoplasty into its own, ethically speaking," it has "created a great demand for surgical workers. . . . The time seems auspicious . . . for all cosmetic surgery and cosmetic rhinoplasty in particular, to be elevated to its proper dignity in the profession, to be popularized and made available for the large number of individuals in civil life who could be benefited in mind no less than in feature." Ferris Smith of Grand Rapids, Michigan, echoed Oppenheimer's hopes for the future. He prophesied that with the knowledge and techniques developed during the war, and with "restored function with pleasing cosmetic results as an inspiration, there is presented a large, new field of vitally essential and true surgery in one's daily practice." The sense of a process that has been begun but not completed—that is, of a profession trying to establish itself—is evident in these surgeons' words. As evident is the conviction that surgeons intent on practicing plastic surgery would have to convince colleagues and prospective patients that there was a place for such surgery.[38]

As they turned their sights toward the civilian practice of plastic surgery, American surgeons began to address questions that would occupy their profession for years to come. One of the most pressing was which physicians should perform plastic surgery. Before the American Board of Plastic Surgery (ABPS) was established in the late 1930s, those who practiced plastic surgery were trained in a number of different fields. In an important article in 1916, John Staige Davis made perhaps the first significant case for plastic surgery as a separate specialty. Modern surgery had become so vast, Davis argued, that no one surgeon could master the entire field, and at times it had been recognized as necessary to separate from general surgery "special branches which demanded special training, and better facilities for their full development. . . . I feel that the time has come for the separation of [plastic surgery] from the general surgical tree."[39]

Separation was necessary, Davis argued, because plastic and reconstructive surgical operations were particularly difficult and thus were "consistently 'botched.'" Citing Sir Frederick Treves, who in his famous *Manual of Operative Surgery* had stated that "no branch of operative surgery demands more ingenuity, more patience, more forethought, or more attention to detail," Davis wrote, "Plastic surgery is done by nearly every general surgeon in his routine work, and is often attempted by eye, ear, nose and throat specialists, and by those physicians who 'operate only occasionally.' I do not believe that it should be done as a routine by any one of these groups of operators." Rather, Davis believed, plastic surgery should be performed only by specialists with a "definite aptitude" and "a certain amount of imagination," qualities that were requisite to success in this field. Other surgeons agreed. As Ralph St. J. Perry of Minnesota put it, plastic surgery is particularly demanding because the results are visible. Unlike abdominal or other surgery, where the results were hidden, Perry wrote, "the work of the cosmetician is palpable and paraded before the world where it speaks for itself." With such claims, surgeons with their sights set on turning specialists tried to create a perception of legitimacy and expertise to bolster their tenuous position.[40]

In describing their competitors, surgeons pointed to practitioners like Charles C. Miller more often than to "beauty specialists." In 1915, Ralph St. J. Perry had complained that these practitioners "draw many of their patients from our territory—mine and yours." Five years later, Gustav Tieck observed that "the greater part of this work has been performed by quacks of the medical profession and laymen without surgical training." Seymour Oppenheimer, in a virtual "call to arms," urged his colleagues to fight back. It was "all-important," he asserted, "to rescue this class of surgery from the clutches of the charlatan and the advertising 'beauty doctor' whose conspicuous signs and blatant advertisements have long preyed upon and ensnared the credulous among the laity." But while they may have been reluctant to acknowledge publicly that they were competing with beauty parlors for patients, their words—and the overlap that clearly existed between the exuberant world of early beauty culture and the chaos that characterized American medicine as it began to organize—suggest that they were reacting to both.[41]

The realization that beauty, as a business, offered seemingly limitless potential, and that American women would spend as much time and effort, and significantly more money, in the quest for beauty than even the most severely injured soldiers, drove surgeons to confront the most important question that emerged from the war: Was there a difference between reconstructive plastic surgery and cosmetic plastic surgery, and if so, where was the dividing line? Surgeons did not immediately resolve this question (and have not resolved it yet). But as they attempted to define the parameters that would enable them to feel comfortable and confident about their status as medical specialists, while still acknowledging and responding to patients' needs and demands, the basic lines along which the specialty would develop emerged.[42]

Reflecting the wartime emphasis on self-sufficiency, surgeons generally agreed that the need for economic independence was one of the factors that made a patient's condition worthy of medical attention. In his 1916 article, John Staige Davis outlined the three goals he believed surgeons should share: relief of pain and deformity, restoration of function, "and, last but not least, [ensuring] the ability to earn a living." On this last, Davis meditated, "One occasionally hears the term 'beauty doctor' applied to those doing plastic surgery. Although this term may have some foundation, . . . a very small part of legitimate plastic surgery is done for cosmetic reasons only. A number of patients have been under my care who previously were unable to secure even the humblest position on account of hideous facial deformities, and who, having been rendered presentable by a series of plastic operations, are now making a good living. If this is being a 'beauty doctor,' the title is worthwhile." Davis affirmed the significance of appearance in relation to patients' sense of self-worth and economic independence; it was in this sense that he claimed the term "beauty doctor" as a mark of honor. In another sense, however, Davis by implication linked legitimate plastic surgery with deformity or lack of function, and thus with reconstructive work, while relegating surgery "done for cosmetic reasons only" to a lesser rank.[43]

There is clearly a gendered value judgment implicit in Davis's words; as this and other articles suggest, in his view the deformity or lack of function that might limit economic independence (and which reconstructive surgery could remedy) might occur in men or women, but only a woman would request surgery "for cosmetic reasons only." For other surgeons, however, this line was not as clear. Marriage had long been enshrined as worthy work for women. As the home was transformed from a locus of production to a haven from it, America's consuming culture redefined the nature and meaning of marriage. By the 1920s, heterosexual companionate marriage achieved widespread acceptance as the ideal, and the work of marriage was redefined to mean companionship and shared consumption and leisure, outside the home as well as within it. This development strengthened the prevailing conviction that in the marriage market, a woman's face was her currency. As historian Kathy Peiss notes, the 1907 silent film *The Veiled Beauty* makes the nature of this exchange explicit. A woman, her face hidden behind a veil, allows a young man to treat her to a day of rides and attractions at Coney Island's Dreamland amusement park only to reveal at dinner that what is behind the veil is an ugly face—this, the film implies, is what she has to trade for the day of treats, and it is not worth the investment the suitor has made. That in this modern dating- and marriage-market women's looks might be assigned something very much like a dollar value challenged surgeons as they attempted to define the limits of their specialty, and some, like Gustav Tieck, found that consideration of gender blurred the boundaries: "Men and women in business and professional life know the value of good appearance. Young women of marriageable age, particularly, feel keenly the disadvantage of distorted features. . . . If the surgeon can . . . improve facial appearance in such cases, he is ministering to a legitimate and important demand, worthy of his best efforts."[44]

Tieck was careful to specify, however, that he was concerned only about disfigurements striking enough to cause "serious social or business embarrassment"; he sympathized with those physicians who felt it was their duty "to heal rather than beautify." Dr. Joseph C. Beck of Chicago similarly distinguished between deserving and frivolous cases. While he endorsed surgery for serious deformities, Beck held "that type of plastic surgery which has to do with cosmetics or beautifying as, for instance, taking off a hump or filling up a saddle defect of the nose" in low esteem, because it "really calls for very little surgical skill." He asserted, "It is the duty of every physician and surgeon to try and argue with [patients], to convince them that correction is unnecessary." Anticipating the interest in psychology that would soon become common among plastic surgeons, Seymour Oppenheimer used the mind as a measuring stick. The mental anguish caused by disfigurement, he wrote, "often restricts the activities of the individual sufficiently to reduce his worth to the community to a serious degree," and in these cases surgery was warranted.[45]

Although they struggled to define limits, surgeons quickly found that it was as impossible to quantify concepts like "serious social or business embarrassment" as it was to define what degree of irregularity in appearance might preclude economic self-sufficiency or psychological well-being. The fact that some surgeons were uneasy at the thought of performing cosmetic operations meant not only that "beauty surgery" would remain specifically gendered female for many years to come but also that the full-fledged sanction of surgery to beautify would have to wait. At the same time, however, the fact that others felt no such qualms meant that the process was already under way. Portland, Oregon, surgeon Adalbert G. Bettman was one of these. "Whenever I see a group of people," Bettman noted, "I am struck with the fact that there is offered a great field for practicing the beautifying and practical, I might say grateful art of plastic surgery." He asserted that "removing wrinkles of the face and neck, double chins and such like deformities" is "probably the most interesting work in plastic surgery" and urged his colleagues to accept such patients. "Persons with these cruel deformities (for they certainly are more cruel than the loss of a leg, for instance)," Bettman wrote, "can and should be relieved."[46]

Bettman was an innovative, as well as enthusiastic, proponent of cosmetic surgery. In a 1919 presentation to the Alumni Association of the University of Oregon Medical School in Portland, he introduced the extensive face-lift incision that, with modifications, is still used today (and may have been the first to demonstrate such an operation using before and after pictures). He made extravagant claims for his work. It was practically painless: "One woman after having this operation done proceeded immediately to a local department store, where she purchased a new hat suitable to her now youthful appearance, certainly an amusement not indulged in when one is in pain." It could be kept secret, even from close relatives: "Another woman," he reported, went home to her husband, mother, and grown daughter and "not one of these noticed the dressings." But perhaps most significant was the new terminology Bettman pioneered.[47]

Although Charles C. Miller took his clients' beauty problems very seriously, he defined them as defects, or, in one case, as "featural imperfections which are not actual deformities." Bettman, in contrast, who specifically referred to wrinkles and double chins as deformities, was apparently a pioneer not only in surgical technique but also in what critics have termed the medicalization of nonmedical conditions. His followers

have not yet arrived at a common answer to the question of what constitutes a deformity, but over the course of the twentieth century they
have moved toward, rather than away from, his definition.[48]

The three men who met at the Chicago Athletic Club on August 8,
1921, to found the first plastic surgical organization in North America
did not then know that "they were laying the foundation for what has
become the oldest existing organization of its kind in the world." According to one surgeon, they simply felt the need for a forum "to interchange
their experiences." They must have been aware, however, that their
meeting was an important step. Plastic surgeons since then have certainly
regarded the meeting as the first step toward the establishment of what
is now one of the largest medical specialties in the United States.[49]

This meeting was held in an atmosphere of transition, as surgeons
who had found their interest piqued and their skills challenged during
the war attempted to translate that experience into satisfying postwar
careers. The year 1921 was transitional not just in medical terms but in
cultural terms as well. Some Americans had learned of plastic surgery
before the war, and many others had become aware of it as the decade
progressed. An exchange that appeared in the *New York Times* in the summer of 1920 suggests something of what they might have heard. On
August 4, the paper introduced its readers to a Parisian woman who
had come to New York for a face-lift and was ecstatic. "I'm just crazy
with joy," Madame confided, "but I daren't smile. That would start the
wrinkles all over again. I would never have needed an operation if I
hadn't gone around laughing and crying over nothing all my life." The
lift would last eight to ten years, she explained, after which the patient
would grow old again. "But by then she will be nearly 59, and laughter
may seem preferable to the complexion of 25." Two days later, a crisply
worded editorial left readers in no doubt about where the *Times* stood
on the issue of laugh lines and face-lifts. Like Hamlet, the editor asserted,
the sensible man "scorns all who, God having given them one face,
make themselves another."[50]

A scant six months later, the paper interviewed Dr. Julian Bourguet,
a Parisian plastic surgeon visiting New York. The reporter had mixed feelings about Dr. Bourguet's wrinkle-removing techniques, which apparently recalled those of Charles C. Miller. About the nose operations in
which Dr. Bourguet specialized, however, the reporter was persuaded.
Dr. Bourguet explained, "People do not laugh at other deformities but

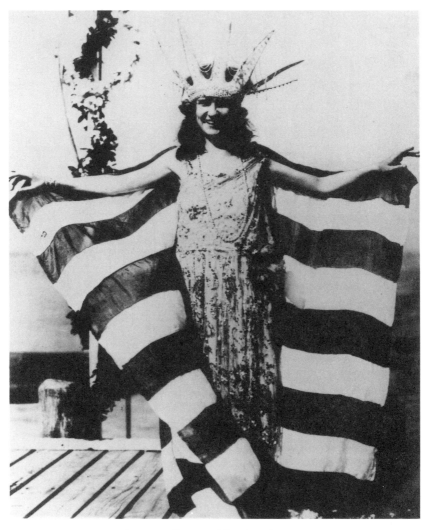

Margaret Gorman, Miss America 1921.

they will laugh at a nose. Most of my patients do not come, necessarily, to be made beautiful. They want to be made inconspicuous . . . they just hope to be unnoticed." To this reporter, being inconspicuous was a more acceptable goal than looking younger: "This is the aspect of his work that leads one to cease scoffing at the beauty cures."[51]

Many Americans did not read the *New York Times*, and plastic surgery, as a specific way of achieving beauty, probably remained outside many Americans' consciousness. But the transformation in American culture that had occurred in the several decades preceding 1921 had made beauty, at least for women, seem not just desirable but necessary. A select few, their images endlessly replicated in films, in the posters that advertised them, and in the magazines that publicized them, became icons for the many, even as growing numbers of increasingly sophisticated advertisements for new products and processes promised that beauty could be, and ought to be, achieved through artificial, external means.

Like the first association meeting, the first Miss America contest was just a beginning. In a bow to already outdated Victorian conventions, the definition of beauty upon which judges relied included a moral component: contestants were valued for appearing both natural and innocent; bobbed hair and cosmetics were prohibited; and many observers commented on the striking resemblance winner Margaret Gorman of Washington, D.C., bore to Mary Pickford, America's cinema sweetheart. But if the 1921 contest was but a shadow of its future self, like the first association meeting, it set a precedent. For perhaps the first time on a national level, it confirmed that beauty was one, if not the primary, criterion by which American women would be judged and would judge themselves. The emphasis on natural beauty recalled an earlier era, but American women understood this for what it was and continued their efforts to improve their looks and their chances for success in the world through artifice. Like the cosmetics and hair care products on which women increasingly relied, plastic surgery, by 1921, had entered the American scene and in the years to come would emerge as an important ally in the war against ugliness in all its forms. Although many surgeons attempted to hold out, by 1921 an adventurous few had enlisted wholeheartedly, and the battle lines were drawn.[52]

CHAPTER TWO

The Specialty Takes Shape

In August of 1923, comedienne and Ziegfeld Follies star Fanny Brice had a nose job and plastic surgeon Henry Junius Schireson became famous. In her memoirs, Brice was less than enthusiastic about her erstwhile surgeon: "I was the beginning of this guy's career," she recalled. "I posed for him for 'before and after' pictures. He made a big nose on the 'before' picture. He was crazy. . . . He'd cut you if you had dandruff." At the time, however, Brice proclaimed her appreciation, and for Schireson, then forty-two years old with a dubious educational background and a less-than-illustrious career, the benefits were clear. Brice's nose job, according to one of her biographers, generated more press attention "than any other medical event until the birth of the Dionne quintuplets," and Schireson, practically overnight, became one of the most renowned plastic surgeons in the United States.

In his 1938 book *As Others See You: The Story of Plastic Surgery,* Schireson proclaimed his admiration for a long list of plastic surgeons, including Vilray Blair and Jerome Webster, all of whom were founding members of the American Board of Plastic Surgery, the specialty board whose organization was already well under way. By then, however, repeated scandals and lawsuits (one of which was immortalized in a 1932 film called *False Faces,* in which a patient shoots her surgeon when it seems she will lose her lawsuit against him) had made Schireson infamous rather than famous, and a veritable posse of medical professionals, journalists, law enforcement agencies, and plastic surgeons were tracking his every move. In 1949, just two years after the state of Pennsylvania had finally prevailed in its effort to revoke his license, Schireson died. The paper trail he left behind locates him clearly at one extreme of the spectrum of professional respectability: the man dubbed "King of Quacks" provided plastic surgeons bent on claiming a place at the opposite end of this spectrum with a compelling reason to organize. That Schireson, to the public, was plastic surgery personified meant that he was also the organizers' nemesis as they did so.

The career of Jerome Pierce Webster offers a very different picture of plastic surgery. Webster was born in New Hampshire in 1888. He studied at Trinity College and the Johns Hopkins University, served with distinction in World War I, and in 1928 headed south to Barnes Hospital, in St. Louis, where Vilray Blair taught and practiced. He was elected to the American Association of Plastic Surgeons in 1929 and in 1931 was asked to organize the Division of Plastic Surgery at the new Columbia Presbyterian Medical Center; he would train forty-four surgeons during the next two decades. During World War II, in conjunction with his residency program, he established one of several three-month intensive army courses that trained surgeons and dentists in primary care of maxillofacial injuries. He was a founding member of the American Board of Plastic Surgery and served as chair from 1947 to 1949. In addition, Webster was an avid collector of antiquarian medical books and a respected writer: *The Life and Times of Gaspare Tagliacozzi*, which he coauthored with Martha Teach Gnudi, won the American Association for the History of Medicine's William H. Welch medal in 1950.

Jerome Webster performed numerous operations, such as nose jobs, that were and are generally considered cosmetic. He prided himself, however, on being a "conservative" surgeon; he spoke to young people "like a Dutch uncle" and told them to concentrate on life's important challenges rather than on their own noses; he routinely advised aging women to stop "mirror-gazing" with "wishful thinking." Webster never achieved anything approaching Schireson's fame, but in professional circles he was well respected. Many patients sought him out because of his reputation, and many more came because their letters and inquiries were referred to him as head of Columbia Presbyterian's division. As a result, he knew, at least by reputation, most of those practicing in New York and many of those who practiced elsewhere; his correspondence with and about those, like Blair, he claimed as colleagues and those, like Schireson, he disclaimed illuminates the sifting process the specialty undertook as it began to mark its boundaries. Webster died in 1974, the recipient of special honorary citations from both the AAPS and the American Society of Plastic and Reconstructive Surgeons, Inc. (ASPRS) for long years of respected service to the specialty he helped found.[1]

The efforts of plastic surgeons like Jerome Webster to rid their specialty of "quacks" like Henry Schireson reflected a broad-based commitment, inherited from the Progressive era and earlier, to bringing order out of the chaos that was American medicine. We will return to Henry Schireson later in this chapter and to Jerome Webster in subsequent chapters. Here their stories offer a path into the tangled thicket of professionalization and organization.

The reorganization of the American Medical Association (AMA) in 1900, which rerouted AMA membership through county and state medical societies, had begun to bring a degree of coherence to the profession, as well as a measure of meaning to the phrase "organized medicine." By 1920 the AMA counted 60 percent of the nation's physicians as members, up from 50 percent in 1910 and fewer than 10 percent in 1900, when only 8,000 doctors had belonged. During the 1930s, the AMA joined with other medical groups to form a "coordinating body" which, as the American Board for Medical Specialties, "set general standards for the examining boards and settled jurisdictional disputes" among the twelve examining boards that existed then (eight more were added later). The reform of medical education, which the AMA had made a top priority following its own reorganization, had also resulted in greater control and standardization within the profession. Educator Abraham Flexner's 1910 report on the nation's medical schools, prepared on behalf of the Carnegie Corporation, accelerated the consolidation of medical education that had begun in the early nineteenth century and thus contributed to the process of "gathering" the medical profession.[2]

As part of this process, the AMA had launched a major campaign against quacks in 1905 under the energetic leadership of a physician with the unlikely name of Arthur J. Cramp. The association republished, as a book entitled *The Great American Fraud,* muckraker Samuel Hopkins Adams's magazine series on patent medicines and medical quacks and distributed more than 150,000 copies. In 1911 it followed up with the 500-page *Nostrums and Quackery*; this and a second, longer edition sold out quickly and were followed, in 1921, by a volume of more than 800 pages that Cramp called "a veritable 'Who's Who in Quackdom.'" The federal government joined the campaign, charging practitioners with false advertising and postal fraud and passing the Pure Food and Drug Act of 1906 (and, eventually, the Food, Drug, and Cosmetic Act of 1936). Patent-medicine manufacturers were the main targets, but practitioners came under fire as well.[3]

The founding, in 1921, of the American Association of Plastic Surgeons, which signaled the beginning of the end of the free-for-all in plastic surgery, can thus be seen as part of a nationwide trend toward professionalization and organization. This first association was joined by the American Society of Plastic and Reconstructive Surgeons in 1931 and by the American Board of Plastic Surgery in 1937. In the four years between 1937 and 1941, plastic surgery achieved recognition as an independent specialty; initially recognized only as a subsidiary of the American Board of Surgery, by 1941 the American Board of Plastic Surgery led a major specialty in its own right. After differentiating among those already practicing, admitting some and excluding others, plastic surgeons began to define a standardized program of education and training that would prepare young surgeons to enter the field and adopted a rigorous qualifying examination. *The Directory of Medical Specialists Certified by American Boards,* published in 1942, testified to the magnitude of their achievement. According to this listing, 120 men from twenty-six states were certified to practice plastic surgery; Canada accounted for another 4. That certification was an option only for those who practiced strictly within the boundaries of organized medicine testifies to the effectiveness of the AMA's publicity campaign: graduation from an AMA-recognized school was required, as was AMA membership and, more broadly, "satisfactory moral character and ethical standing in the profession." In his preface to a 1926 series on plastic surgery, the editor of *Hygeia,* the association's consumer magazine, offered consumers another means to identify those "on the border lines of sound medical practice. . . . The reliable cosmetic and plastic surgeon is usually associated with a hospital that has been classified by both the American Medical Association and the American College of Surgeons as a reputable institution."[4]

Given the fluidity of medicine in general and of plastic surgery in particular in these years, the formation of the ABPS was a spectacular achievement. But until 1941, attempts at organization and control were just that—attempts. Standards for academic accreditation and professional recognition were hazy at best, and until education and training were standardized, plastic surgery drew from a wide variety of related fields, including general surgery, thoracic surgery, dermatology, otolaryngology, opthalmology, dentistry, and oral surgery. Gustave Aufricht, one of the specialty's founding members, recalled that when he arrived in New York in 1923, the four or five plastic surgeons practicing there divided their time with other specialties: otolaryngology, general surgery, opthalmology, even gynecology. Those who had participated in the wartime plastic surgical services created a network of sorts, but many aspiring plastic surgeons continued to travel to Europe to apprentice with masters like Berlin's Jacques Joseph. Others simply tried to be "in the right place at the right time when older surgeons needed someone to help out with their practices." By the 1930s some students were apprenticing with Vilray Blair at Barnes Hospital in St. Louis and John Staige Davis at the Johns Hopkins University in Baltimore, but most continued to forge their own paths. According to New York surgeon Joseph C. Beck, as late as 1933, only two of the thirty-two self-proclaimed cosmetic surgeons in one unidentified city were members of the regular local medical societies. During the 1920s and 1930s, in short, most of those who called themselves plastic surgeons remained unaffected by professional organization.[5]

In the field of plastic surgery, the task of professional organization was complicated by issues of publicity and profit, and those who were working to define the new specialty seriously considered ceding the cosmetic, or beautifying, territory to others, reserving as their own only the more conservative field of reconstructive surgery. They realized, however, that Americans who were discontented with their features far outnumbered those born with congenital deformities or injured in later life, and that enterprising practitioners, with varying degrees of training and imagination, were busy staking claims in this growth industry. They advertised in phone directories and newspapers, gave public demonstrations of their work at beauty conventions and in department stores, published books and pamphlets extolling their skills, and generally conducted themselves in a manner abhorred by most physicians who considered themselves professional. Precisely because of this conduct, however, it was these practitioners whom the American public knew and accepted as plastic surgeons. Even the most conservative surgeons came to understand that to define the specialty only in terms of reconstructive surgery would be to give up, both professionally and economically, the largest piece of the pie.

To support their move toward cosmetic surgery, plastic surgeons developed a theoretical framework that drew, first, on sociological and historical interpretations of the changes the nation was undergoing, and, second, on the insights offered by the new sciences of psychology and psychiatry; both these subjects are covered in the next chapter. In this chapter, we shall see how surgeons began to answer the more elemental questions that the decision to incorporate cosmetic surgery forced them to confront: What qualities and qualifications made someone a plastic surgeon? By what authority might this title be claimed, and for what reasons might it be withheld? As the comparison of Schireson and Webster suggests, some cases were clear-cut. But despite instinctive agreement on the definition of "quack" and "surgeon," the plastic surgeons who set out to organize the American Board of Plastic Surgery had trouble drawing the line. A look at the careers of six surgeons—Vilray Papin Blair, Jacques W. Maliniak, Joseph Eastman Sheehan, Maxwell Maltz, John Howard Crum, and Henry Junius Schireson—offers a revealing perspective on the world plastic surgeons inhabited in these formative years. Of these, only Blair practiced entirely outside New York; Jerome Webster, whom Blair trained, became his eyes and ears there. All were actively operating during the years from 1921 to 1941, all were relatively well known, and all played key roles in shaping the profession, as well as the public's perception of it, during these crucial years.[6]

As with other professional organizations, the formation of the ABPS constituted an attempt on the part of some plastic surgeons to seize control of the specialty by defining its boundaries and identifying those qualified to claim membership. In this sense, it was an exclusionary move, and a successful one at that. Many practitioners—thirty of the thirty-two Joseph Beck had identified, and three of the six named above—were judged ineligible, and as the cachet of board certification became more widely known in lay as well as medical circles, some practices undoubtedly dwindled. From another perspective, however, professionalization in plastic surgery seems an inclusionary move, and it is this perspective that is more significant to the shape the specialty eventually took. In moving to incorporate cosmetic surgery, plastic surgeons were acting on public, as well as professional, ideas about the shape the specialty should take. This decision ultimately transformed the specialty from within, even as those who were excluded continued to shape the specialty from without, demonstrating that at least as far as cosmetic surgery was concerned, good press was as important as good professional standing. By 1941, the Board's organizers had emerged as the specialty's leaders, but those who found their leader in the public, rather than the profession, did just as much to shape the field and to make it what it is today.

Because plastic surgery was taking shape in the public as well as the professional realm, before turning to our six surgeons, let us examine the lens through which the public viewed them. In 1927, responding to the stream of lurid stories appearing in "yellow" newspapers, writer Richard J. Walsh attempted to explain the beauty business to readers of *Woman's Home Companion*: "On one flank are the reputable plastic surgeons and dermatologists. On the other flank is the vast and growing array of beauty shops for the most part conducted by conscientious hard-working women who confine themselves to such harmless and proper work as bobbing hair and giving facial massage, permanent waves and marcels. In between is a horde of charlatans." The problem, Walsh asserted, was that distinguishing between these practitioners was as difficult for the professional as it was for the layperson. "The borderline between the legitimate and the illegitimate in facial operations is very narrow and hard to define," he wrote. "There is no uniform standard which determines who is a doctor and who is not." State laws differed, Walsh noted, not only as to who was licensed for what but who could claim what title in the phone directory; a greater problem was that "the old-timey family doctor simply does not exist anymore," and people were increasingly likely to choose doctors from directory listings and advertisements, which were unregulated.[7]

Dr. Joseph Colt Bloodgood, a professor of clinical surgery at Johns Hopkins, believed that the way a surgeon balanced professional judgment and medical responsibility with commercial interest could reveal where he fell on the spectrum Walsh described. "As far as I can learn," Bloodgood told the *Delineator,* another popular women's magazine, in 1927, "a beauty surgeon works strictly on a commercial basis. For example, he would be willing to perform on any set of ears, providing that the individual was not satisfied with them." A plastic surgeon, in contrast, was "a trained member of the medical profession, one who has the ideals and education of that profession"; he "would be willing to operate only when the deformity was sufficient to justify it, and when he knew there would be real improvement." Journalist Maxine Davis, like Bloodgood, saw commercialism as a litmus test of sorts. "Lots of quacks

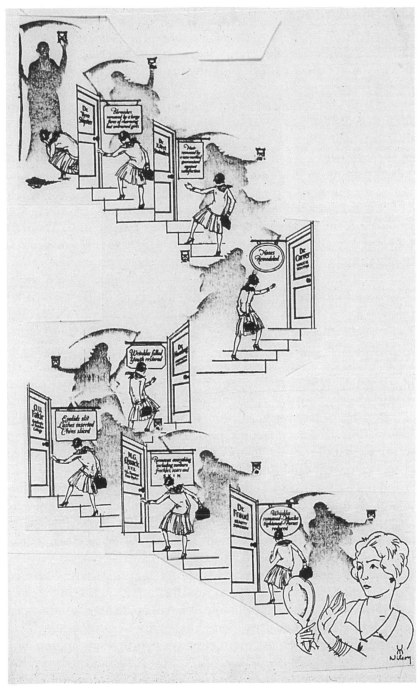

This 1927 illustration from the *Woman's Home Companion* warned women about the dangers of the beauty business.

exist. They charge fabulous prices. They operate in their offices, and sometimes even in beauty parlors. Big cities are full of such men," she cautioned in *Pictorial Review*. Reputable plastic surgeons, in contrast,
shared with other physicians a commitment to providing medical care
regardless of cost—an assertion Davis supported with a story about a
little girl, badly burned in a childhood accident and helped by a plastic surgeon who, "like most great scientists, . . . took the case for a fee
Adele's parents could afford. . . . It's those quack 'beauty surgeons' who
charge the outrageous prices—payable in advance!"[8]

Other commentators believed that quacks were simply those who
would perform cosmetic operations. Reporter Thyra Samter Winslow
told *New Republic* readers in 1931 that "conservative surgeons are still
holding aloof from all connections with the beauty racket. Plastic surgeons connected with the larger hospitals will accept only cases which
will correct serious defects, such as disfiguring birth marks, or, after
injuries, the restoration of faces. . . . These surgeons will not accept cases
that are concerned only with women's vanity." *Popular Mechanics* writer
Boyden Sparkes made the same distinction. While he was heartened by
the fact that the recent world war was "paying back to humanity thin
but accumulating dividends in the form of a new craftsmanship . . . called
plastic surgery," Sparkes cautioned readers against confusing plastic
surgery with beauty surgery. "None of the men from whom I sought
information are beauty doctors," he noted. "All of them uttered solemn
warnings that the beauty doctors make extravagant and unsupported
claims as to what can be done."[9]

For Dorothy Cocks, who tackled the topic for *Good Housekeeping*
in 1930, attitude toward and use of advertising and self-promotion were
the primary criteria that divided "flagrant charlatans," "semi-charlatans,"
and "truly ethical surgeons." Flagrant charlatans, Cocks asserted, "advertise in the newspapers as 'cosmetic surgeons,' 'plastic specialists,' etc. The
very fact that these men advertise is proof that they have discarded
their professional standards, have declared themselves outlaws of the medical world, have abandoned all hope of having patients recommended
to them by ethical physicians." Semi-charlatans, Cocks continued, "do
not actually advertise," but promoted themselves in ways almost as blatant and equally as offensive. These men "use the subtler methods of newspaper publicity . . . attach themselves to motion picture colonies . . . [and]
offer commissions to barbers, milliners, casting directors, and others,

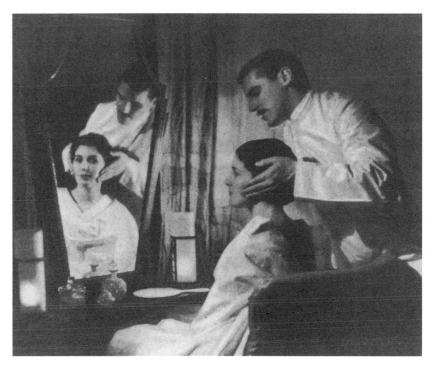

In 1930, *Good Housekeeping* cautioned women to beware of "smooth operators."

for patients recommended. [They] are trying to hang on to their professional reputation as a cloak for their ignorance and lack of professional standing." "The circle of truly ethical surgeons," Cocks concluded, was made up of "not more than six" men, who had achieved their status through their appointment by war-time authorities to handle army hospital patients. These men, whom Cocks deemed "the only real plastic surgeons in the country," were distinguished not only by the fact that they "would rather turn coal-heavers than be thought of as 'beauty doctors'" but also by their total abstinence from self-promotion. These surgeons, "who never talk except before medical societies, who never advertise in any way . . . are elevating plastic surgery to a level of technical skill which will make it feasible and safe for any woman who needs such an operation."[10]

In 1930, even the most conservative plastic surgeons would have found Cocks's definition too strict. The American Association of Plastic

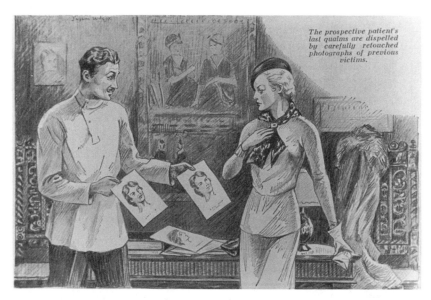

The American Medical Association warned women to be careful through *Hygeia*, its family health magazine.

Surgeons had a full complement of forty members by then (not including senior members), and some plastic surgeons were already planning a second, larger professional society. Taken together, however, these pronouncements suggest something of how Americans defined quacks in the specialty of plastic surgery during the period in which the specialty was defining itself. First, quacks were motivated by profit. Subordinating professional judgment to patient desire, they let the prospective patient decide whether an operation was warranted, and they charged high, fixed fees, payable in advance. Second, quacks performed cosmetic surgery. Unlike those who confined their efforts to remedying deformities, quacks catered to women's vanity, and as a result engaged in riskier procedures. Third, quacks operated quite literally outside the boundaries of organized medicine. Unable to obtain hospital privileges, quacks operated in their own quarters, or in beauty parlors; unable to obtain referrals from colleagues, they actively recruited patients in the public domain. Finally, rather than confine discussion of their work to the rarefied atmosphere of medical societies, quacks talked— through intermediaries, through apparently legitimate articles, and, of course, through patently illegitimate advertisements—to anyone who would listen.

This broad consensus suggests that Americans had become familiar with the professional aura with which the American Medical Association was endeavoring to surround medicine and with the various rules and requirements the AMA was attempting to promulgate. It also suggests that at least a certain group of literate Americans shared with those who were leading plastic surgery's organizing drive a general prejudice against cosmetic surgery and those who practiced it. Yet as we turn to our six surgeons, let us keep in mind that while they occupied a range of positions on the spectrum Dorothy Cocks and others described, the differences between them were not as clear as one might expect. More important, while Americans may have lauded the great doctor who performed the serious work of reconstruction as the ideal, in reality they lionized his despised colleague, the "beauty doctor."

Vilray Blair and Jacques Maliniak are today remembered as among the most important of the specialty's founders: Blair for his contribution to organizing the American Board of Plastic Surgery, and Maliniak for founding the American Society of Plastic and Reconstructive Surgeons, the specialty's largest and most influential professional organization. At first glance, they appear to have little in common. Maliniak trained at the best universities in Europe and in the Russian Army during World War I. He appears never to have wavered from his commitment to plastic surgery and was more comfortable than many of his contemporaries with its cosmetic applications. Blair, the son of a prominent St. Louis family, dabbled in several fields before settling on medicine. His education was not particularly rigorous, and his training occurred mostly on the job. Throughout his long career, he remained uncomfortable with cosmetic surgery and was reluctant to call himself a plastic surgeon. Both men, however, worked entirely within the ranks of organized medicine, teaching at medical schools, writing clinical books, and publishing numerous articles in medical journals, and their early differences have been largely forgotten.

Vilray Papin Blair (1871–1955)

Vilray Blair was born in 1871 to Edmund Harrison Blair and Mary Clementine Papin, whose family had been among the earliest settlers of

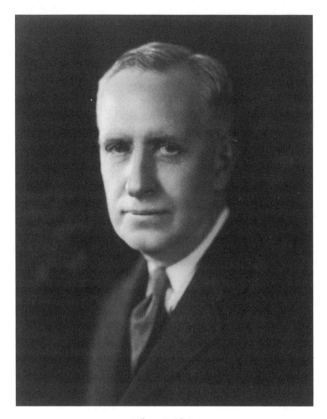

Vilray P. Blair

St. Louis, Missouri. He graduated from Christian Brothers' College in 1890. After spending a year at the St. Louis Medical College, which was among those targeted in the 1910 Flexner report, Blair left to string telephone wires in the Rocky Mountains. When he returned to St. Louis he wanted to give up medicine in favor of a program at the Westinghouse Electrical Engineering School, but his family disapproved. Blair returned to the St. Louis Medical College and received his medical degree in 1893. A year later, he earned a masters, again from Christian Brothers' College.[11]

Blair held various positions at the Washington University schools of medicine and dentistry from 1894, when he was hired as an instructor in practical anatomy, to 1941, when he became professor emeritus of both clinical and oral surgery, but his career took several unusual twists and turns along the way. Five years into his medical career, Blair, as he later put it, "'broke flat'... went to sea and found out that life was really worth living." He worked on tramp ships in the Mediterranean, went up to Edinburgh Medical School, and then obtained a position as a surgeon on a South American voyage, which he followed with a trip up the Gold and Ivory coasts of West Africa. Then thirty years old, Blair returned to St. Louis; again he contemplated leaving medicine, again his family encouraged him to pursue a practice. He spent some time at the London General Hospital in 1903, married and had a family, and prepared his clinical text, *Surgery and Diseases of the Mouth and Jaws*, which was published in 1912 and is still regarded as a classic. The text greatly improved Blair's standing in the profession and led to his appointment as head of the section of Oral and Plastic Surgery and chief consultant in Maxillofacial Surgery with the American Expeditionary Forces during World War I. By 1917, Blair's text had gone through three editions, and he had published thirty-two articles on plastic surgery.[12]

Blair returned to St. Louis and to Washington University after the war. As a professor of both clinical and oral surgery, he trained a number of surgeons who later became famous, including James Barrett Brown, who organized the army's plastic surgical services for World War II, and Jerome Pierce Webster, who would go on to establish a veritable plastic surgical dynasty at Columbia Presbyterian. As Webster later recalled, Blair's growing reputation "led also to the performance of what Blair laughingly called 'beauty surgery,' although he was most insistent that he be called a general surgeon and not a plastic surgeon." Blair was invited to be a founding member of the American Association of Plastic Surgeons in 1921, and was one of only two men for whom the double degree requirement (medical and dental) was waived.[13]

Blair is best remembered for organizing the American Board of Plastic Surgery, to which he began to devote attention in 1935. "It is evident we are due to engage in some radical housecleaning before some well-intentioned neighbor undertakes to do it for us," he warned his colleagues. The ABPS's founding documents reflect Blair's conviction that plastic surgery's poor public image was largely deserved, as well as his belief that its new popularity called for an organized response: "An increasing prevalence of defacing and deforming accidents added to natural contour vagaries, in a people who have become almost universally appearance-conscious, have combined to create an even greater need," Blair emphasized. "We have an increasing multitude demanding surgery that might better their social, business, or industrial circumstances, or what is more important, their self-confidence." Blair was above all a reformer, who believed it was essential that reputable surgeons devise a fair method of judging and credentialing candidates so that other doctors, and prospective patients, would be able to differentiate between those who deserved their trust and those who did not. He also hoped to improve the field generally by standardizing education, and by steering candidates into internships and other programs that provided adequate preparation through clinical experience.[14]

In 1936 and 1937, Blair traveled around the country, observing and interviewing surgeons and discussing the formation of a specialty board. His paper, "A Plastic Surgery Board: Is Its Formation Now Desirable and Opportune?" formed the basis for meetings in Boston, Philadelphia, Houston, San Francisco, and Los Angeles. In 1937, Blair held the first organizational meeting for what would become the American Board of Plastic Surgery at his home in St. Louis. John Staige Davis agreed to serve as chairman, while Blair accepted the post of secretary-treasurer.[15]

The first, and most difficult, problem Blair confronted was how to distinguish among the surgeons then practicing. Future generations of would-be plastic surgeons would have to demonstrate their competence according to objective standards: grades in approved medical schools, time in recognized residency programs, and a passing grade on a comprehensive examination. Founding members, however, were to be identified by their colleagues' recommendations and invited to join on the basis of their reputations and experience. Jerome Webster, to whom Blair turned for information about New York, was initially dubious about undertaking this project: "There are so many off-color men in this field and those who hover about the line dividing the ethical from the unethical that it is getting to be extremely hard to decide who shall and shall not be eligible," he wrote to Blair in March 1937. "I admire your courage and agree with you in principle, but I am sure the formation of such a Board at this time would stir up a great deal of heartburns and hot tempers."[16]

Webster complied with Blair's request for names, but his response raised more questions than it answered. In a letter to John Staige Davis, Blair noted, "What Webster put on his list is beside the mark. The names he did not put on is [*sic*] what interests me." Because of their numbers, Blair mused, New York was a particularly competitive market for plastic surgeons, and hard feelings were inevitable. Still, he stressed to Davis, it was important that "good men" not be excluded simply because of "local prejudice." A later letter from Blair to Davis suggests that the difference with Webster was not a matter of prejudice or competition, but rather a misunderstanding (or an honest difference of opinion) over the Board's purpose. Blair wrote, "I am strongly impressed with the idea that for the present the Board can make itself as useful by exerting pressure upon capable and otherwise well-intentioned men, who may have shown more energy than judgment in their way of getting practice, as will be accomplished by official selection of the 'lily-whites.' The former type are going to continue in practice. Much I have observed along that line has been due more to lack of proper association than anything else, and if they are not essentially vicious more real good and protection might be given to the public by making it worthwhile for them to behave" than by excluding them altogether.[17]

Although the situation in New York continued to be touchy—almost a year later Blair told Davis "we are getting no leads in New York"—Blair remained committed to the idea that the Board could be more successful by including, rather than excluding, borderline practitioners. In notes he jotted during the sixth meeting of the Board's executive committee, held November 27, 1938, Blair commented, "Local prejudice or favoritism must both be avoided. Embarrassment to local member. To have real authority it must enroll most all worthwhile men. The really wrong ones are harmful, but Board cannot be run as gentlemen's club."[18]

Convinced that exclusivity could jeopardize the Board's existence and render it powerless, Blair was less likely than many of his colleagues to condemn practitioners for past behavior. Plastic surgery's image needed to be improved, he agreed, but that could best be achieved by bringing as many practitioners as possible under a central authority. Blair himself, however, seems to have retained the impression of the specialty the Board was organized to combat; he eschewed the title of "plastic surgeon" throughout his life. Not until just before the Board's organization did he expand his definition of plastic surgery to include cosmetic surgery, and as plastic surgeon Kathryn Lyle Stephenson later recalled, although Blair did perform operations that were cosmetic in nature, he "did not consider it worthy of reporting."[19]

Jacques W. Maliniak (1889–1976)

Ironically, Jacques Maliniak, who is remembered not only as a skilled surgeon and dedicated educator but as the founder of the American Society of Plastic and Reconstructive Surgeons, posed one of the thorniest problems Blair and Webster faced in selecting among New York's many surgeons. Maliniak was born Jacob Maliniac in Warsaw, Poland, and educated at the universities of Nancy and Paris. Poland was then part of Russia, and as a Russian national Maliniak was called into the Russian Army during World War I. He was decorated twice during the four years he served on the Balkan front and in Kiev as a medical officer; after the war he worked with both Hippolyte Morestin in Paris and Jacques Joseph in Berlin (Joseph had changed his name years earlier; his example evidently inspired Maliniak, who also took the name Jacques). In 1923 he arrived in Cincinnati, where he spent two years; in 1925 he opened a private practice in New York.[20]

Maliniak was not a member of the American Association of Plastic Surgeons, which required that all members have both a dental and a medical degree, limited its membership to forty, and confined its activities to one meeting a year. Maliniak believed there were many more surgeons practicing plastic surgery who could benefit not only from the camaraderie and scholarly exchange an association would provide but also from an expanded agenda of activities, including meetings, conferences, and roundtable discussions. His experience organizing a plastic surgical service at New York's City Hospital on Welfare Island (the first such service in a municipal hospital) had convinced him that a broader organization of the specialty was necessary. Rather than limit membership to an arbitrary number of men holding a particular degree, Maliniak believed interest in and commitment to the "ethical practice of plastic and reconstructive surgery" was the main criterion by which potential members should be judged.[21]

In 1931, Maliniak held an invitational dinner in New York at which the ASPRS was formed. Interested physicians from all eastern states and from all fields in which "plastic problems" were encountered were invited. Some who considered themselves plastic surgeons disdained Maliniak's efforts, believing that he had included "borderline specialists, such as eye surgeons, otolaryngologists, oral surgeons, and dermatologists." By one account, surgeon Clarence Straatsma initially joined as a "sort of secret agent" to find out what was afoot, while his colleague

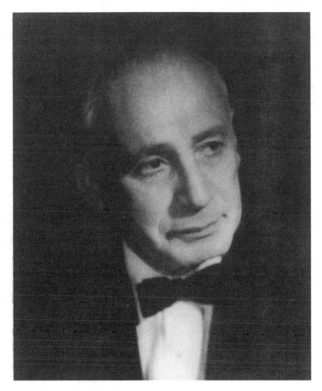

Jacques W. Maliniak

Lyndon Peer joined a year later "to help Clarence tone Maliniac down a bit, and to establish high standards for this new society." Despite this rocky start, the ASPRS quickly become the largest and most influential organization in the specialty.[22]

Although Maliniak believed that the AAPS was unduly restrictive, he by no means advocated an open door policy. Membership in the ASPRS was extended by invitation only to those who could offer an impressive record of both education and experience. Neither was Maliniak particularly liberal in the image of plastic surgery that, under his guidance, the new society presented to the public. At its first annual meeting, in 1932, Maliniak told the *New York Times* explicitly that the society's members were not "beauty specialists." A year later, the ASPRS passed resolutions condemning beauty parlor surgery and deploring the sensationalization of plastic surgery; "plastic surgery," the society emphasized, "is a regular surgical specialty designed to remedy defects and malformations rather than a cosmetic device."[23]

Maliniak's involvement in New York City's clinic project, which occasioned a public debate on the morality of plastic surgery, probably sensitized him to the problems of bringing plastic surgery to the public. On January 27, 1930, Dr. J. William Greefe, then commissioner of hospitals, first told the *New York Times* of his plan to provide plastic surgical services for "persons of limited means." "Persons facially disfigured have been at the mercy of quacks and so-called beauty specialists, who have victimized them without remedying their defects," the *Times* reported. Whether inherited or acquired, Greefe believed that disfigurements "are rarely the fault of the person suffering from them" and thus should not prevent the afflicted person from obtaining work. Greefe's emphasis was clearly on severe disfigurement, but New Yorkers, who had been following plastic surgery's progress ever since Fanny Brice's nose job in 1923, had a different idea. "Women Who Want Faces Beautified Are First to Appeal to City's New Plastic Surgery Unit," the *Times* reported just two days later. Typical of the applicants was a commercial artist, who explained, "Fate has bestowed on me an unusually prominent nose that people cannot ignore and it just ruins everything for me."[24]

Under the headline "Beauty Seekers Scorned," Greefe quickly explained that the city-run clinics (plural because several were planned, although only one actually opened, and that temporarily) would not lift faces or provide other cosmetic procedures. "Those who want to improve a face not disfigured will be definitely advised against any such foolish procedures," the *Times* warned. Problems that would fall within the clinics' purview were disfigurements resulting from injury, disease, burns, and congenital deformities. Greefe clarified this statement in an extended explanation that the *Times* quoted in full: "These deformities . . . must be determined on the basis of surgical experience and judgment and not upon the opinion of the patient. This last sentence contains the distinction between cosmetic or beauty surgery and real plastic surgery. . . . Plastic surgery, like any other surgery, is aimed at changing an abnormal condition back to normal. . . . Now as to beauty surgery. It is taking a reasonably normal part of the face or body and attempting to create an improvement which is against the dictates of surgical judgment. The Department of Hospitals is interested in this work only in so far as it can persuade people against this unnecessary attempt at improving upon the average natural feature."[25]

After helping to organize the clinic service, Maliniak established surgical services at Beth Israel Hospital in Newark, New Jersey, and St. Peter's Hospital in New Brunswick, New Jersey, and served as clinical professor of plastic surgery at the New York Polyclinic Hospital. He wrote three well-regarded books on plastic surgery: *Sculpture in the Living* (1934), *Rhinoplasty and Restoration of Facial Contour* (1947), and *Breast Deformities and Their Repair* (1950). Although he published primarily in medical journals, his expertise was hailed in lay circles as well. *Sculpture in the Living* circulated among prospective patients; Rose Brumberg told Jerome Webster that she had been thinking about a nose job for a long time but that Maliniak's book had made up her mind. Maliniak figured prominently in a story that ran in *Literary Digest* in 1937 about a woman who had suffered a bad car accident. "Three weeks after I returned home," "Miss H.C." recounted, "my doctor pronounced me medically fit and horribly enough disfigured to consult a plastic surgeon. He sent me to Dr. Jacques W. Maliniak, a consummate artist whose work should bear his signature as any sculptor's in marble does. I learned that had a different procedure been followed, rather than hasty emergency treatment, I might now be finished with the experience rather than just beginning a painful, tedious and expensive repair job. . . . The jagged edges of my cuts had not been trimmed to straight lines, nor was subcuticular horsehair suturing employed, according to the best plastic surgical practice." Maliniak also published frequently in *Hygeia*, the American Medical Association's consumer health magazine.[26]

Despite his reputation and the contribution he had made to the specialty by organizing the ASPRS, to the organizers of the American Board of Plastic Surgery, Maliniak was a problem rather than an asset. According to the minutes of the executive committee meeting of October 16, 1939, a decision on Maliniak's membership—along with those of Keith Kahn, Joseph Eastman Sheehan, and Howard Updegraff—was postponed. In June 1941 the Board again deferred action on Maliniak's application. The cryptic notation recorded in the minutes—"Board said to tell him we cannot give dual certification. (We have given a number of dual certifications, hence we cannot say that)"—suggests that board members were having trouble coming up with a supportable reason for their reluctance, or that they were loath to state their real reasons. Correspondence on the matter continued over the course of that summer until finally, in August 1941, John Staige Davis notified Blair, "We talked over Maliniac at great length, as he has been pressing the matter hard with Webster, and with considerable reluctance have come to the conclusion that he was no worse than dozens already certified, and that he would do less harm in than out. . . . Sheehan was also discussed and my impression is that when this matter is brought up again that the New York members will recommend his certification also." On September 21, 1941, the Board carried a motion made by Vilray Blair and seconded by Ferris Smith that Joseph Eastman Sheehan and Jacques Maliniak be accepted into the founders' group.[27]

Just what so troubled Maliniak's colleagues is not clear. They may have found him lacking in tact, but his behavior was not out of line with prevailing professional standards. True, by the end of the decade, plastic surgeons, along with their colleagues in the wider medical profession, were moving toward a more stringent prohibition on public exposure. A 1939 article in *Ladies Home Journal,* for example, carried the following note from the editor: "Names of individual surgeons are not used in this article, because of the profession's dislike of anything verging on advertising. Its statements have been approved by medical authorities." Before the decade's late years, however, publicity alone would not have precluded board certification. Only if an article stepped over the commonly accepted (if ill-defined) boundaries of propriety did it become a source of censure for the surgeon. Maliniak's name appeared in the popular press, but so did those of many others, including Vilray Blair, whose talents *Popular Science* extolled at length in a 1934 article.[28]

It seems likely that Maliniak fell victim to precisely the "local prejudice" Blair was so anxious to avoid, particularly as Jerome Webster was his main opponent at every turn. In the long run, however, he won out, and a letter that the Board preserved suggests that his colleagues eventually came to share his patients' conviction that Maliniak was a credit to the profession. On April 2, 1949, Mrs. A.F. wrote to the Board, describing her experience. About ten years previously, she had requested a list of surgeons in her area who could reduce her pendulous breasts. She consulted with two, but as she was then just a housewife, she could not justify the expense. In 1943, however, she had to return to work. Desperate for help, she picked Maliniak at random from the list, and he agreed to a price she could afford. "I have been through the 2 stages of the operation and to me it seems as if he performed a miracle, he treated me perfectly wonderful," the woman continued. "Dr. Maliniac worked hard on me, each operation took 5 hours and now I know why the fees are so high. I can never thank Dr. Maliniac enough so I thought you would be interested in knowing how much good Dr. Maliniac is doing. I'll be forever grateful to him." In the years after 1948, Maliniak devoted most of his attention to the Educational Foundation of the ASPRS, which he had organized to encourage the worldwide exchange of ideas and techniques in plastic surgery, in part by providing traveling fellowships to students. He retired to Florida in 1964 but remained involved in the Educational Foundation until his death in 1976.[29]

If Vilray Blair and Jacques Maliniak represented one end of the spectrum Dorothy Cocks had described, Joseph Eastman Sheehan and Maxwell Maltz fell somewhere in the middle. Both came from respectable but impoverished families; both attended Ivy League schools; both continued their training in Europe; both set up practice in New York. Their careers, in fact, appear to have followed similar paths, but for one significant difference. Despite a shared penchant for the spectacular, Sheehan is remembered with pride as a founding member of the profession, while Maltz is almost never mentioned.

Joseph Eastman Sheehan (1885–1951)

As a child, J. Eastman Sheehan emigrated with his family from Dublin, Ireland, to Wallingford, Connecticut. His father's early death impoverished the family, and Sheehan reportedly waited on tables to finance his graduation, in 1908, from Yale Medical School. Sheehan then traveled and studied in Berlin, Vienna, Heidelberg, Budapest, Paris, London, and Oxford, returning to New York in 1912. He worked with Sir Harold Gillies at Sidcup during World War I and again returned to New York. Sheehan was a dedicated teacher and held posts at the New York Polyclinic Medical School and Columbia University; for years he was chief of plastic surgery at Post Graduate Hospital (later University Hospital of the New York University Medical Center). In 1925, along with Gillies and Ferris Smith of Michigan, he was one of three chief instructors at the first International Clinic of Facio-Maxillary Surgery, held in Paris.[30]

Sheehan had a knack for attracting attention and controversy. In 1927, in what was then reportedly the largest suit ever brought against a physician, Rhea Huston Stevens (actor Walter Huston's ex-wife) sued him for $100,000 over a face-lift. Stevens charged that Sheehan had made incisions in places she had specifically told him not to; as a result she was disfigured and suffered from impaired sight in one eye. Sheehan's lawyers told the press that he had had to alter his original surgical plan upon finding that Mrs. Stevens had already had a face-lift (she had assured him that she had not) and that in any case she had signed a consent form. Had Sheehan not been a member of the AMA and of the American Association of Plastic Surgeons, the suit might have jeopardized his career; as it was, it was eventually settled out of court.[31]

Despite this inauspicious episode, Sheehan prospered and in 1935 was elected president of the AAPS. The arrest and death, that year, of outlaw John Dillinger—and the arrest of the plastic surgeon who had attempted to disguise Dillinger's identity with a nose job and face-lift—generated a surge of interest in plastic surgery among journalists and the public and indirectly caused more problems for Sheehan. In 1925, when a burglar was captured in Vermont, a $450 receipt found in his pocket led police to a plastic surgeon. In 1928, Chicago bandit Willie Jackson's plastic surgery (allegedly undertaken not to evade the police but the gangsters he had double-crossed) had been well publicized. Because of the public attention given crime and criminals during the Depression (not to mention that already given to the connection between crime and plastic surgery), the stakes were higher by the time the Dillinger case broke in 1935. J. Edgar Hoover, director of the Federal Bureau of Investigation, responded by vociferously warning surgeons about their civic responsibilities, and tabloids and respectable papers alike were having a field day.[32]

All this publicity worried New York City Police Commissioner Lewis Valentine, who summoned Sheehan to educate the police force on what was and was not possible with plastic surgery. The talk apparently came off well, but Sheehan made the tactical error of inviting the *Time* reporter who attended the lecture to accompany him back to his office. The resulting article infuriated Sheehan's colleagues. Within the walls of "the world's most gorgeous consultation establishment," the article reported, the devoted ministrations of two butlers, a manager, secretary, and housekeeper ensured that "at any moment the Doctor may have his whittled asparagus, hamburgers or sausages, toast, strawberry jam and tea." Hilda, the housekeeper, also pressed Sheehan's suits ("25 at a time," the magazine exclaimed). Under a photograph of an extremely dapper Sheehan, wearing a bowler and sporting a white carnation, it was noted that operations could cost as much as $10,000. All but ten members of the AAPS resigned to protest the image of the specialty Sheehan had

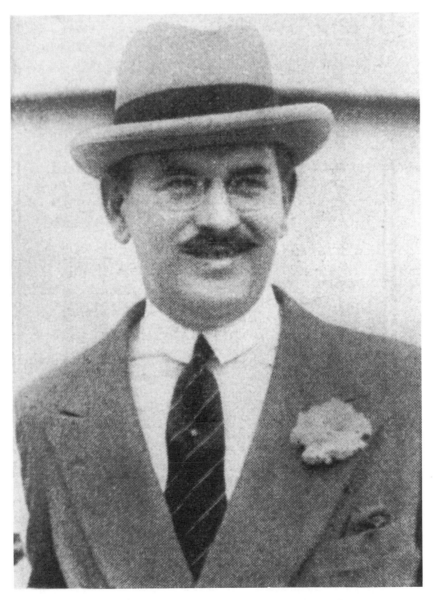

This photograph of J. Eastman Sheehan scandalized his colleagues.

presented. Sheehan agreed to resign as trustee, at which point the members agreed to rejoin and to allow him to finish his term as president.[33]

The brouhaha over the *Time* article suggests that organized medicine was prepared to censure its own, as well as those outside its control, for improper behavior. Plastic surgeons, already very sensitive about their public image, were especially prone to take umbrage. In this case, however, the issue was apparently the nature—not the fact—of the press coverage. Surgeons were commonly mentioned by name in popular magazine articles, and the mention of Sheehan's name in a 1927 article had generated no comment. What was at issue in 1935 was the image of the profession Sheehan had presented to the public. An article about a rich, dapper, society surgeon who lived and worked in a fabulous penthouse, kept servants, dined on "whittled asparagus," and charged as much as $10,000 for a single operation, his colleagues concluded, could significantly damage the fledgling specialty's credibility.[34]

The lack of judgment Sheehan exhibited in 1935 troubled the Board's organizers as they began to select founding members. At the October 1939 executive committee meeting, Sheehan's name was among those deferred for consideration at a later date, and in his case, as in Maliniak's, reputation—not technical competence—seems to have been the issue. In a letter to Vilray Blair dated January 24, 1940, John Staige Davis wrote, "I have never seen Keith Kahn work. . . . In my opinion, he belongs in the group with Sheehan and Maliniac, although I doubt if he is nearly as good technically as either of these men." Clearly, Sheehan's colleagues were dubious about his character if not his surgical technique.[35]

The issue of board certification came up again in 1941, and again the question of character was raised. In February 1941, a number of New York plastic surgeons, including Jerome Webster and J. Eastman Sheehan, received invitations from a plastic surgeon named Herbert Pomerantz to become contributing editors of his new publication, the *Journal of Plastic Surgery*. Only Sheehan and a Brooklyn surgeon named Walter Coakley accepted the invitation outright; the others notified Blair, who marshaled the troops to investigate the situation. As the reports came in, they suggested that once again Sheehan had shown poor judgment. On April 1, Webster informed Blair that Pomerantz had graduated from New York University Medical School in 1904 but was not a member of any of the local medical societies; he had written the historical introduction to plastic surgeon Joseph Safian's book on rhinoplasty and "got the facts wrong." Two days later, Clarence Straatsma tipped Blair that the journal was backed by Louis Sunshine, "who until recently was our leading abortionist" and who was now giving "weekly talks on plastic surgery over some obscure radio station." On April 4, Gustave Aufricht informed Blair that Pomerantz was currently sharing an office with Safian; neither surgeon was connected with any of the New York hospitals. Finally, on May 9, Sheehan was asked to explain himself. In his response, dated May 24, he apologized for his lack of judgment and stated that he had already resigned the editorship. "What I did not allow for, sufficiently, when I accepted the editorship," he mused, "was that [the journal's] quality might fall below my concept of it." Four months later, on September 21, 1941, Sheehan was admitted to the founders' group.[36]

Sheehan's penchant for controversy continued throughout his life. His ties with Europe, and particularly with Spain, were strong; he counted many members of the nobility among his friends and for years maintained a summer practice in London. In 1928, he had helped train Spanish surgeons who were treating soldiers injured in the Morocco uprising. During the Spanish Civil War, he was again invited to help organize hospitals and train surgeons; as a sign of appreciation, he was made an honorary colonel in Franco's army. This honor later cost Sheehan an endowed chair in plastic surgery at Oxford. Although at the request of the chair's sponsors, Lord and Lady Nuffield, Winston Churchill intervened and Sheehan was eventually allowed to enter England, the taint of fascism led Oxford's Board of Overseers to select another candidate. Sheehan returned to New York, where he mended fences with his New York colleagues and continued an active private practice until his death in 1951 (asked to testify against Sheehan in a 1948 malpractice suit, Jerome Webster noted that "luckily" he would be in China during that time). Although some of his equally controversial colleagues are remembered only as quacks or publicity hounds, Sheehan is remembered indulgently as a talented surgeon with a particular talent for publicity. His obituary noted tactfully that he "had a flair for showmanship and the spectacular which was frequently misunderstood by his associates."[37]

Maxwell Maltz (1899–1975)

Maxwell Maltz was born in New York in 1899, fourteen years after J. Eastman Sheehan. He graduated from Columbia in 1919 and received his M.D. degree from the Columbia College of Physicians and Surgeons in 1923. Like Sheehan, Maltz went to Europe to study with Sir Harold Gillies and

Jacques Joseph. When he returned, he later recalled, he had some trouble establishing a practice and getting hospital privileges because most physicians regarded his work as "vanity surgery." Maltz undertook his own mini-publicity campaign, in medical meetings and in less formal conversations with others. He soon opened a fourteen-room penthouse combination home and office and evidently had little trouble maintaining a practice.[38]

Maltz held posts at Beth Israel Hospital from 1925 to 1935, at Metropolitan Hospital from 1930 to 1936, and at Beth David Hospital from 1930 to 1939; he also served as director of plastic and reconstructive surgery at West Side Hospital. In 1930 he was one of the eleven surgeons involved in J. William Greefe's charity project, and he helped start a similar program that provided plastic surgery for criminals, especially juveniles. Articles in *Cosmopolitan* and *Esquire* publicized his work and helped to create a receptive audience for his first book. Published in 1936, *New Faces, New Futures: Rebuilding Character with Plastic Surgery* eclipsed other books on plastic surgery published in the 1930s, garnering favorable reviews from the *New York Times,* the *Scientific Book Club Review,* and *Booklist.* A number of New York surgeons, including Jerome Webster, benefited from the publicity Maltz generated, as new patients, often clutching copies of articles or of Maltz's book, came to ask if the transformations Maltz had wrought for others might be recreated for them.[39]

Although Maltz was apparently a responsible, if not a model, surgeon, a brief look at the neighborhood in which he practiced illuminates the world he inhabited. For most of his professional life, Maltz kept an office at 57 West Fifty-seventh Street in New York City. During the 1920s and 1930s, his most active years of practice as a plastic surgeon in the United States, Maltz enjoyed an interesting selection of neighbors. "A new method of plastic correction of the bust" was available a few blocks away at 205 West Fifty-seventh; an institution that advertised itself as offering "Chirurgie Plastique Moderne" was at 205 West Fifty-fourth. Madame Mays, who promised "Spend 12 days with Madame Mays. Freckles, wrinkles, puffs scientifically removed . . . Physicians' endorsements," operated out of 38 West Fifty-third. Mme. Louise Hermance, "the one and only originator of the scientific method of face lifting without surgery or operation," was probably a more serious competitor, at 62 West Fifty-seventh, with the "Plastic Surgery Institute," Fifth Avenue at Fifty-eighth, a close second. Natalie Tovim, registered nurse, advertised electrolysis (the barer fashions of the 1920s ensured this new hair-removal technique's popularity); her office was located in Maltz's building. At 162 West Fifty-sixth, "Faceyouth Rejuvenation" required more of a walk, but some women undoubtedly made the trek. Dr. James Stotter—like Maltz, author of an enthusiastic 1936 consumer guide to plastic surgery, and, like Maltz, a thorn in Jerome Webster's side—was just blocks away on Forty-second. Surrounding buildings were filled with businesses and professional offices offering hair removal (by electrolysis, X-rays, or unspecified methods), facial massages and peels, facials, cosmetic makeovers, and a variety of beauty products.[40]

This, *Vogue* advised, was the essential neighborhood for all women interested in beauty. All of these practitioners advertised in the magazine's back section, first called the "Shoppers' and Buyers' Guide" and, later, the "Address Book," and all, readers were assured, were "thoroughly reliable." Introductions like this one, which appeared in the February 1, 1935, issue, emphasized the magazine's endorsement:

> STOP puzzling over where to find
> That something new you have in mind!
> GO to the shops on these two pages,
> For finds you'd never find in ages,
> Except that VOGUE, your tireless friend,
> Will always tell you where to spend![41]

Maltz did not, in fact, advertise in *Vogue,* but he did seek publicity in ways that offended his colleagues. Early on, Maltz joined the new ASPRS; he appears in the photograph of the group's October 28, 1932, meeting, which now hangs in the National Archives of Plastic Surgery. He is absent, however, from the 1934 annual meeting photograph, probably because he sponsored a rival society. The American Society of Plastic Surgeons of the City of New York met only once, on March 6, 1934, but it was enough to ruin Maltz's chances for board certification.

According to Jerome Webster, who forwarded this information to Vilray Blair in connection with the Board's organization, Maltz founded the new society with Walter Coakley (who, with Sheehan, had accepted the journal post without clarifying its sponsors' status) and Keith Kahn. Kahn had come to New York from New Orleans, where he had been practicing cosmetic surgery. When Webster refused to put him on staff, he went to Europe; upon returning he established an office in the theater district's Hotel Taft, which he advertised as the Keith Kahn Hospital for Plastic Surgery. One of the officers of the *New York State*

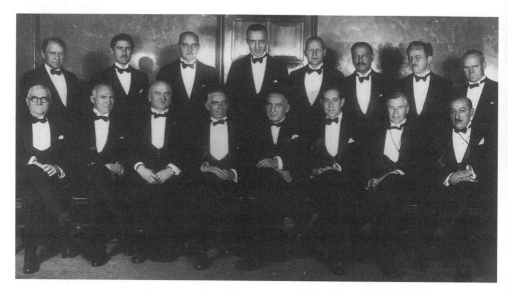

The first meeting (October 28, 1932) of what would become the American Society of Plastic and Reconstructive Surgeons, Inc. *Standing, left to right:* H. Lyons Hunt, Maxwell Maltz, Arthur Palmer, Charles M. Gratz, Clarence Straatsma, Gaston Labat, William Bierman, Ralph Waldron; *seated, left to right:* Leon T. Lewald, Harold S. Vaughan, Fred Albee, Robert Ivy, Jacques W. Maliniak, Harry Finkelstein, Carl Burdick, Isidore Goldstein.

Medical Journal had confided to Webster that he "had a very difficult time keeping Keith Kahn on the upper side of the ethical line," and that Maltz, who "used his title in this society to sign articles in lay literature to considerable monetary advantage," was no better.[42]

Maltz, as surgeon Joseph Tamerin recalled, was a master of publicity. He started the new society "because of his pique at Maliniac who was getting publicity with his society," and at least one of the surgeons who joined Maltz's society did so simply because he "was always at sword's point with Maliniac." Maltz had secured his colleagues' participation by promising that he envisioned a professional organization and would not seek publicity, but then "laid out a publicity campaign that was the daddy of them all." Whether Coakley and Joseph Safian, who had also joined, faced any repercussions is not clear, but it is likely that they were not severe; both men, after all, had been on the original founders' group list in 1939. The correspondence regarding Maltz's application to the Board is incomplete, and the minutes of the 1942 executive committee meeting, at which his membership was discussed and denied, are missing, but the information that remains concerning Kahn and Maltz clearly implies that their colleagues were dismayed by what they considered unethical behavior. Their decision is recorded in a crisp notation: on May 31, 1942, "the Board voted not to issue its certificate to the following: Dr. Keith Kahn, Dr. R. C. Pearlman, Dr. Curt J. Englemann, Dr. Maxwell Maltz."[43]

At some point—possibly in 1944, although it may have been earlier—Maltz operated on the daughter of President Trujillo of the Dominican Republic. His success made him a celebrity throughout Latin America; he eventually became an honorary professor at the universities of Santo Domingo, Nicaragua, Honduras, El Salvador, and Guatemala, as well as Athens. He was a fellow of both the International College of Surgeons and the Latin American Society of Plastic Surgeons and an honorary fellow in several other Latin American medical societies. Maltz continued to publish technical articles on plastic surgery through the mid-1940s.[44]

In his middle years, Maltz apparently concentrated on writing, dividing his time between fiction and self-help books. A proposed television series based on his life never materialized, but *The Magic Scalpel,* a paperback novel about a plastic surgeon, appeared in 1960. In 1963 he wrote and produced a play about plastic surgery entitled *Hidden Stranger,* which received scathing reviews and closed after only seven performances. (The *New Yorker*'s John McCarten called it a "sorry affair. . . . The most mysterious thing about it is why it ever got written"; while *Newsweek* thought it a "vanity production . . . [an] outrageously foolish melodrama," and nominated Maltz's "surgeon-hero, who scrupulously shuns both ethics and morals" as "the worst doctor of the year.") Just before he died, Maltz published a florid novel entitled *The Time Is Now,* a fictionalized account of the life of Gasparo Tagliacozzi, sixteenth-century Italian pioneer in plastic surgery, which critic Frank Slaughter, author of the heroic doctor novels so popular in the post–World War II years, described as "a richly colored tapestry, a fine, gutsy recreation in fiction of one of the most exciting periods of history, Renaissance Italy, and above all, of one man's towering struggles."[45]

Although he achieved some fame as a novelist and playwright, Maltz is best known as the founder and main publicizer of psycho-cybernetics, a self-help program that combined self-image psychology and self-hypnosis with an emphasis on programming suggestions

Maxwell Maltz, *The Magic Scalpel*

into the unconscious. In addition to his four autobiographical works on plastic surgery (*New Faces, New Futures* [1936], *The Evolution of Plastic Surgery* [1946], *Dr. Pygmalion: The Autobiography of a Plastic Surgeon* [1953], and *Adventures in Staying Young* [1955]), Maltz published at least ten self-help books between 1960 and 1975, including *Psycho-Cybernetics: A New Way to Get More Living Out of Life* (1960), *The Magic Power of Self-Image Psychology: The New Way to a Bright, Full Life* (1964), and *Power Psycho-Cybernetics for Youth: A New Dimension in Personal Freedom* (1971). *Psycho-Cybernetics* became so popular during the 1960s that *Readers Digest,* for the first time, devoted two issues of the book section to a single book; by 1966 it had gone through several editions and had sold more than six hundred thousand copies.[46]

Broadly speaking, Maxwell Maltz and Joseph Eastman Sheehan were both reputable members of the medical profession. Both were fellows of the International College of Surgeons, and both maintained their memberships in the New York state and county medical societies and the AMA until they died. They shared a commitment to international travel and professional and educational exchange: both claimed membership in several international plastic surgical and medical societies and held various visiting professor- and lectureships overseas. Both were prolific writers, and both are remembered as charismatic self-promoters who in the process promoted plastic surgery.

The careers of Maxwell Maltz and Joseph Eastman Sheehan, in short, followed similar paths, with one significant exception. Sheehan joined the American plastic surgical associations and was certified by the American Board of Plastic Surgery; Maltz did not and was not. According to the standards of the American Medical Association, this should have been reversed. In his later years, Maltz became a self-help guru, but in 1941 he could boast a flawless, if somewhat flamboyant, reputation as a plastic surgeon; Sheehan's record, in contrast, was tainted by a major malpractice suit, two significant professional flaps suggesting at best a lack of judgment, and the suggestion of fascism. Given the similarities between their careers, this divergence is almost impossible to explain, and it becomes more curious given the profiles of others who were certified. In addition to Sheehan, Coakley, and Safian, the Board admitted Adalbert G. Bettman, a Portland, Oregon, surgeon whose supervisor at the University of Oregon was "most positive that Bettman was no plastic surgeon," and Herbert O. Bames, who was (his Los Angeles colleagues discreetly informed the Board) a cosmetic surgery "enthusiast." Perhaps more than anything else, the case of Maltz and Sheehan suggests that the criteria that divided surgeon from quack in these years were often arbitrary.[47]

In some cases, however, the differences that divided surgeons are crystal clear. J. Howard Crum and Henry Junius Schireson are the quintessential examples of the so-called "advertising" plastic surgeons of the 1920s and 1930s. Crum practiced in New York from 1928 until his death sometime in the 1970s. Schireson, in contrast, moved around. He reportedly began practicing in Chicago (although the date is unknown), moved through Philadelphia in the early teens, then through New York, and ended up back in Philadelphia in the early 1940s; he is known to have obtained medical licenses in at least eight states. No evidence suggests that the two surgeons knew each other, although because each dominated headlines at one time, they probably were aware of each other's existence. In addition to a love of publicity and of showman-ship, Crum and Schireson shared a high regard for the profession of plastic surgery, a fervent belief in its ability to improve the world, and a commitment to furthering its development. Neither is listed in the medical literature or in the histories of plastic surgery that surgeons have published; instead, they operated in the public realm of commercial beauty culture. Ironically, although these men remained outside the self-defined boundaries of organizing professional medicine, neither join-ing medical societies nor publishing in medical journals, together they did more to shape the public image of plastic surgery than almost any other physicians.

John Howard Crum (1888–197?)

On March 12, 1931, J. Howard Crum, plastic surgeon and author of *The Making of a Beautiful Face; or, Face Lifting Unveiled,* provided the high-light of the 1931 International Beauty Shop Owners' Convention when he performed "the first public face-lifting operation on record" in the Grand Ballroom of New York City's Pennsylvania Hotel. Mrs. Martha Petelle, a sixty-year-old character actress, submitted to the operation "vol-untarily and with much apparent joy," explaining that her employment opportunities would be enhanced if some of her wrinkles were removed.

The *New York Times* reported that more than six hundred women attended, but a later article in the *New Republic* put the crowd at fifteen hundred.[48]

In accordance with its strict reporting style, the *Times* refrained from commenting on the operation, but the *New Republic* described it with relish. According to reporter Thyra Samter Winslow, "the operation, as publicly performed, appeared amazingly simple—about as easy as peeling a banana. Areas in front of the ear and on the back of the neck . . . were marked off with iodine. A solution of novocaine was injected. . . . The surgeon drew up the sagging face. Snipped it. Sewed it together into a semblance of youth. He bandaged the two long, narrow wounds. And the old lady, much younger looking, certainly, had her hair waved and her photograph taken!" Winslow's article was not entirely positive in tone. She warned women about pain and scarring, as well as the possibility that the operation could leave them "more than a bit lopsided. Or with a set expression. Or entirely disfigured." She acknowledged, however, that many women would be willing to take the risk: "But if you're getting on, and are beginning to be psychopathic about your appearance, regaining a semblance of youth may mean more to you than anything else in the world. And an operation including many injections of novocaine, cutting, fifty stitches or so, five hundred to a thousand dollars, very real danger of infection and the chance of being disfigured for life, may seem a small price to pay for the possibility of looking younger again."[49]

Crum clearly believed these risks were worth taking. In *The Making of a Beautiful Face*, he admitted that plastic surgery could be seen as "an encroachment upon the province of Mother Nature" but justified his career on simple grounds. "An aging and unattractive face will often have as disastrous an effect on a woman's life as would some physical deformity," he claimed, and plastic surgery offered "the one reliable method whereby time and age may be pushed back and the happiness of woman advanced." Much like advertisers, who played on American fears about everything from insufficient brain power to body odor, Crum played on women's fears about being ugly and old. Despite the "present world-wide emancipation of woman," he asserted, "a beautiful face is still reckoned as one of woman's most valuable assets"; it "frequently decides the matter of marriage for her." Making explicit his definition of what constituted waged work for women, Crum continued: "'Face Value' is more than a mere phrase—it is a distinct asset and a moral obligation. You can not afford to look anything less than the best. . . . Your own success and happiness may depend upon this factor more than you realize."[50]

More conservative plastic surgeons were not impressed with Crum's performance at the beautician's conference. Jacques Maliniak was so disgusted he penned a scathing rebuke, which appeared in *Hygeia*: "The operation should be performed only by legitimate surgeons under the most sanitary conditions. . . . It is hard to picture a more blatant disregard of the elementary rules of asepsis than occurred at a recent meeting of cosmeticians when a face-lifting operation was demonstrated in an ordinary assembly hall before a large group of spectators." That Crum styled himself a plastic surgeon and received a great deal of publicity also incensed Jerome Webster; Webster saw a number of patients who were dissatisfied with Crum's work, and he was at least as concerned as Maliniak about the effect practitioners like Crum had on the specialty's image. Little is known about the aspects of Crum's life that did not make the papers, but the available information suggests that he consistently disregarded the proprieties promulgated by organized medicine; he was, in fact, exactly the type of practitioner Maliniak and Webster were trying to put out of business.[51]

Crum was born in 1888 and graduated from Bennett Medical College in Illinois in 1909. The school, which was not approved by the AMA, had just assumed the name; since its founding in 1868 it had borne the more descriptive name of the Bennett College of Eclectic Medicine and Surgery. Among its more famous, or infamous, students the school counted John R. Brinkley, goat-gland huckster extraordinaire, whose tenure overlapped slightly with Crum's. Crum received his New York license in 1928, when he was forty years old, and published his book that same year. Liberally illustrated with photographs of beautiful women— the implication being that such beauty can be created through surgery— *The Making of a Beautiful Face* promises miracles but contains no details of how they will be achieved. Crum sought further publicity through magazine articles and newspaper and phone directory advertisements, and by touring department stores and giving lectures. These strategies brought him recognition and a steady string of patients. Well into the 1950s, Jerome Webster saw patients who had gone to Crum years, sometimes decades, earlier.[52]

Crum lost no sleep over his colleagues' displeasure. In 1932 he again provided the highlight of the International Beauty Shop Owners'

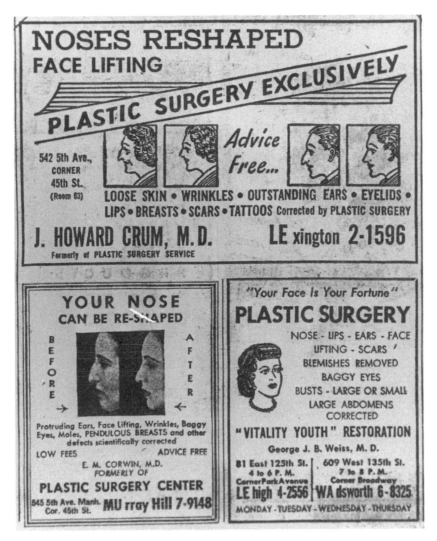

J. Howard Crum's listing, with others, in the Manhattan Yellow Pages, 1952.

Convention, this time with a "type-changing" operation. Crum's patient had allegedly just been released from jail after serving twenty years on a manslaughter charge. Perhaps reflecting then-current ideas promulgated in Cesare Lombroso's widely read works on criminology and by a host of phrenologists, Crum promised that by changing her face he could change her personality (or "type") and ensure that she would become a law-abiding citizen. More than a thousand women reportedly witnessed the operation; the audience was so enthusiastic that twelve extra police guards were required to keep order. Four women fainted and one was hit by a falling lamp, but the audience appeared to appreciate Crum's theatrical approach. Crum made the papers again in 1937 when five women and ten men fainted during his performance of "three nose operations done in the manner of vaudeville turns" on three members of a Honduran family.[53]

His 1937 operation may have been Crum's last bid for publicity, but he or someone much like him performed another public operation in 1938 or 1939. In a 1939 article in the journal *Medical Times,* San Francisco surgeon Albert D. Davis complained about the public "personality operation" that a New York surgeon had recently performed in front of one thousand beauty experts on stage at the Hotel Roosevelt. According to Davis, the patient entered the "personality shop" and selected a face to suit her personality; the doctor made a model, and the operation—"unique in medical practice"—began: "Klieg lights blazed, and press photographers let off great flashes. . . . The Doctor worked away, making incisions here, removing long strips of flesh there—following the ideal model which a nurse held up. . . . Meanwhile the pianist rendered such appropriate tunes as, 'As You Desire Me,' 'I'll See You Again,' and ended up with 'Beautiful Lady.'" After the operation, the doctor explained, "You see I'm an artist rather than a surgeon. I model in human flesh. If this thing succeeds, plastic surgery will have reached perfection!" Never a member of the AMA or of any state or local medical society, Crum listed himself in the American medical directory as a general practitioner rather than a surgeon or plastic surgeon. He apparently died sometime between the 1973 edition, in which he is listed as retired, and the 1979 edition, in which he is not listed.[54]

Surgeons who meticulously maintained their membership in the American Medical Association and sought to bolster their professional credentials through the new plastic surgical societies despised Crum; in their view, his active pursuit of publicity and showmanship did nothing for the profession save exemplify what it was not. But the outcry Crum's antics inspired in medical circles had little effect on his career or his reputation. Only library assistant Alice Rogers's curiosity—and Jerome Webster's quick work—saved the New Orleans Lions Club from embarrassment in 1937. Attempting to write up a program featuring Crum as the scheduled speaker, Rogers turned to Webster when she could find no information in standard medical sources. Wary of being sued (which had happened in a similar case), Webster wrote Iago Galdston at the New York Academy of Medicine; Galdston wired Rogers: "Person concerning whom you inquired from Dr. Webster is not in good standing, not a member of the county society, and flagrantly violates professional ethics." Even the *Saturday Review of Literature* remained ignorant of his disrepute among professionals. In its review of his 1941 book *Beauty and Health,* the magazine noted that "many readers may not agree with Dr. Crum's calmly acquiescent attitude towards face lifting and other plastic surgery," but otherwise gave his "course in loveliness"—complete with a series of exercises for the facial muscles called "crumacises"—a glowing recommendation. And to the general public, Crum was plastic surgery personified. Thousands of women, and some men, flocked to his performances, where the link he forged between plastic surgery and beauty was indelibly imprinted in the public mind; as late as 1951, women wrote to the American Board of Plastic Surgery to inquire about his status.[55]

Henry Junius Schireson (1881–1949)

Those who were trying to make plastic surgery respectable found even more infuriating the career of Henry Junius Schireson. Instead of staging showy operations, Schireson recruited famous patients to impart an aura of glamour to his practice. In this he was successful, but in the process he brushed up against the law and became the target of the AMA's commitment to clean house. Some of the details of Schireson's life and career are sketchy, and little is known about his childhood. Even with these limitations, however, a review of his career is instructive.[56]

Schireson was born in Russia; his parents emigrated to the United States when he was eight. He attended public schools and Cooper Union in New York, as well as an unidentified academy in Baltimore, Maryland. After a short stint as a drugstore clerk, he enrolled at the University of Maryland School of Medicine in 1903, but left less than a year later after flunking all but two subjects. In 1906, after a year's work, Schireson received a diploma from Maryland Medical College in Baltimore, which was not AMA approved. He was licensed to practice in Philadelphia in 1910; he practiced there from 1910 to 1913 and again from 1932 to 1947. In 1915 Schireson reportedly practiced in New York, perhaps abandoning his practice when his methods were questioned by the County

Medical Society. In 1922 he received a diploma from the nonaccredited Kansas City College of Medicine and Surgery in St. Louis, Missouri, at that time the home of numerous diploma-mill medical schools and, by one account, "more illegal doctors in proportion to population than any other city of its size in the United States." Schireson eventually obtained licenses in Vermont, Massachusetts, Connecticut, New Jersey, Pennsylvania, Ohio, Michigan, and Illinois. His first successful practice, although he never obtained a license there, was in New York, also the site of his first major publicity stunt—the nose job he performed in Fanny Brice's apartment at the New York Ritz in August 1923.[57]

Schireson's first brush with the law came just a year later. In early 1924, a lawyer named Walter E. Boerger asked that Schireson's Illinois license be revoked on the grounds that he was not a graduate of a medical school in good standing. No action on the petition was taken, and he remained popular in Chicago. That same year, press agent Victor Rubin (who had recruited Brice, among others) sued Schireson for failing to pay him, as promised, $500 per month for three years and a 25 percent commission on all business he generated. In 1927 Schireson again made headlines when he sued British actress Lady Diana Manners and her mother, the Dowager Duchess of Rutland, for failing to pay him for face-lifts he had performed. Lady Diana emphatically denied the charges and posed for photographs to disprove his story; she said that Schireson had simply treated her mother's eyes. Jacques Maliniak believed that the entire episode was a publicity stunt. Schireson, Maliniak charged, had originally agreed to perform the surgery for free, believing that Manners's title and reputation would be reward enough. Later, fearing that he would not be able to capitalize sufficiently on this, he "had hit upon this expedient for extracting the last measure of publicity from the operation."[58]

Schireson's next celebrity client was "the notorious Peaches Browning," a showgirl whose legs he allegedly reshaped. In 1928, however, a similar operation went awry, sparking an investigation by the AMA and the beginning of a trend toward less-than-favorable publicity. Under the headline "Schireson—The Disgrace of Illinois," the *Journal of the American Medical Association* (*JAMA*) reported that Schireson had promised a Miss Sadye Holland that he could correct her bow legs through surgery. Unfortunately, gangrene had set in and the young woman was now in critical condition, with both legs amputated above the knee. The disgrace, according to *JAMA*, lay not in the fact that a malpractice suit had been filed; such suits were not unusual. Rather, it lay in Schireson's irresponsible conduct. The vast majority of practitioners at that time deemed leg operations too dangerous; Schireson had erred by promising the impossible and by minimizing the risks involved.[59]

This incident marked the beginning of Schireson's long battle with organized medicine. Among other things, the article revealed that Schireson had been denied a license to practice in Illinois in 1911 and had not succeeded in getting one until late 1921 or early 1922, "during the incumbency of the notorious ... W.H.H. Miller, who later was convicted of the fraudulent sale of medical licenses, fined $1,000, and removed from his position." Many patients had complained to the AMA and to state authorities. The article concluded with the question, "How much longer will Illinois tolerate Henry Junius Schireson?"[60]

Illinois did not in fact tolerate Schireson much longer. In June 1930, a year after settling the Holland case out of court, the "self-styled dealer in beauty to fading womankind" lost his Illinois license on the grounds of "fraud, character unbecoming to a physician, and gross malpractice." The following May, Schireson voluntarily surrendered his Ohio license, probably to avoid a special meeting the state medical board had scheduled to discuss its revocation.[61]

The sad case of Sadye Holland had attracted enough publicity that some viewers probably recognized Schireson in the 1932 film *False Faces*, but he was not named in the film, and it did not generate much publicity. Schireson dropped out of sight until 1938, when his book appeared, and the hiatus in publicity evidently helped him, as his previous reputation did not affect his book's reception. *Science News Letter* quoted from it in both 1938 and 1939, identifying him only as Dr. Henry J. Schireson, "plastic surgeon of Philadelphia," and noting that his book was filled with "fascinating details."[62]

In early 1939, Schireson's name cropped up on *JAMA*'s list of quacks who were undercutting the medical profession, but no new information on his career was included; the association had apparently lost track of him. In June of that year, however, *JAMA* picked up the scent of an investigation the *Philadelphia Inquirer* had begun to conduct into Schireson's career in Pennsylvania. The inquiry had been sparked by a grand jury indictment for fraud and perjury. Facing a string of lawsuits and bad debts that threatened to disrupt his fancy Spruce Street practice, the *Inquirer* reported, Schireson had declared bankruptcy in 1937, claiming to be single with assets of only $334. In fact, investigators found, he was married and had concealed assets of $130,000 in his wife's name. On March 27, 1940, Schireson was convicted on both counts and on May 8 was sentenced to two concurrent terms of eighteen months at Lewisburg Federal Penitentiary.

His appeal kept the case in the press, and, during the months before a decision was announced, Philadelphians were treated to a review of the surgeon's criminal record, as disclosed by the paper's intrepid reporters. First convicted of selling narcotics illegally in Baltimore (whether or not he served time for this charge is not clear), Schireson had then spent ten months in the Allegheny County Workhouse for conspiracy to cheat and defraud and six months on Rikers Island for practicing medicine illegally (in New York, where he was not licensed). In addition, Philadelphians (and physicians, through *JAMA*'s bulletins) found out that, although his Illinois license had been revoked in 1930, the Illinois Supreme Court had restored it in 1933, holding that "incompetent testimony was permitted at the hearing before the medical board." On October 18, 1941, Schireson finally began serving two concurrent sentences of one year and one day, after having pled *nolo contendere* to both charges.[63]

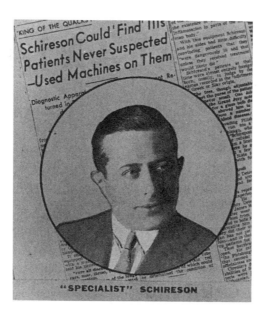

The "King of Quacks," as depicted in *Hygeia*'s 1944 exposé.

At this point, New Jersey attempted to revoke his license on grounds of moral turpitude, but—just as he had in Illinois—Schireson countersued, asserting that because a plea of *nolo contendere* did not acknowledge guilt, the state had no right to revoke his license on such grounds. On September 24, 1943, the New Jersey State Court of Appeals and Pardons upheld his case, setting aside the state board of medical examiners' April 1942 revocation of his license. In November, *JAMA* again decried authorities' obvious inability to deal effectively with Schireson, bemoaning the New Jersey court's verdict and asking plaintively, "Who is to protect the public now?"[64]

The *Philadelphia Record* and the AMA, along with other news agents and law enforcement organizations, continued to pursue Schireson, and his notoriety grew. *Time* dubbed him "King of Quacks" in May 1944, and *Hygeia* ran a similar article the following month. Schireson, however, was seemingly unstoppable. Organized medicine lacked effective enforcement capabilities, and Schireson's impressive ability to manipulate the legal system prevented his pursuers from closing in on him. In 1944, eleven years after the Philadelphia County Medical Society had begun demanding revocation of his license, Schireson was still in practice. And, according to the *Record*, the recent investigation

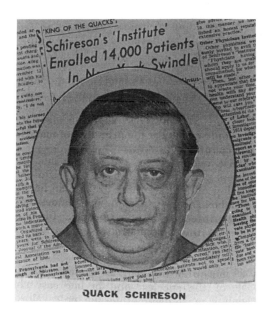

QUACK SCHIRESON

allegedly conducted by the state board was useless. Not only had the board's senior investigator failed to investigate, but he had also attempted to intimidate anti-Schireson witnesses.[65]

Despite these disclosures, the story continued for several more years. In June 1944, Schireson faced both a grand jury indictment for falsely obtaining fees from a patient (whom he had assured that he was on the staff of a naval hospital) and a hearing to consider revoking his Pennsylvania license on the grounds that it had been obtained fraudulently. Once again he outmaneuvered his opponents. In September, Schireson convinced the Dauphin County Court to issue a temporary injunction barring the state board from holding a hearing on his license, contending that the state had no authority to revoke a license for fraud. In November 1945, Judge Karl E. Richards indignantly declared that the state has "the inherent right to revoke a license obtained by fraud," but Schireson again appealed, and the case went to the Pennsylvania Supreme Court. In June 1946, the court declared in favor of the state and dismissed Schireson's appeal at his cost. The Pennsylvania license he had received on June 29, 1910, was finally revoked in August 1947. Two years later, on March 27, 1949, Schireson died of chronic myocarditis. He was sixty-eight years old.[66]

If nothing else, Schireson's story clearly demonstrates the limits of organized medicine's power in these years. As *Hygeia* noted in 1944, this "lord of all his loathsome brethren" had a "preposterous career" that spanned forty years. "Trailing him, but always too far behind, has been the pitiful wake of his victims." Plastic surgeons were especially preoccupied with decorum because of their sensitivity to publicity and, until 1941, the marginality of their field. Given this orientation, J. Howard Crum, who seems simply to have behaved in a manner his colleagues judged unbefitting a respectable physician, was bad enough. Schireson, in contrast, posed a clear danger to his patients, but even so, the combined efforts of the American Medical Association, indignant journalists, and local, state, and federal law enforcement officials succeeded only in slowing him down. As he had with Crum, Jerome Webster ran interference, steering patients who came in asking about Schireson to more reputable surgeons and cautioning practitioners about him, but for those who came to see him after they had seen Schireson, he could do little.[67]

More significant is what Schireson's career suggests about the state of plastic surgery in these years. Not only did the many disclosures fail to end his career, they did little, if anything, to undermine his reputation as a famous plastic surgeon. For much of his career, Schireson, like Crum, dominated news coverage of plastic surgery. From 1923 through the final revocation of his license in 1947, Schireson managed to escape not only the AMA but also his own reputation. His services were much in demand, as was his opinion. Even in the late 1930s, as the American Board of Plastic Surgery began to coalesce, popular magazines looking for commentary on plastic surgery turned to Schireson as readily as to the Board's founders, and into the 1940s potential patients wrote to the Board asking whether they should trust him.[68]

Henry Junius Schireson, J. Howard Crum, Maxwell Maltz, J. Eastman Sheehan, Jacques Maliniak, and Vilray Blair represent the full range of practicing plastic surgeons during the years between the two world wars, yet they had much in common. All played important roles in shaping plastic surgery's professional and public image during the specialty's organizing years, and all saw themselves as pioneers, participants in the glory days of plastic surgery's emergence as a recognized medical specialty.

Commentators both within and outside the medical profession, during these years, concurred about the need for professional organization and generally agreed on the criteria that should be employed to determine a plastic surgeon's standing. Plastic surgery, they believed, was not a business. It was a specialty within the larger medical profession, and its practitioners should abide by certain rules of behavior and principles of practice. Plastic surgeons themselves generally subscribed to this view. For them, the problem arose not when they considered general principles but when they considered individual practitioners. When the general principles are applied to these six surgeons' careers, some of the complexities surgeons faced as they selected the specialty's founding members emerge.

To writer Dorothy Cocks, who considered publicity the most significant criterion, Schireson and Crum would have been "flagrant charlatans." In addition to publishing self-aggrandizing books and contriving elaborate publicity stunts, they advertised in newspapers and magazines. Maltz and Sheehan, just as clearly, would have been "semi-charlatans." They did not actually advertise, but their self-promotional efforts were only slightly less blatant. Maliniak and Blair are examples of the "truly ethical surgeons" Cocks admired. They had acquired their experience in the war, they preferred reconstructive surgery to cosmetic surgery, and they confined their interactions to medical circles. Even publicity, however, could not have functioned as a litmus test in these years. Unlike Maltz, Crum, and Schireson, who not only gravitated toward publicity but actively created it, Blair and Maliniak eschewed publicity in other than medical circles, and even Sheehan, burned by his early experience and the professional scandal it sparked, thereafter toed the line. All six of these surgeons, however, were mentioned in the popular press at one time or another and often in highly complimentary terms.

No matter what criteria were employed, differentiating among these men was problematic. Commentators generally agreed that quacks were motivated by profit, performed cosmetic surgery, and moved outside the boundaries of organized medicine. The individual financial practices of these men are unknown, but to the extent that all were trying to support themselves and their families through plastic surgery, all were motivated by profit. Sheehan, in particular, publicly acknowledged charging what was then considered an outrageous amount. Figures on the relative proportion of cosmetic and reconstructive operations they performed are not available, but again, the information that is available suggests that all of them performed some surgery that would have been considered cosmetic. Even Jerome Webster, who prided himself on being a conservative surgeon, relied on cosmetic surgery for a significant part of his practice. The issue of professionalism is also murky. Before 1941, a connection with organized medicine meant, loosely speaking, a good education, a license, hospital privileges, and membership in medical societies. All of these physicians were licensed, some several times over. Maltz, Maliniak, and Sheehan attended excellent schools, but Blair, like Crum and Schireson, had graduated from a disreputable school. Sheehan, Maltz, Maliniak, and Blair had hospital privileges, often at several different institutions. These same four maintained memberships in the AMA through their county and state societies and in various other professional organizations as well.

The founding of the American Board of Plastic Surgery provided, for the first time, a litmus test for plastic surgeons. Before 1941, who received recognition as a plastic surgeon was as much a matter of luck and public opinion as anything else. After 1941, those who were certified became the "real" plastic surgeons, while those who were not became quacks. The Board's founders were aware that this would occur, and they took their responsibility seriously. They agreed, not surprisingly, to include the men they judged to be skilled, reputable surgeons like

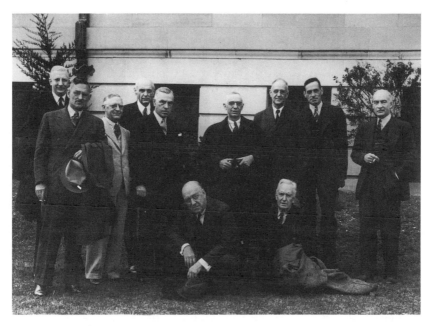

The first annual meeting of the American Board of Plastic Surgery, 1938. *Standing, left to right:* William S. Kiskadden, George W. Pierce, Ferris Smith, William E. Ladd, E. Fulton Risdon, Robert Ivy, John Staige Davis, Harold L. D. Kirkham, Jerome Pierce Webster; *kneeling:* George M. Dorrance, Vilray Blair (*absent:* James Barrett Brown, Sumner L. Koch, John M. Wheeler, Gordon B. New).

themselves; by any standard, Blair's behavior and reputation would have ensured his certification. Predictably, they also decided to exclude those known to be incompetent or irretrievably immoral, and it is not surprising that the antics of J. Howard Crum and Henry Junius Schireson precluded their certification. It was those in between—and most of the surgeons then practicing fell into this category—who presented problems; and it seems clear that in this category, in some cases, the Board's decision was arbitrary. The biggest difference between Maliniak, Maltz, and Sheehan seems to be that in 1941, when the first list of certified specialists in plastic surgery was published, two of them made the cut, while one did not.

The trouble the Board's organizers had in selecting members suggests that to some extent the "local prejudice" Vilray Blair feared did in fact come into play. On a deeper level, however, it reflects the extent to which Board members were divided over the shape the specialty would take. For many surgeons, the urge toward professionalization was sparked in part by a desire to remove plastic surgery from the public realm of beauty conventions and place it where they thought it belonged: in the professional realm of organized medicine, in the hospital. The process of organization was problematic because quacks and surgeons trod similar career paths, behaved in similar ways, and voiced similar sentiments. And this confusion was exacerbated by the fact that, although Americans found reconstructive surgery interesting and admirable, they found cosmetic surgery absolutely absorbing. Only by embracing the practice of cosmetic surgery could plastic surgeons enlist the public's support in their attempt to assert control over their specialty.

By 1941, when plastic surgery was brought under the ever-expanding umbrella of organized medicine, the specialty looked quite different than it had twenty years earlier. In the process of organizing, the field transformed itself in unexpected ways, and the line that Commissioner Greefe had so confidently drawn between "cosmetic or beauty surgeons" and "real plastic surgeons" was erased. The American Board of Plastic Surgery succeeded in excluding some practitioners, but it succeeded only by incorporating their essence: their values, their practices, and to some extent their relationship to the public. While board-certified surgeons were among the most strident critics of the unashamed self-promotion practiced by their less restrained colleagues, they benefited from it in the end. Americans whose interest had been piqued by Crum's antics or by Maltz's or Schireson's books helped provide the impetus and financial support for plastic surgery's emergence as a recognized specialty.

CHAPTER THREE

Consumer Culture and the Inferiority Complex

In 1927, Hazel Rawson Cades, long-time beauty editor of *Woman's Home Companion* and Girl Scout booster, published *Any Girl Can Be Good Looking,* a beauty guide for young women. The book opens with a warning that even a reasonably confident teenager might have found alarming: "Everybody is thinking more these days about good looks. The bar has been raised for the jump. The passing mark is higher. Being good looking is no longer optional. . . . There is no place in the world for women who are not." Those less confident would have found little reassurance in the description of the world that awaited them: "Competition is so keen and . . . the world moves so fast that we simply can't afford not to sell ourselves on sight. What if we are kind? And quick-witted? And make wonderful biscuits? . . . People who pass us on the street can't know that we're clever and charming unless we look it." Women coming of age in the 1920s, Cades cautioned, were entering a very different world than the one their mothers and grandmothers had faced—more distant, more anonymous, more competitive, and far less forgiving.[1]

Between 1921 and 1941, plastic surgeons organized and defined their specialty in the context of a rapidly changing culture. The vagaries of birth and nature continued to produce a wide variety of congenital abnormalities, and traumatic defects increased as bicycles, motorcycles, and especially automobiles became more popular. But the biggest change was that American eyes became more critical. As they paged through advertisements and papered their walls with pictures of movie stars,

Americans created and participated in a new, visual culture, where appearance seemed to rank ever higher in importance.

Evidence that this development was being exploited by increasing numbers of practitioners whose enthusiasm outstripped their skill provided a compelling reason to bring cosmetic surgery under the umbrella of plastic surgery. Newspapers and magazines frequently ran stories about practitioners like "beauty doctor" Gertrude Steele, who fled to Germany in 1925 after autopsies on two of the patients whose faces she had peeled revealed traces of phenol poisoning in the brain. It was the menace of "beauty doctors" like Steele that made up Ohio surgeon George Schaeffer's mind: "There is a certain amount of cosmetic surgery that is legitimate and that should be done by competent plastic surgeons," Schaeffer wrote in 1925. "If the surgical profession will recognize this as legitimate work and do it, there will be less chance for the quack to exploit the people."[2]

There were, however, equally strong countervailing currents. The relaxation of Victorian strictures against vanity had fueled the prodigious growth of the beauty business, but most Americans drew a clear line between going to the beauty parlor and having surgery. Fashion and beauty advisors often counseled against surgery. "If you are badly disfigured, certainly I advise seeking surgical aid," Hazel Rawson Cades wrote. "But if it's just a whim about a nose, or an idea that your face is too wide or your chin is too short, I beg of you, try to forget it." A 1926 article in the *Delineator* made the point most clearly; to the question, "What about plastic surgery?" advice columnist Celia Caroline Cole answered, "*No!*"—in general, such surgery was too dangerous, too impermanent, too likely to fail to justify the silly pursuit of vanity. *Photoplay* advice columnist Carolyn Van Wyck cautioned a Dallas, Texas, teenager who wrote her in the early 1920s, "I would, personally, think twice about undergoing an operation upon a feature that is nearly satisfactory."[3]

Film director Florenz Ziegfeld objected to plastic surgery because "you never know how it will turn out." And surgeons, too, had doubts. The American Medical Association's campaign to distance itself from those it termed quacks and irregular practitioners was in full swing. Cosmetic surgery's association—if only in the public mind—with vendors of patent medicines, mail-order cosmetic miracles, and medical "devices" of dubious value had tainted cosmetic surgery's image, and the distrust and disrespect Americans felt for beauty doctors often extended to rep-

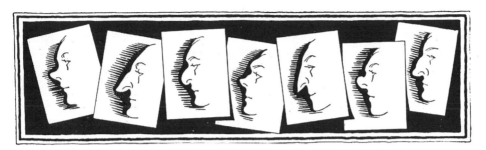

In 1926, surgeon Joseph Beck warned, "It is best to leave well enough alone when it comes to noses. Surgical attempts at improving their shape are full of risk."

utable surgeons as well. "Uncle Henry," *Collier's* folksy commentator on American life, mocked Americans' fascination with cosmetic surgery in a 1929 article entitled "Hi-Jacking the Face" and warned his readers, "almost any beauty doctor can skin you."[4]

The most significant hurdle plastic surgeons faced, however, was the one they had constructed themselves. Many surgeons continued to believe that medicine was meant to heal rather than to beautify. This barrier was built into individual practices: as surgeon Joseph Beck noted in 1921, "I have refused to operate on many more cases of this . . . type than I have accepted, because I have always felt that in most instances the correction was unnecessary and only giving in to a neurotic or self-centered, vain individual." It was also a cornerstone of the emerging specialty's philosophy. In an influential article entitled "The Art and Science of Plastic Surgery," published in 1926, surgeon John Staige Davis asked rhetorically, "What is the ethical difference between doing an abdominal operation and removing wrinkles from a sagging face?" The answer, he responded, was simple: "The abdominal operation is necessary to the health of the patient, the operation for removal of wrinkles is unessential and is simply decorative surgery." "True plastic surgery," he continued, "without question . . . is absolutely distinct and separate from what is known as cosmetic or decorative surgery." Vilray Blair also looked askance at cosmetic surgery. Blair's reluctance to operate on what he termed minor defects was due in part to a "feeling of resentment at being called on to belittle our profession by catering to the vanities and frivolities of life," but in larger part to a belief that the practice of cosmetic surgery went against the medical profession's fundamental principles.

"I was reared in the most orthodox medical surroundings," Blair explained, "with an unquestioning belief in the correctness of the underlying ethics and rules of practice of the profession."[5]

But the social and cultural changes that occurred during the interwar years gave new impetus to the practice of cosmetic surgery. The urge toward self-improvement, which had deep roots in American culture, took on new meaning as Americans struggled to win friends and influence people in a society where competition seemed fierce and survival unsure. A host of voices—like that of actress Edith Nelson, who told *Photoplay*'s readers, "Attention to personal appearance is nowadays essential if you expect to succeed in life. You must 'look your best' at all times"— encouraged Americans to see the scalpel as an ally. The new emphasis on looks forced surgeons to confront troubling questions: Which of these defects, if any, were to be judged worthy of their time and effort? Upon what criteria should these decisions be based? And who would judge— the patient, the surgeon, or someone else altogether?[6]

As they attempted to formulate a collective response to the new demand for their services, surgeons found a compelling conceptual framework in the psychological concept that came to be called the inferiority complex. In the 1920s and 1930s, Americans became fascinated with the new science of psychology in all its various incarnations. They learned about it from books, magazines, newspapers, and even radio broadcasts and were quickly persuaded of its relevance to their lives. The inferiority complex received a particularly enthusiastic reception in the United States. Formulated by Viennese psychologist Alfred Adler before World War I, the inferiority complex, by the mid-1920s, had become common currency in both lay and medical circles. Unlike Freudian psychoanalysis, which struck many Americans as mysterious, depressing, and overly concerned with sex, the inferiority complex seemed uniquely accessible—and particularly relevant to the practice of plastic surgery.

The inferiority complex, in fact, became the final link in the self-reflexive argument plastic surgeons formulated to justify the practice of cosmetic surgery. Patients who developed inferiority complexes because of physical defects would find their economic status adversely affected, because those suffering from such complexes were unable to present themselves with the confidence necessary to ensure success in a competitive world. Conversely, those who could not obtain work because of their appearance would find that their psychic health was at risk: unable to support themselves and their dependents, they would develop inferiority complexes. In either case, surgery could make an important, even key, contribution.

This is not to say that surgeons incorporated psychology in a calculated attempt to increase their patient lists, although a few surgeons did do this. The notorious Henry Schireson, for example, included lengthy discussions of psychology in his 1938 book, presumably in an attempt to bolster a questionable reputation. Most surgeons, however, were captives, as well as captains, of the new enthusiasm for psychology. They responded with alacrity because the theories shed light on questions they had been unable to answer or rendered answers unnecessary.

During the 1920s and 1930s, increasing numbers of Americans came to believe that looks were crucial to social and economic success, as well as to mental health. As a result, their demands for surgical attention became more insistent at the same time as the new language of psychology made these demands more persuasive. Surgeons, too, were affected by this development; they began to invest surgery undertaken solely for the improvement of appearance with this larger medical and societal importance. Some adventurous surgeons had, of course, believed this all along. What changed during these years was that even the most conservative surgeons—those who had originally formulated a justification that covered soldiers and only grudgingly expanded it to cover movie stars—began to extend this understanding to normal, average, everyday Americans. In breaking down the barrier restricting them to reconstruction, surgeons laid claim to the whole body and mind of healthy individuals by linking physical abnormalities to psychological problems for which cosmetic surgical intervention was the prescribed cure. And by 1941, when the first list of diplomates in plastic surgery was published, most plastic surgeons had incorporated cosmetic surgery into their practices.

The Public Eye

In 1930, writer Cecil Barton described for the readers of *Vogue* the new world that had taken shape in the California town that was now known as Hollywood: "Nowhere else in the world are there gathered together so many conventionally beautiful people. This is a town inhabited almost entirely by gods and goddesses of beauty. The girl shutting the window is Venus disguised as a most exquisite Madonna.

The newspaper boy is a fair young Apollo. Every cashier with golden sausage curls is even prettier than Mary Pickford. Every sales man is a John Gilbert. After a time, one loses one's sense of proportion, and nothing remains to stare at. And here, good looks and artifice go hand in hand, for feathery eyelashes are never left unmascaraed, or blond hair unbleached." The American preoccupation with beauty was nowhere more evident than in this sun-baked corner of the City of Angels. The 1920s marked the beginning of America's movie boom. In New York alone, the capacity of movie theaters increased by a factor of eight between 1910 and 1930, while the population merely doubled. In the 1920s, middle-class Americans spent more of their recreation dollars on the movies than on anything else and avidly consumed news about and images of their favorite stars in the pages of the new and numerous fan magazines.[7]

Not everyone found this world as charming as Barton obviously did. In 1923 Mrs. Nesta E. Harris had complained to *Photoplay* that movie stars were "too beautiful" and beauty too much emphasized in the magazine's pages: "If Will Rogers can make good on the screen why not a chance for some other ordinary faces?" Harris asked. "I am watching for a plain girl star, who yet can win her way by her ability and personality without the help of a pretty face." But Harris's voice was drowned out by the chorus of commentators who insisted that a pretty face was paramount. The pages of the nation's magazines and tabloids demonstrate incontrovertibly that Americans preferred their stars pretty and had few, if any, qualms about the various artifices on which they relied to appear so.[8]

Even cosmetic surgery was considered acceptable for those in the public eye of stage and screen. In 1923, speculation about why Jewish comedienne Fanny Brice had decided on a nose job was widespread, and Dorothy Parker's quip that Brice had "cut off her nose to spite her race" was widely quoted. But if Americans enjoyed speculating, most accepted and approved of the reason Brice herself gave most often: she had done it for career reasons, to enable her to play a wider range of roles. "Everything about me has stopped growing except my nose," Brice explained to the *New York Times*. "No woman on the stage of today can afford to have a nose that is likely to keep on growing until she can swallow it." The *Times* wholeheartedly endorsed Brice's conviction that she could "change her style by changing her nose," concluding, "Hurrah for the intrepid Fannie, whose motto is all for art and a nose well lost." Americans so widely accepted the fact that appearance was important to their stage and screen idols that in 1929 the *New York Daily News* and *Literary Digest* could run very sympathetic articles about a man's nose job. According to these reports, when screen idol Rudolph Valentino died, his older brother Albert Guglielmi, with encouragement from highly placed sources in Hollywood, decided to try his hand. Four years and seven nose jobs later, he still lacked "a nose that the camera will like," and the hope of the family, and their friends in Hollywood, had come to rest on his thirteen-year-old son Jean.[9]

Cosmetic surgery was not routine, even in Hollywood. Sylvia Ullback, a beauty advisor and masseuse who published and broadcast under the name Sylvia of Hollywood, was more positive ("If you can afford it and *if* you get a really fine doctor, it's wonderful and by all means have it done") than Hazel Cades, but even so, she advised extreme caution: "I've seen some terrible butchery," she wrote in 1935. In warning women, these counselors were making not a moral judgment but rather an educated guess that the chances of finding a reputable, experienced surgeon (particularly when the potential patient was a naive, screen-struck young woman) were small. Beauty advisors were aware that the younger and barer fashions of the 1920s had raised the stakes. In addition to patients who had received paraffin injections, physicians were beginning to see increasing numbers of women who had undergone the new carbolic acid and phenol face peels, or who had been burned or scarred after undergoing X-ray treatment, which was then being advertised as a solution for everything from moles to undesired body hair. Calls for federal regulation of these procedures went unheeded. Surgeon Jacques Maliniak, speaking before the Society of Medical Jurisprudence at the New York Academy of Medicine in 1933, acknowledged that the pursuit of beauty had a long history, but stressed that modern technologies and new inventions had raised the debate to a new level. "If there is any striking difference between the old and the new ways [of enhancing beauty], it is that on the whole the old were safer," he commented dryly.[10]

Americans of the 1920s and 1930s who defined beauty as an acquired, rather than an inherited, characteristic invested the quest for beauty with a new, and sometimes desperate, urgency. Journalists and advertisers both reflected and encouraged this preoccupation, and they fed the public's fascination with the transformative possibilities of cosmetic surgery. The *New York Daily Mirror's* 1924 Homely Girl contest offers a particularly illustrative example. Each day during the

Homely Girl Contest

Who is the homeliest girl in New York?

Daily Mirror wants to find her—for a great opportunity awaits her.

A plastic surgeon has offered to take the homeliest girl in the biggest city in the country and to make a beauty of her.

Daily Mirror will select competent judges to pass upon the qualities of the contestants.

All you have to do is to send your photograph with name and address to Homeliest Girl Contest Editor. We will not print names, and the photographs will be "masked." Our art department will paint the masks on the photographs to obviate identification.

Here is the chance for New York's homeliest girl. Her misfortune may make a fortune for her.

Send in your photographs right away.

The *New York Daily Mirror* announced the "Homely Girl Contest" on December 1, 1924.

month of December, the paper featured a contestant's photograph, along with a first-person account of the trials and tribulations homeliness had wrought. The winner, sweatshop worker Rosa Travers, received a surgical makeover from Dr. W. A. Pratt, owner and sole proprietor of the Pratt Feature and Speciality Company of Brooklyn, and an opera audition (what happened afterwards was not reported).[11]

Because confusion about what was and was not possible and safe—either in the beauty parlor or in the operating room—was widespread, even would-be cautionary voices sometimes inspired fantasies about miraculous transformations. In 1926, for example, the *Delineator* explained that "each day's mail brought questions . . . to [beauty editor] Celia Caroline Cole, and everywhere she turned she met conflicting opinions. So she marched off to get some first-hand, scientific information on plastic surgery." The advice Cole offered her readers, allegedly from the horse's mouth by way of William Bayard Long, chief of the dermatological clinic at St. Luke's Hospital in New York, is almost bizarre, given her warnings against plastic surgery. "'Skinning?' Allright . . . but be careful who does it. There are skinning, peeling lotions—acids—that are all right, but the ultra-violet ray is better, only have a good skin specialist use the ray. It's like having a sunburn, no worse, and the outer layer peels off and there's your baby-skin." *Literary Digest,* in a 1934 article about criminal John Dillinger, noted that while the story about Dillinger's plastic surgery was "probably a romantic fantasy, its premises are not by any means incredible. Even before the war, when plastic surgery made prodigious strides, it was capable of completely disguising a personality, including the stature by bone graft and the color of the eyes by injection of coloring fluid." And as was the case with Cole's *Delineator* article, often the fantastic information was included in what was, overall, a fairly balanced account. In an otherwise judicious 1939 article in the *Ladies Home Journal* entitled "When Plastic Surgery Is Justified," writer Gretta Palmer told women, "No hospitalization is required for widening the eyes, changing them from round to oval, shortening the eyelids, lengthening or shortening the mouth or varying the width of the lips."[12]

Many Americans were disturbed by the national preoccupation with appearance, which they took as proof of the superficiality of American culture. Others, however, took it in stride. The *New York Times,* in 1927, responded to the mounting chorus of jeremiads with an editorial asserting that the nation's half-billion-dollar cosmetics and beauty parlor industry was not a cause for alarm but a source of national strength; it had democratized beauty by making the means of self-improvement and transformation available to all. The American tradition of self-improvement provided the fabric into which these new beliefs about beauty were woven. Seventeenth- and eighteenth-century Americans had defined the project of self-improvement primarily in religious terms; John Bunyan's *Pilgrim's Progress,* first published in London in 1684, offers perhaps the quintessential example. During his journey to the Celestial City, pilgrim Christian is beset by a series of temptations, most of which represent some aspect of the physical or material world which would dissuade him from his higher moral purpose. Happily, he perseveres, and with his spiritual conviction strengthened by the testing he has undergone, he reaches his destination.

As religion became less important in the secularizing world of nineteenth-century America, the religious emphasis was replaced by a broader conception of moral self-improvement, whose goal was understood as a better character. Throughout the nineteenth century, self-appointed advisors offered conflicting advice; some emphasized material gain, while others urged a more philosophical focus. But although they differed in emphasis, all of these advisors shared a conception of self-improvement that downplayed the religious emphasis on the soul in favor of a broader conception of a moral life embedded in the concept of character. Character, which Ralph Waldo Emerson defined as "moral order through the medium of individual nature," was denoted in the popular imagination by words such as "citizenship, duty, democracy, work, building, golden deeds, outdoor life, conquest, honor, reputation, morals, manners, integrity, and above all, manhood." It was a more holistic concept than soul, encompassing a broader range of beliefs and actions.[13]

As historian Warren Susman has shown, the emphasis on character gave way in the early years of the twentieth century to the still broader goal of a sterling personality. Personality—described by words such as "fascinating, stunning, attractive, magnetic, glowing, masterful, creative, dominant, forceful" and widely defined as "the quality of being Somebody"—was even more expansive in concept than character. Not only did personality encompass a wide range of attitudes, beliefs, and behaviors, fundamentally it emphasized presentation of the self, with the goal of standing out in the crowded, competitive society of twentieth-century America. In this it differed strikingly from character. A good character, it was assumed, would do for itself. Personality, in contrast, was implicitly social rather than autonomous; it cried out for external ornamentation and promotion in the form of appropriate speech, dress, and manners.[14]

Clearly, as Americans had originally defined it, self-improvement did not mean learning new makeup techniques, nor did it encompass cosmetic surgery. But the concept of self-improvement was malleable: while conserving an essential meaning, Americans altered its particulars to reflect new circumstances. With the progression from the spiritual quality of soul to the moral quality of character to the all-encompassing quality of personality, traditional boundaries between mind and body began to blur: mental (or moral) qualities no longer seemed distinct from physical ones.

Sylvia of Hollywood made this link explicit. She defined personality as "a combination of brains, character, charm, physical attractiveness, manner and manners," insisting that "your physical appearance has so much to do with your personality that it's difficult to tell where one leaves off and the other begins." Personality "gets jobs, it wins friends, it draws beaux like a magnet; it keeps husbands in love with you." Most important, it could be acquired: "You don't have to be born with it. You can develop it. . . . Work for what you want. You must have will power, courage and determination." Once diets, exercise, cosmetics, and hair color were deemed acceptable steps in the pursuit of beauty, and physical appearance came to be conflated with personality, the line that separated cosmetic surgery from other forms of self-improvement and self-culture became more difficult to draw.[15]

The conviction that appearance was crucial to success in modern life was reinforced by what Roland Marchand has identified as one of the "great parables" of modern advertising—the Parable of the First Impression. Beginning in the late 1920s, numerous advertising tableaux told American consumers that first impressions could bring immediate success or failure. From Dr. West's toothbrushes (which promised a "magic road to popularity in that first winning smile") to Sherwin-Williams paint (which warned, "many a man has been rated as lacking in community spirit . . . even as a business failure—merely because of a paint-starved house"), advertisements alternately promised and warned Americans that others' first impressions—of themselves, their houses, even their bathroom fixtures—could determine the course of their lives.[16]

As Marchand has noted, while many of the stories advertisers recounted were "clearly fantastical," the strategy was effective because it "drew much of its persuasive power from its grounding in readers' perceptions of contemporary realities." Just as Cades warned her "twelve to twenties" that they had to look as if they made good biscuits, advertisers warned prospective buyers that in an increasingly mobile and individualistic society, personal presentation counted for more than ever before. Business organizations were ever larger, family members distant, and neighbors perhaps unknown. Hiring and promotion decisions often appeared arbitrary and impersonal, and personal interactions were "fleeting and unlikely to be repeated." In this atmosphere, the idea that a first impression might make the crucial difference was not as far-fetched as it once might have seemed.[17]

Throughout the 1920s and 1930s, advertisers preached the parable of the first impression with more intensity than did any other medium of popular culture. Movies and comic strips often questioned the accuracy of first impressions, even offering moral lessons on hasty judgment as they revealed that first impressions were incorrect. Advertising, however, stressed that although first impressions might be incorrect (i.e., a man with body odor might be a potentially hardworking employee), important decisions were nevertheless often based upon them, and Americans should deodorize (or brush, or wash) accordingly. The Great Depression only increased the parable's effectiveness. In 1931 Dorothy Dix told *Ladies Home Journal* readers that they could increase their self-confidence, thus more effectively preparing for that crucial first impression, by using Lux laundry detergent: "a lovely frock, washed in Lux, would enable any woman to overcome an inferiority complex and feel a 'deep, sure, inner conviction of being charming.'" Williams Shaving Cream company similarly told readers in 1932 that keeping "face-fit" was not vanity, but "good business—more so in these keenly competitive days than ever before." The Depression impoverished many Americans, but it did not slow the growth of the cosmetics industry, which, through advertising, played on the conviction that personal grooming was key to securing employment. The *New Republic* noted in 1931 that the cosmetics industry accounted for $750 million per year, and beauty shops still employed more than one hundred thousand women, demonstrating that "No matter what the condition of international affairs, beauty must go on."[18]

The world evoked by this parable—an anonymous world in which one's fate was determined not by one's character and ability but by one's face—was not without basis in reality. Ushered in by a census that showed, for the first time, a society more urban than rural, the decade of the 1920s heralded a new kind of America: urban, mobile, individualistic, and competitive. In this new world, the idea that looks could determine success (or lack of it) made instinctive sense. Advertisers invoked this idea to sell products; Americans bought it along with their toothpaste and deodorant. And plastic surgeons came, increasingly, to see their work in this new context.[19]

For many surgeons, the irresponsible practitioners who wielded scalpels and applied caustic chemicals with a free hand in the back rooms of beauty parlors constituted a compelling reason for performing cosmetic surgery. As *New York Times* reporter Rose C. Feld noted in 1927, "many reputable practitioners are changing their attitude" because of the damage done by irregulars. "When an actress who is dependent upon her beauty for her livelihood asks to have her wrinkles removed, the fear that she will go to someone less skillful" was forcing reputable surgeons to think twice before refusing her request. Yet the reluctance of the medical profession to accept cosmetic surgery as an appropriate expenditure of reputable physicians' time and energy was prodigious.[20]

During the 1920s, most surgeons drew clear distinctions between cosmetic and reconstructive surgery, believed that terms such as *deformity* and *disfigurement* were self-explanatory, and tended to defend the specialty only on reconstructive grounds. "When possible," John Staige Davis noted in 1926, "I even avoid the use of the word cosmetic in my reports. . . . It has little place in true plastic surgery, whose main objective is the correction of actual deformities. . . . Personally, I have never cared to do cosmetic surgery, as its aims do not coincide with my conception of what true plastic surgery should be. . . . At the Johns Hopkins Hospital we are not interested in either the development or the performance of cosmetic surgery." Even those who accepted cosmetic work played down its significance. As H. Lyons Hunt of New York noted in 1934, "Even in the medical profession, few realize that the cosmetic branch of plastic surgery is indeed what I have called, a *branch only*. . . . Though the facial work is of great validity and value, it is but a branch of an intricate, difficult, and most interesting type of surgery." In 1939 the *New York Times* similarly deemphasized the cosmetic side of the field. "Most of us think of plastic surgery as a sop to vanity. Actually the plastic surgeon is kept busy more by the victims of accidents who need rehabilitation than by motion picture celebrities who do not like their noses or their ears or whose jowls are beginning to sag." As these comments suggest, Americans viewed plastic surgery as a gendered spectrum, with the reconstructive work men needed at one end and the cosmetic or aesthetic work women desired at the other.[21]

Even before World War I, however, surgeons had begun to formulate a justification for their work that included appearance as well as function. During the war, physicians and others had argued that soldiers deserved faces that would enable them to achieve economic self-sufficiency, and the American public had agreed. By expanding the definition of their work to include appearance, surgeons relied upon and reinforced the increasing cultural conviction about the social and economic importance of appearance. In theory, drawing limits according to this criterion seemed easy, but in practice, surgeons found it impossible. If appearance was crucial for a man who needed to support himself (and perhaps others as well), why not for a single woman or widow? What about a wife, the continuance of whose homemaking career might well depend on keeping her husband from straying to a younger woman? What about actors, dancers, and movie stars, whose livelihood really did depend upon their looks? And what about the millions of Americans—not movie stars, and often not even anything important—who were nevertheless becoming increasingly convinced that their appearance played a key role in determining their access to the good things in life?

Like their potential patients, surgeons in these years were becoming more familiar with the concept of the public eye and more convinced that that eye was exacting in its requirements. They were also—again, like their patients—beginning to equate the condition of being in the public eye with existing in the modern world. Some plastic surgeons had proclaimed this for years in order to justify the practice of cosmetic surgery. In the 1920s and 1930s, however, such statements were as likely to emanate from those who considered themselves reputable members of the medical profession as from those who advertised in the back pages of *Vogue*, and for the first time they were seen as applicable to a wide range of Americans rather than to a specific, privileged group.[22]

Surgeons related the changes in their thinking directly to the changes they observed in American society. In 1925, J. Eastman Sheehan admonished his colleagues to "be mindful of the fact that in the modern world it is vitally true that one's face is his fortune. Rather, it is often very palpably his misfortune, and against this he is entitled to remedy." George D. Wolf of New York agreed. In 1929, at the annual convention of the American Medical Association, Wolf asserted that while some minor deformities were "better off if left alone," patients who suffered "socially or economically" because of their physical appearance "should receive the same degree of consideration from the serious-minded physician as those afflicted with an organic disease." Even Joseph Beck, who had consistently voiced his disapproval of cosmetic surgery, conceded that "social and economic conditions may be such as to necessitate a plastic operation."[23]

For plastic surgeons, as for advertisers, the advent of the Depression reinforced this link. The October 1929 crash ushered in more than a decade during which Americans' economic prospects were increasingly bleak. By early 1933, more than one-fourth of the nation's workers were unemployed, and while the election of Franklin Delano Roosevelt raised the country's hopes, the New Deal could not provide enough jobs to turn the tide. Sharing in and reflecting the national mood of anxiety, surgeons conjured an increasingly Darwinian worldview, as they stressed that appearance had taken on new importance in this ever more competitive world. In 1929, face-lifting pioneer Adalbert G. Bettman wrote: "People are more sensitive at this time regarding their appearance . . . for the reason that the present day individual has harder competition in the race of life." Just a year later, H. O. Bames asserted that the "striving for enhancement or maintenance of good looks is therefore evidence . . . of a serious determination, born of necessity, to let no remedial [*sic*] defect stand between success and failure in the struggle for existence." George D. Wolf, in 1931, admonished *Hygeia* readers: "In this highly progressive twentieth century in which we live, in this age of high-powered efficiency when every possible advantage must be grasped for success in social or business life, personal appearance plays an important part." In 1932, New York surgeon Clarence Straatsma noted, "During this present depression the economic importance of . . . appearance has been especially stressed, and we are constantly besieged by patients who want all sorts of physical defects repaired, the reason . . . being that they cannot obtain work because of their appearance." Detroit surgeon Claire L. Straith observed, "The struggle for existence has reached new heights . . . competition is ruthless. . . . In this struggle for the survival of the fittest it is not surprising to note an increasing interest in the acquisition of every available asset, [including] good physical appearance." Jacques Maliniak believed that "there has never been a period when the competition of life was as intense as it is today."[24]

Personal appearance was so important, surgeons agreed, because first impressions now counted for so much. George Wolf, for example, believed nasal surgery deserved particular attention because "the nose, the most prominent feature of the face, is a powerful factor in creating favorable first impressions." In *Beauty Unmasked*, published in 1936, James Stotter asserted that first impressions were particularly crucial at job interviews. "This fact has become increasingly evident," he noted, "with the growing competition for positions and the economic hardships which have prevented applicants from appearing at their best." Ugly people, Stotter conceded, did sometimes succeed, but beauty "serves to smooth the path of life and aids considerably in the attainment of any reasonable goal. . . . The importance of first impressions cannot be overemphasized."[25]

Surgeons who came to believe fervently in the importance of physical appearance, and who enthusiastically endorsed surgery as a solution, probably helped to spread the gospel of self-improvement through plastic surgery. All of their pronouncements, however, would have amounted to nothing had they not hit a nerve in the American consciousness. All Americans, many from personal experience, realized that the world was a tougher place in the mid-1930s than it had been in the mid-1920s. The Depression so shook Americans' views of their society that many who had until then resisted any government involvement in daily life demanded it or at least welcomed it when it arrived. Given this, it is not surprising that some Americans, admittedly grasping at straws, held fast to the idea that control over the limited arena of physical appearance at least offered a chance for social and economic security, and that others simply acted on the belief that it couldn't hurt.

The various interpretations historians have offered of the changed and changing meaning of the body in twentieth-century America suggest that the idea of control can illuminate American attitudes toward cosmetic surgery in these years. T. J. Jackson Lears, for example, has suggested that the paradigm of progressive liberation from Puritanism and Victorianism that has dominated historical interpretations of the body is inadequate: "As the public world outside the self becomes diffuse, distant, governed by institutions we cannot control or even influence, the body remains important as an arena we actually can control—or think we can. It becomes a domain of self-expression, a field for developing one's own set of cultural meanings, and a source, quite naturally, of anxiety." Modernism, Lears asserts, brought with it its own set of anxieties and constraints, as well as urges toward action. Like Lears, Roland Marchand acknowledges multiple meanings: the parable of the first impression may have intensified some Americans' sense of social insecurity, but it also offered the possibility of a new liberation. Anonymity had benefits as well as drawbacks in that history, in the sense of family, heritage, and character, was no longer requisite to success. Instead, all that was necessary was a pretty face, which was available for sale.[26]

The records of New York surgeon Jerome Webster, who organized the new Division of Plastic Surgery at Columbia Presbyterian Hospital in 1931, suggest that some Americans turned to cosmetic surgery as a means to security. Discouraged and out of work, interior decorator Muriel Johnson came to see Webster in 1931, wondering if a face-lift would help her secure clients. Richard Thomas, the following year, thought a new nose would help his career. In 1933, photographic model Lily Pells came in because one of the photographers she worked for had complained about her nose. Seventeen-year-old Betty Hogan hoped to go into commercial photography in 1936 and believed her nose would be "detrimental." In 1941, Lucy Wolf's modeling instructor told her her nose was too broad; Jane Hatch, recently arrived from England with two children, hoped a new nose would help her get a better position. Webster refused several of these patients. He told Richard Thomas that while his concern "might have more excuse in a woman, a man is judged more by what he does than what he looks like," and Muriel Johnson that at thirty-five she was too young for a face-lift, but in general he sympathized with patients' concerns.[27]

While surgeons continued to guard their turf, insisting that they would operate only when they, in their professional capacity, decided a problem was significant enough to warrant surgical intervention, the new social and economic justification for cosmetic surgery persuaded them to listen to prospective patients' complaints with new sympathy. Jacques Maliniak believed a malformation "must be sufficiently conspicuous to mar the appearance of the face or threaten social and economic opportunity." Joseph C. Beck wrote: "It is generally conceded that an abnormality that is sufficient to impair function or interfere with social intercourse or economic endeavor, not only is admissible but is actually desireable of repair." Widespread acknowledgment of the importance of economic security was among the factors that persuaded even stalwarts like Vilray Blair to change their minds. Reflecting on his career, Blair noted in 1936, "I now feel that I neglected more opportunities to do good than otherwise" and had since come to endorse cosmetic surgery. San Francisco surgeon Albert D. Davis similarly wrote in 1939 that understanding of the "economic value of personal appearance" had led him to include minor deformities, as well as blatant ones, "within the scope of dignified practice." To those in daily competition, Davis noted, "personal appearance becomes the keynote to success. . . . If therefore, they seek a more direct method [of winning], every effort should be made . . . to meet their demands."[28]

The widely held conviction that beauty had, in the modern world, assumed a social and economic value helped to persuade surgeons to reevaluate their attitudes toward cosmetic surgery. By itself, however, this justification was tainted by a clear link to consumer culture. Surgeons like Jerome Webster sympathized with patients who requested cosmetic operations. But, trained and accustomed to defining their work in terms of medicine, they resisted any line of reasoning that seemed to place them on a par with hairdressers and beauticians. Plastic surgeons confronted this dilemma at the clinical level as they met with patients and at the philosophical level as they attempted to make a place for their specialty in the wider context of medicine. They found their way out of this quandary with the help of the new science of psychology, and, specifically, the inferiority complex.

Psychology offered surgeons a new way to think and talk about their patients, their specialty, and themselves. The psychological interpretation linked plastic surgery to a new science that was quickly gaining national credibility. It enabled surgeons to portray their specialty as a more serious, and more medically necessary, practice than it might otherwise have seemed. No longer was it merely vanity surgery; instead, it was "psychiatry with a scalpel," vital to mental health. Applying psychological theories enabled surgeons to bypass many of the most troubling questions the specialty faced in the years following World War I. Demarcations that had once loomed large—such as the difference between cosmetic and reconstructive surgery or between a deformity and a malformation and a simple case of ugliness—seemed less significant when viewed through the lens of psychology. Finally, focusing on the mind, at a time when every American was presumed to have a complex, enabled plastic surgeons to claim the largest possible target audience for their specialty.

Enter the Inferiority Complex

Plastic surgeons had begun to think about and discuss the psychological aspects of their work well before the advent of the inferiority complex. During World War I, they had commented with particular pride on the psychological effect their work produced, and as Americans at home learned of the miracles surgeons were performing overseas, they were apprised also of the psychological transformations the surgeons effected. In these discussions, surgeons tended to invoke commonsense terms about unhappiness or insecurity rather than specific psychological concepts. In 1920, for example, Seymour Oppenheimer had noted that a person's "mental attitude toward his disfigurement" might become a problem; Gustav Tieck, similarly, wrote that an obvious disfigurement was a "real and potential cause for unhappiness." In 1929, Portland, Oregon, surgeon Adalbert G. Bettman, an early cosmetic surgery enthusiast, asserted that "the ancient art of plastic surgery has been perfected to such a degree that it is now available for the improvement of patients' mental well-being, their pursuit of happiness."[29]

Faith in the link between plastic surgery and psychology was so widespread that some surgeons began to see surgery as a cure-all, capable of entirely remaking people, even criminals, who had been adversely affected by physical anomalies. In 1927 a pilot project to test the rehabilitative effects of plastic surgery on prisoners at San Quentin received an enthusiastic review. Convicts themselves, the *New York Times* noted, were responsible for initiating this program, "which is intended to give them a better chance to go straight." As an example, the newspaper cited the case of a fifty-year-old convict who, just before his release, took literally the chaplain's advice to become a "new man" and requested surgery. In his case, the surgery included the repair of a cauliflower ear, a dented nose, and wrinkles. "With a blond, unlined complexion and delicately formed features . . . he is certain to be a different person," the *Times* enthused, concluding that while experiments with mood-altering drugs were interesting, "they hardly compare with the thrill of reform through facelifting."[30]

Popular magazines, too, began to take note of surgery's potential to effect psychological change. In 1926, for example, even as she cautioned women against plastic surgery, *Delineator* beauty editor Celia Caroline Cole acknowledged that it might be appropriate in cases where the patient's psychological health was at stake. "Suppose you have some really hideous feature that's spoiling your life—not for a moment are you free from the consciousness of it," she wrote. "Then go to the most reputable plastic surgeon you know of and take a chance on an operation."[31]

By the 1920s, psychology, psychiatry, psychoanalysis, and mental hygiene were generating ever-increasing levels of interest in the United States, among philosophers, academics, practitioners, and the general public, as well as plastic surgeons. Those in the upper echelons of medical and academic circles commonly decried the fact that popular knowledge of these sciences tended to be shallow and simplistic, and by academic standards, it was. It is clear, however, that Americans thought they understood the new psychology and applied these theories to their daily lives.[32]

Americans had begun to explore the mind during the nineteenth century through fads like spiritualism, mesmerism, and even phrenology, which purported to explain personality traits through the study of skull size and shape. In the early years of the twentieth century, interest focused on the new sciences of psychology and psychiatry. Both the 1893 Columbian World Exhibition in Chicago and the 1904 Louisiana Purchase Exposition in St. Louis included exhibits on psychology and featured public lectures. In 1909, at the invitation of Clark University psychologist G. Stanley Hall, Sigmund Freud and Carl Jung visited the United States. The wave of interest sparked by Freud's visit was temporarily interrupted by the war, during which German theories of the mind—like German books, German food, and German dogs—fell out of favor, but quickly revived afterward. In the six years between 1912 and 1918, American medical journals published almost two hundred articles about psychoanalysis. Psychologist and journalist Henry Addington Bruce, who between 1903 and 1917 published sixty-three articles in magazines such as *Good Housekeeping*, the *Delineator*, *American Magazine*, *Outlook*, and *McClures* (in addition to seven books), introduced lay readers to concepts like the subconscious and the power of suggestion.[33]

As prominent figures in psychology and psychiatry made regular appearances in the nation's dailies, psychology became a fad. It was in part defense attorney Clarence Darrow's reliance on psychiatric evaluations that secured the Leopold-Loeb case's place on the front page of every major newspaper in the country throughout 1924. The three terms used most frequently in newspaper stories about Freud—"unconscious," "repression," and "Oedipus complex"—became staples of American conversations. Marjorie Nicolson, the venerable dean of Smith College, found the new national mania troubling. "The jargon of pseudo-psychology or psychoanalysis has put into the mouths of adolescents a vocabulary at which their elders stand aghast," she complained in 1930. "In their eagerness to exhibit superior knowledge, they magnify by large, mouth-filling names conditions in themselves normal, simple, universal." But Americans were hooked. As teenager Elizabeth Benson recalled: "We studied Freud, argued Jung, checked out dreams by Havelock Ellis, and toyed lightly with Adler, . . . and all these authorities warned us of the danger in repressing our normal instincts and drives."[34]

To some Americans, Freud's emphasis on sex and evocation of the primitive, uncontrollable forces of the unconscious offered an intriguing alternative to the spiritual vacuity of postwar life. Max Eastman, in 1915, noted that Americans perceived psychoanalysis as "a kind of 'magic,'" and psychoanalyst Walter Bromberg later recalled, "The freedom to investigate sexual matters cast a special glamour over the new profession; the opportunity to explore the hitherto muted sexual experience of men and (especially) women was now clothed in scientific respectability." Others, however—self-proclaimed proud members of an increasingly urban, consumerist society—were troubled by the "dreary picture" Freud drew of humankind and found a kindred spirit in Alfred Adler. In the 1920s and 1930s, Adler's system of individual psychology was as widely known as Freudian psychoanalysis and as widely misunderstood. But even the most superficial acquaintance with Adler's teachings produced the impression that he "restored to man a sense of dignity and worth that psychoanalysis had pretty largely destroyed." Americans found this orientation compelling. As the *New Yorker* noted in 1928, they "eat up—like the good Rotarians they are—the fundamental hopefulness, courage, and drive in his individual psychology."[35]

Adler began to formulate the concept that Americans would come to know as the inferiority complex early in the century. By 1910 he had moved from his initial emphasis on organ inferiority to a theory that took into consideration not only biological conditions but the social environment as well, based on his conviction that power, not sex, was at the center of human psychology. Adler's basic thesis was that feelings of inferiority were inherent and natural in infants and young children, who were constantly made aware of their lack of power in relation to the larger, competent adults in their lives, as well as to older, more able siblings. These feelings were negative only if they became twisted in the process of growing up. If, for example, a child was continually frustrated by undertaking (and failing at) tasks that were beyond his ability, the child might withdraw into himself, becoming timid, indecisive, and cowardly, and use his sense of inferiority as an alibi to explain his failure. Alternatively, that same child might overcompensate for these feelings, hiding them under a defensive, defiant, aggressive attitude. If, however, the maturation process was healthy and normal, with challenges appropriately geared to the child's increasing abilities, initial feelings of inferiority would result in a "goal-directed striving for mastery," or successful adaptation to the social environment. Adler's work offered a means to bridge not only the debate over heredity and environment but also the "chasm between physical and mental developments." Some American psychoanalysts reportedly thought Adler's system "superficial and oversimplified," and some readers were confused by his initial focus on "organ inferiority" (largely because Freud had introduced a sexual focus, and they misread Adler's work as a supplement to Freud rather than as an independent alternative to the Freudian model). To most American readers, however, Adler's "easy colloquial style and democratic interest in the mental health of school children" were assets. His identification of mental health with action would prove particularly appealing to the American public.[36]

Although he is best remembered for the inferiority complex, Adler himself did not invent the term; until the late 1920s he used the terms *feelings of inferiority, sense of inferiority,* and *inferiority feelings* interchangeably. Freud and Jung both used the term *complex*; its application to Adler's system probably reflects the fact that Adler's early association (and 1911 break) with Freud was well known, as well as the fluidity that characterized the public's response in these years; lay readers (like some practitioners themselves) tended to collate ideas from various sources with ease. At any rate, by 1926, when he began to visit the United States regularly, the term had become widely known and generally acknowledged as Adler's greatest contribution to the study of the human psyche. Adler himself accepted this convention enthusiastically, and Greenberg Publishers astutely invoked the term to propel his 1927 book *Understanding Human Nature* to best-seller status.[37]

If Adler was the father of the inferiority complex, the American public was its mother. It was the American public who named it, endowed it with special meaning, and made it an icon of popular knowledge and popular culture. With the advent of the Depression, the inferiority complex began to make particularly good sense. Psychologists all over the country noticed that during the 1930s Americans suffered more from feelings of inferiority than ever before. In 1932, Douglas A. Thom, director of Massachusetts's division of mental hygiene, wrote that the pre-Depression national mood, which he characterized as "extreme optimism and exaltation," had given way to widespread feelings of anxiety, insecurity, and inferiority. A report of the council of social agencies of Rochester, New York, similarly concluded that in a national depression, "feelings of security and personal adequacy give way to feelings of insecurity and inferiority." Advertisers, too, took note of these widespread feelings, successfully focusing on insecurity and inferiority as drives to consumption. As *Review of Reviews* explained in 1935, Americans' buying patterns were generated, in part, by the desire to overcome feelings of inferiority (or, to "be more adequate"); salesmen and advertising men would thus do well to acquire "an appreciation of these unconscious forces."[38]

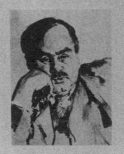

Greenberg Publisher's advertisement for Alfred Adler's *Understanding Human Nature.*

A few examples from the pages of popular magazines suggest the extent of the American fascination with the inferiority complex. *Collier's* pioneered in 1924 with a story about young Anne Sheldon, who almost married Gordon Hale because she feared Perry Osborne, the man she really loved, had an inferiority complex and would never amount to anything. That same year, *American Magazine* described "The Four Commonest Complexes and How to Get Rid of Them." The *Delineator*, in a 1927 article entitled "Your Child and That Fashionable Complex," explained to mothers what could cause an inferiority complex in children (almost anything, including teasing, ridicule or sarcasm, comparing one child to another, a bad family reputation, overprotection from parents, a physical defect or shortcoming) and how to prevent or cure one. *Hygeia,* in 1931, similarly warned parents of the many possible causes of such a complex. The *Literary Digest,* in 1932, encouraged Americans to fight their inferiority complexes. Paul Popenoe noted in a 1939 issue of *Scientific American* that the inferiority complex had "in recent years . . . become a part of the common vocabulary" and urged Americans to take stock of their disabilities and overcome them.[39]

The American tendency to interpret everything in terms of an inferiority complex reached new heights with a *New York Times* article that explained the popular song "Yes, We Have No Bananas" as a metaphor for a national inferiority complex resulting from the Depression. So widespread was knowledge of the inferiority complex that in 1939 *Collier's* could run an article with the headline "How's Your Old I.C.?" Readers with inferiority complexes, the magazine informed them, were in good company. Abraham Lincoln, Napoleon Bonaparte, Theodore Roosevelt, "probably Thomas A. Edison, almost certainly William Shakespeare" had all suffered from the same thing. "So . . . if you have a big, husky, ingrowing inferiority complex you're . . . about as lucky as you could hope to be," the editors concluded, "provided you have the . . . backbone along with it."[40]

The speed with which the "inferiority complex" became a mainstay of the medical literature dealing with plastic surgery and the frequency with which it was invoked suggest that plastic surgeons found it an equally compelling concept. Vilray Blair, in 1926, was one of the first to use the term. "Anything that attracts notice to a child in an unpleasant way is, as a rule, bad for the child," Blair wrote. "Only those who have dealt with a great number of such children can appreciate how unhappy they can be and how great a permanent damage may result from an inferiority complex." In 1930, New York surgeon William Wesley Carter noted that "a fair portion of the misery of this world is borne by those whose prospects and happiness are blighted by the possession of a misshapen nose. . . . The subjective sensation of inferiority in appearance constitutes the real menace which has wrecked innumerable lives." San Francisco's George Warren Pierce agreed, citing plastic surgery as the best solution. "It is interesting to note almost a change of character which often comes to patients after the correction of a facial deformity," he mused. "Increased attention to personal appearance and dress, an infusion of confidence evident in bearing, and a losing of sensitiveness which sometimes amounts to an inferiority complex." Clarence R. Straatsma in 1932 asserted that plastic surgery's goal should be "to alleviate or remedy illnesses which in many cases are far more serious than bodily pain; namely mental anguish due to the patient's constant realization of the defect which in turn causes the development of an inferiority complex, resulting in an attempt of the individual to withdraw from society. . . . Many dependent persons are made self-respecting and self-supporting members of society by the removal of physical and resulting mental handicaps."[41]

Surgeon Jacques Maliniak placed so much importance on the link between plastic surgery and psychology that he enshrined it in the founding principles of the ASPRS. According to the provisional constitution adopted at the first annual meeting, held in October 1932, the society's objectives were: "To promote and further medical and surgical research pertaining to the study and treatment of congenital and acquired deformities . . . ; to keep the medical profession informed of the scientific progress and the possibilities of plastic and reconstructive surgery . . . ; and to stress the great social, economic, and psychological importance of this surgical specialty."[42]

Maliniak discussed the psychological effects of ugliness and deformity at length in his 1934 book *Sculpture in the Living*, and he used *Hygeia* to bring the message to parents: "Once the child is aware of his disfigurement, the postponement of reconstructive procedures places him at a functional disadvantage and predisposes to the development of grave psychological disturbances as a result of the curiosity and taunting of other children," Maliniak warned in 1935. Correction "helps to restore a normal psychic balance. It is not necessary to point out the social and economic opportunities that depend on a pleasing appearance." Maliniak was so convinced of plastic surgery's value in promoting mental health that he used terms like *deformity* more freely than many of his colleagues and advocated free plastic surgery for all. Just as Americans recognized a societal debt to citizens' physical welfare, "Should it not offer relief when psychic health is threatened by a congenital or acquired deformity that stands between the individual and normal living?" he asked. "Free clinics for plastic surgery are to a certain extent an index of a community's civilization."[43]

Newspapers and magazines carried news of this link to a wider audience. In 1927, for example, *New York Times* reporter Rose Feld offered readers two stories that illustrated plastic surgery's psychological significance. In one, a new nose made a woman happy that her suicide attempt had failed and got her a new husband; in the other, a new nose enabled a man to get a job; in both, Feld explained, the patients got "a new lease on life" or, in psychological terms, "the cause of the inferiority complex is removed." Alfred Adler himself helped to cement the link plastic surgeons were forging between his theories and their work. In 1936 he supplied an enthusiastic introductory essay for New York surgeon Maxwell Maltz's book *New Faces, New Futures: Rebuilding Character with Plastic Surgery.* "As we live in a group and are judged by the group, and as this group objects to any departure from normal appearance, . . . a facial deformity can have a very deleterious effect on behavior," Adler wrote. Following Adler, Maltz described how surgery could help: "the surgeon . . . seeks to ease the mind by remolding the . . . features to a conformity with the normal. Once normality is attained, the mind throws off its burden of inferiority, of fear of ridicule and of economic insecurity. . . . The personality relaxes into naturalness and character is transformed." For both Maltz and Adler, normality meant successful adjustment to adult life in modern America. The elusive state of mental normality could not be achieved if physical abnormality clouded the picture, because observers' reactions to physical abnormality would result in mental aberration. Surgery, however, could remove this obstacle: "Now and in the future," Maltz insisted, "the plastic surgeon is an integral force in the unceasing battle of human beings for normality."[44]

"Advertising" plastic surgeons, too, helped spread this message to the public. The notorious Henry Schireson laced his 1938 book *As Others See You* with statements such as, "The psychological reaction [to a nose job] is nearly always an entirely new outlook on life." Like Maltz, Schireson referred specifically to Adler's work: "Self-consciousness," he stated definitively, "is the basis of the inferiority complex." New York surgeon James Stotter, who advertised in the back pages of *Vogue* in the 1930s, similarly emphasized the psychological import of his work in *Beauty Unmasked*, published in 1936.[45]

Surgeons' published writings suggest that the inferiority concept offered them a new way to think about the practice of cosmetic surgery. The cultural record, similarly, demonstrates that at least a certain segment of literate Americans would have been familiar with the term and the concept it represented, if only at a basic level. While the limited availability of patient records makes it impossible to quantify the effect this concept had on surgeons' daily practice or on patients' outlooks on a large scale, surgeon Jerome Webster's records offer anecdotal evidence of how this concept worked at the level of clinical practice.

Like many plastic surgeons, Webster cited the inferiority complex in his published writings, and it figures in his records as well. He used this term frequently, commenting approvingly that a patient did not appear to have an inferiority complex or, with concern, that another seemed in danger of developing one. He used it in corresponding with other physicians, and they used it in referring patients to him for surgery. Dr. Iago Galdston of the New York Academy of Medicine, for example, referred a female patient and then wrote to affirm Webster's decision to operate: "With all the talk of complexes, a bulky bridge, reduced to normal proportions, may be just that much weight lifted to put the scales back in balance." Dr. Estella M. Strayer cited similar terms in one of her referrals. The patient's scar, she wrote, "has given her a definite inferiority complex. . . . [She] will not participate in parties, dates or even go out with her girl friends because she is so sensitive of the marring of her appearance."[46]

Significantly, patients also used this term to explain or justify their requests for surgery, and whether or not Webster believed that a patient suffered from an inferiority complex was often what determined his decision. Alicia Martin was seventeen when her father brought her to see Webster in 1939. She had been saving money for three years for a nose job that an uncle had promised would lead to a screen test in California. Webster proudly described himself as a "conservative" surgeon and was, in general, unmoved by dreams of fame and fortune. In this case, as in several similar cases, he refused to perform surgery. When Alicia's father returned alone, however, to plead that the screen test was secondary to the main problem—a severe inferiority complex—Webster agreed

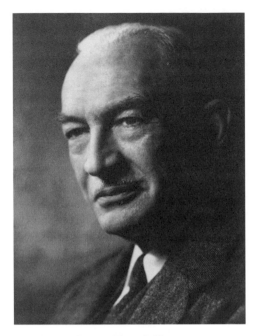

Jerome Pierce Webster

to operate. Diane Davis's request several years later was made on the same grounds. It might seem "selfish, or unpatriotic" to want cosmetic surgery in the middle of a war, she acknowledged. "On the other hand, people who go on and on carrying a load of complexes around with them most probably aren't much good to themselves or anyone else—and I very definitely do seem to be the victim of a very bad inferiority complex."[47]

In one sense, it is surprising that plastic surgeons adopted the psychological viewpoint so quickly. After all, a psychological problem such as an inferiority complex could easily be defined as needing the professional attention of the psychiatrist rather than the plastic surgeon. Plastic surgeons, however, found that they could make an equally strong case that a psychological problem that was the direct result of a correctable physical anomaly was on their turf. As Jacques Maliniak put it, "In many of these cases, self-consciousness over a real or imagined disfigurement plays a part; and the right and duty of physicians [surgeons] to cope with psychological disturbances of this type must be recognized." By such pronouncements, plastic surgeons managed to steal some of their colleagues' fire and, in the process, to use the growing credibility of the psychological profession to bolster their own.[48]

In linking the inferiority complex to physical causes, plastic surgeons were supported by a wide range of experts, including mental hygienists and child psychologists. William E. Carter of Los Angeles wrote in 1926 that "obvious physical defects are of importance because of their tendency to produce feelings of inferiority." W. I. Thomas and Lawson G. Lowrey, both well-known authorities on child guidance, similarly cited physical causes. Thomas tied misbehavior among children to "a sense of social misplacement and personal inadequacy . . . an 'inferiority feeling.'" In sixty cases involving stealing, he continued, all the youthful perpetrators suffered from inferiority feelings, which in turn were often tied to "physical characteristics which stamped the individual as being different." Lowrey noted that physical conditions ranging from a simple departure from the norm to severe disfigurement or illness could result in feelings of inferiority. Childhood nicknames like "limpy" or "four eyes" that originated in connection with "physical stigmata" were among those "chance beginnings" that Edward Strecker, professor of psychiatry at the University of Pennsylvania, believed might result in an inferiority complex. Psychiatrist Karl Menninger also tied such feelings to organic origins, noting that problems such as speech defects and birthmarks often had far-reaching effects. In *The Human Mind,* a best-seller and Literary Guild selection for 1930, Menninger specifically recommended surgery as a solution: "When it is possible by means of medical, surgical, dental, or other devices to correct some of the actual inferiorities, such treatment is, of course, indispensable. The plastic surgeons and orthopoedists and orthodontists have done and are doing much in the direction of mental hygiene." By "actual inferiorities" Menninger would not have meant a slight bump on the nose, but the context in which this comment appeared suggests that he might have meant a significant one. While it is difficult to reconstruct precisely what was meant by terms like these, taken together and in context they indicate that many practitioners were moving toward more expansive definitions.[49]

Psychologists and surgeons agreed on the significance the concept of the inferiority complex bore in relation to plastic surgery, but they found that the very thing that made it so persuasive in theory—its widespread applicability—made it vague, unwieldy, and dangerous in practice. As early as 1928, W. I. Thomas complained that the inferiority complex posed a particularly sticky problem. "All the behavior manifestations of the

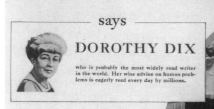
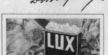

The inferiority complex could sell almost anything.

constitutionally inferior," Thomas asserted, "can be paralleled from the clinical records of children who are organically normal." Lawson Lowrey, too, noted this problem. "There is apt to be confusion as to what an inferiority complex really is," he wrote. "Must the individual actually have an inferiority as the basis for an inferiority complex? Or is it only the individual who has no actual inferiority who can suffer from the inferiority complex?" The faddish aspect was what made social worker Stanley P. Davies uneasy. In 1932 Davies complained that "the inferiority complex and all his little brother and sister complexes are trotted out to do their conversational stuff in drawing-rooms, in dining rooms, in club rooms and hotel lobbies up and down the land." As a result, even "intelligent, reasonably normal people" had fallen victim to "an over-awareness of their mental processes and a tendency to self-analysis and self-excuse in psychiatric terms." The venerable Karl Menninger, who had once found adherents of the inferiority complex a welcome change from "obstreperous and preposterous Freudians," had by 1937 ceased believing in the condition altogether.[50]

Plastic surgeons, too, found the inferiority complex confusing. In 1927 Joseph Colt Bloodgood, professor of clinical surgery at Johns Hopkins, commented on the mental instability he had noted in potential cosmetic surgery patients: "Many of these individuals mentally exaggerate their deformities. . . . Their mental twist makes them easy prey." Los Angeles surgeon Everett S. McCalland voiced similar concerns. For fifteen years, he wrote in 1937, he had performed minor plastic surgery to help patients conquer their inferiority complexes. Despite this experience, he still was not entirely comfortable with the practice. He advised his colleagues to "discourage those who come with trifling defects, such, for example, as a large or humped nose, which should not be a detriment to anyone."[51]

The inferiority complex, then, was not without its drawbacks for surgeons as well as for psychologists. Conceivably caused by anything and everything that men and women experienced in the process of growing up and living in modern America, an inferiority complex began to seem, to some, not a psychological disturbance that could be remedied by plastic surgery but simply a part of being human. As one of Alfred Adler's biographers noted, "The inferiority feeling has assumed overwhelming importance in the field of comparative individual psychology because every human being feels himself directly spoken to by this expression."[52]

Despite the confusion over its prevalence and pathology, the inferiority complex continued for many surgeons not only to provide a compelling explanation of their surgical art but also to shape that art. In
emphasizing the social and economic importance of appearance, surgeons had begun to share the task of making the diagnosis (which most
physicians guarded jealously as a source of power and status) with the
general public. And in emphasizing the psychological importance of
appearance, surgeons increasingly shared this task with patients. Not the
surgeon's objective judgment but the patient's subjective evaluation
became the factor that determined whether a deformity existed and
whether surgery would take place. The inferiority complex encouraged
surgeons to listen to their patients and to allow patients' self-diagnoses
to inform their own. Jerome Webster's records suggest something of how
this worked in practice. Webster prided himself on speaking frankly to
younger patients; he often used sports metaphors, encouraging patients
to stop daydreaming about their looks and "get into the game of life."
He guarded his medical authority: if he believed a patient's dreams
unrealistic or her request frivolous, he did not agree to surgery, whether
or not the patient suffered, or claimed to suffer, from an inferiority complex. But while he reserved the right to make the final decision, Webster
clearly took patients' subjective evaluations into account.

And as they moved toward a definition of plastic surgery that
incorporated the cosmetic work patients desired, surgeons began to
think about terms like *deformity* in new ways. Throughout the 1930s, surgeons used the term to denote an increasingly wide variety of conditions.
"Bulbous, prominent nasal tips" were deformities, according to one
surgeon. Another listed the conditions of "humpnose, pendulous breast,
abnormally prominent ears, receding chin, moles or other small nevi of
the face, lines and wrinkles about the eyes, jowls and neck." According
to another, "wrinkled forehead, baggy eyelids, donkey's ears, wrinkled
face, double chin, and various deformities of the nose, the most common being the hump and hook nose with or without the twist, and
saddle nose" were all "deformities or disfigurements."[53]

Reclassifying such conditions as deformities may have made it
easier for surgeons who saw their function as dealing with serious problems to justify their work, to themselves, to others, and to official bodies such as the American Medical Association and the American Board
of Surgery. Rather than call themselves cosmetic surgeons or beauty doctors, they continued to define themselves as plastic surgeons, merely bring-

ing more conditions under the umbrella of plastic surgery. But however unintentionally, by expanding such definitions surgeons redefined the specialty itself. By the late 1930s, words like *deformity* had come to connote any and every physical attribute that might spark the feelings of inferiority that would threaten an individual's chances for social and economic security and success.

By the late 1930s, too, surgeons were in almost universal agreement about psychology's relevance to their work and proud of themselves for the progress they had made in incorporating these new ideas into their practices. According to surgeon M. Reese Guttman, "one of the basic changes" that had occurred in the specialty was "the broadening of the indications for plastic surgery . . . to include smaller and at times minor defects that are associated with definite evidence of mental reaction that is of psychiatric, social, or economic import." And American newspapers and magazines continued to strengthen the link surgeons and psychologists had forged between physical appearance and psychic health. A 1939 article in *Independent Woman* is typical: "The defect may seem slight, but its psychological consequences may be serious enough to undermine the patient's mental health or economic security," writer Lois Miller explained. Plastic surgery could "banish the feeling of shame and inferiority that is often the worst part of deformity. . . . Psychiatrists are convinced that many cases of mental illness have been cured by the correction of facial abnormality through plastic surgery."[54]

In the 1920s and 1930s, cosmetic surgery was transformed from a suspect practice at the specialty's borders to an approved practice at its center as plastic surgeons, bidding for credibility and recognition, brought the new specialty of plastic surgery under the auspices of the AMA and other professional organizations. For the surgeons who belonged to these organizations, this process involved retaking the field from the assortment of quacks, irregulars, beauty doctors, beauticians, and profiteers who had begun to explore and exploit the growing American faith in appearance as a means to success. As more and more reputable surgeons entered the field, surgeons' anxiety subsided and their confidence grew. "From a humble beginning in barbershops, hotel rooms and beauty parlors," surgeon A. M. Berman reminisced in 1939, "plastic surgery has now come to be a recognized specialty, practiced by men who are thoroughly grounded in the principles of present day aseptic surgery. . . . The quacks and charlatans . . . are rapidly disappearing

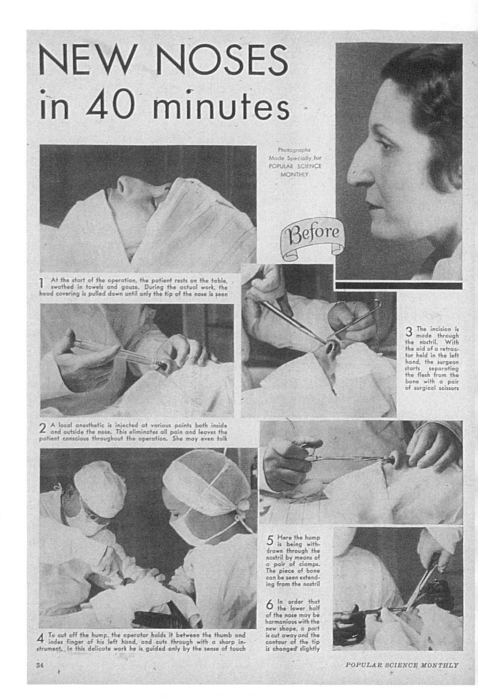

NEW NOSES
in 40 minutes

Photographs
Made Specially for
POPULAR SCIENCE
MONTHLY

Before

1 At the start of the operation, the patient rests on the table, swathed in towels and gauze. During the actual work, the head covering is pulled down until only the tip of the nose is seen

2 A local anesthetic is injected at various points both inside and outside the nose. This eliminates all pain and leaves the patient conscious throughout the operation. She may even talk

3 The incision is made through the nostril. With the aid of a retractor held in the left hand, the surgeon starts separating the flesh from the bone with a pair of surgical scissors

4 To cut off the hump, the operator holds it between the thumb and index finger of his left hand, and cuts through with a sharp instrument. In this delicate work he is guided only by the sense of touch

5 Here the hump is being withdrawn through the nostril by means of a pair of clamps. The piece of bone can be seen extending from the nostril

6 In order that the lower half of the nose may be harmonious with the new shape, a part is cut away and the contour of the tip is changed slightly

In 1937, *Popular Science Monthly* reported that plastic surgeons could create "New Noses in 40 Minutes."

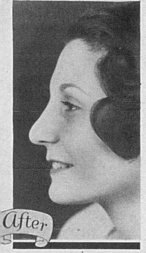

After

IN A forty-minute miracle of modern surgery, an unshapely nose now can be transformed in such a way as to change the owner's face completely. Working entirely through the nostrils in order to leave no unsightly scar, the surgeon's deft hands are guided almost exclusively by the sense of touch as he removes the hump and shortens the nose to normal proportions. Only a local anesthetic is used and the patient is conscious throughout the delicate operation. The complete transformation of the patient's nose is accomplished in about forty minutes. In the accompanying photographs, a high-speed camera has caught the successive steps of the work in one of the most dramatic series of pictures ever made in an operating room.

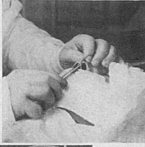

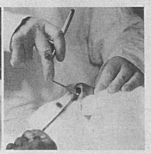

7 The next step in the operation is stitching. The parts that have been severed are sewed up

8 Here the saw is being inserted for narrowing the bridge. The teeth of the saw are at the end of the L-shaped instrument

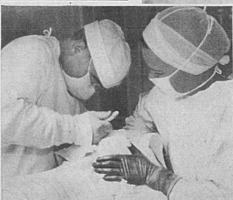

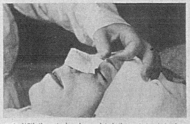

10 With the actual work completed, the next step is to dress the nose. Face coverings are removed and the entire nose is covered with adhesive tape as seen in the photograph above

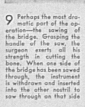

9 Perhaps the most dramatic part of the operation—the sawing of the bridge. Grasping the handle of the saw, the surgeon exerts all his strength in cutting the bone. When one side of the bridge has been sawed through, the instrument is withdrawn and inserted into the other nostril to saw through on that side

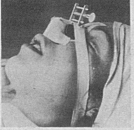

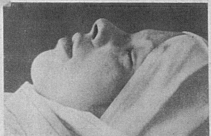

11 Over the tape is placed an adjustable clamp which must be worn for three days to guard the shape of the nose while healing

12 The nose as it appears after all surgical work has been completed. It will not appear normal until all swelling and healing has taken place. Compare this picture with the one at the start

from the horizon, and their places are being taken by thoroughly trained surgeons who are at last really practicing reconstructive surgery as it should be." Those who preferred to trace their specialty's birth to the battlefields and base hospitals of World War I probably would have taken issue with Berman's history, but there is more than a grain of truth in his account. Medical imperatives shaped the specialty of plastic surgery, but cultural pressures were at least as important. By the end of the 1930s, the definition of deformity had expanded to include a much wider variety of conditions, and the number of potential patients seemed limitless. If the line between reconstructive and cosmetic surgery had not disappeared, it had at least been significantly blurred.[55]

Plastic surgeons were and continue to be among the most vociferous supporters of the link between deformity and mental illness (or, conversely, between cosmetic surgery and mental health). During the interwar years, famous surgeons like Adalbert G. Bettman and infamous ones like Henry Schireson pioneered this viewpoint. According to Bettman, vanity was not unhealthy; rather, "the disgrace, if any, is in allowing a manifest deformity to remain." Henry Schireson similarly insisted, "It is not vain for a man or a woman to desire a pleasing appearance. . . . It is, or should be, a matter of pride and self-respect." As John Van Duyn of Columbus, Georgia, put it years later, "the borderline cosmetic defect is often well-worth correcting, because it may not always be what we actually look like to the outside world that most affects our self-confidence and behaviour so much as the way we think we look."[56]

The plastic surgeons who had begun, in these years, to think about cosmetic surgery in new ways were in part simply reflecting changes that had taken place in American culture. Popular magazines offer one path by which this change may be traced. By the mid-1930s, magazines were both reinforcing and reflecting a new attitude toward cosmetic surgery. In 1937, in a pioneering photo essay entitled "New Noses in Forty Minutes," *Popular Science* told its readers that "In a forty-minute miracle of modern surgery, an unshapely nose now can be transformed." *Science News Letter* offered a similar account the following year. "Plastic surgery has an esthetic as well as a reparative objective," the magazine explained in 1938. "It remedies the looks and appearances of individuals who enjoy good physical health but are weighed down psychologically by some deformity of appearance." Even when authors limited their discussions to reconstructive surgery, they waxed euphoric about the miraculous trans-

Cincinnati Ohio

Dear Sir:

I have a slight bump on my nose, which I'd like removed. I am interested in learning the cost of such a procedure.

I obtained your name from the Board of Plastic Surgery.

There is a problem on my mind. A friend had her nose corrected, they administered a local, then broke her nose. Her eyes have been blackened for a whole year, as a result of this. Is this necessary?

Sincerely,

my nose now.   *as I would like my nose*

Letter to Jerome Webster, circa 1940.

formations such operations effected, and it is likely that readers paid more attention to the transformations described than to the physical problems that underlay them. And some explicitly linked plastic surgery to minor problems, as Lois Miller did in her 1939 article for *Independent Woman*.[57]

As the 1930s wound to a close, articles that portrayed inferiority

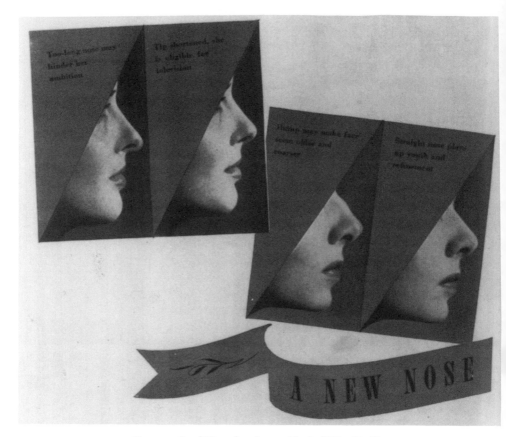

By 1940, *Good Housekeeping* could ask, "Why Not?"

complexes as rational responses to less-than-perfect looks (however that was defined)—and heralded the decision for surgery as healthy—began to supersede less sympathetic ones. The following example, which was used to personalize a *Good Housekeeping* article on the benefits of rhinoplasty, is typical of these poignant tales. "She was just a rather untidy girl with a big nose," the story began, "sitting in the doctor's waiting room. A dusty felt hat pulled down over her eyes, her dowdy dress, and the way she slumped in the chair indicated her indifference to the details of her appearance." Just four weeks later: "The same girl—but how hard to recognize! A saucy hat perched back of her brand-new pompadour, her dress was trim, her bearing confident. Everything about her bespoke a touching new-born vanity. She, who once felt that the world was against her,

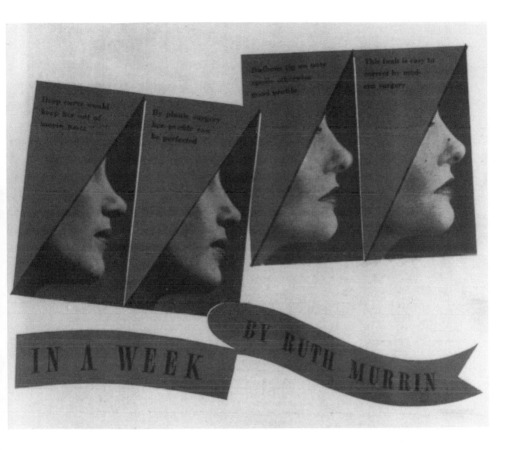

now obviously felt that the world was her oyster. This miracle had followed a brief five days in the hospital, where skilled surgical hands had trimmed down her nose to pleasant proportions." As they perused articles like these, it is not surprising that many Americans developed a faith in the transformative powers of plastic surgery. As physical conditions ranging from deformity to simple ugliness were defined as the cause of an inferiority complex and thus equated with mental illness, cosmetic surgery, once associated with lack of mental balance and overweening vanity, came to be seen as a step toward mental health.[58]

As a psychological or psychiatric concept, the inferiority complex was vague, even simplistic. As a medical concept, it was subjective; it was defined by the patient rather than diagnosed by the surgeon. Above all, it was relative: inferiority could be defined only in relation to others. Seen from another perspective, however, one informed by the nation's new consumer culture, its drawbacks became significant virtues: it could be applied widely, and it was easy to understand. Because it was so subjective, it enabled surgeons to explain why one person with a large nose could laugh about it, while another moped. More important, acceptance of the relative nature of deformity or ugliness released the surgeon from the impossible responsibility of deciding where to draw the line.

As surgeons debated the inferiority complex in the pages of medical journals and tested its applicability in their practices, they redefined their own role as well as the nature of their specialty. Instead of making objective determinations about what constituted a deformity, they listened to their patients' statements about how their faces made them feel. Mediators rather than judges, they weighed this knowledge against the context of an increasingly appearance-conscious society, and they recognized—indeed, enshrined—the comparative, competitive nature of the pursuit of beauty as a factor in American medicine as well as in American culture. Cosmetic surgery was not universally recognized as an acceptable solution. In 1939, for example, a surgeon agreed with Gretta Palmer of the *Ladies Home Journal* that "there has never been a time when so many women have been discontented with their appearance," but insisted, "Nine tenths of these women have no need for surgery. They need, instead, to learn to accept the fact that some other women are more beautiful than they are." But as surgeon Claire L. Straith noted in that same year, Americans had begun to learn "that correctable deformities or even blemishes . . . need not be borne through life with 'patient resignation.'" Supported by a centuries-old tradition of self-improvement, surrounded by an aura of reason and technology, and crowned by the halo of progress, cosmetic surgery had become another tool for success in a competitive world. Thus, by 1940, *Good Housekeeping* could ask rhetorically: "Why should anyone suffer under the handicap of a conspicuously ugly feature? Why not let modern science give him a normal face and an equal chance with other people?" with the obvious expectation that readers would answer, "no reason at all."[59]

CHAPTER FOUR

The Lifting of the Middle Class

AGING IN POST–WORLD WAR II AMERICA

In 1973, Paramount Pictures released *Ash Wednesday*. Featuring the most graphic surgical footage that had ever been included in a Hollywood film, the movie starred Elizabeth Taylor as the middle-aged Barbara Sawyer and Henry Fonda as the straying husband she hoped a face-lift would help her hold. Shortly after the film's release, Taylor told an interviewer that she had little in common with the character she had played: "I don't worry about growing old. . . . We can't stop the inevitable, so why try? I'm forty-one and have never felt better. Plastic surgery isn't for me—simply because I don't base my happiness on the physical aspects of life." Braver words were never spoken. Yet, twenty-some years later, Taylor looked, in columnist Ellen Goodman's words, "thirty-five and holding" and seemed to be haunted by the chance remark of another of the film's characters: no matter what a woman does, "a younger woman will always walk into the room."[1]

Taylor's visibility makes her an obvious example, but she is only one among the growing number of American women who will never be able to answer feminist Germaine Greer's elegantly phrased question, "If a woman never lets herself go, how will she ever know how far she might have gone?" In the early years of the century, aging was regarded as a natural (if less than desirable) process, and women who resisted that process were generally chided, ridiculed, or caricatured as victims of a pathological vanity. In Gertrude Atherton's 1923 novel *Black Oxen*, for example, Viennese youth serum treatments cause the Countess Marie Zattiany (née Mary Ogden) to appear young and radiant, but the treatments cannot transform her old and embittered soul. Cosmetic surgery

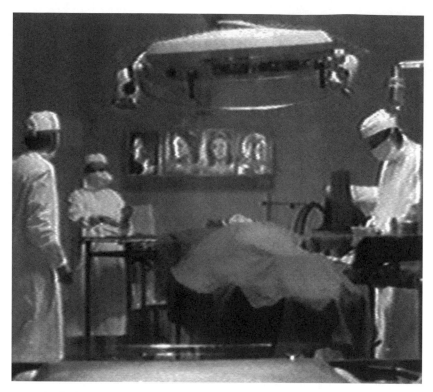

Elizabeth Taylor goes under the knife in *Ash Wednesday* (video frame still).

was redefined as both a rational response to the higher standards set by consumer culture and a way to achieve psychic balance in the interwar years, but the face-lift remained suspect, largely because the techniques then in use were ineffective. After World War II, however, this last barrier was lifted, and the number of face-lifts among middle-class Americans—first women, then men—began a climb that continues to this day.

The postwar surge of interest in face-lifting was sparked, in part, by the enthusiastic coverage wartime plastic surgery received in the popular press. Throughout the war, surgeons warned the press and the public about plastic surgery's limitations: as Lieutenant Colonel James Barrett Brown, a leader in wartime surgery, put it, "We are giving the injured the best modern surgery can provide . . . [but] we cannot duplicate what God has made." Despite such cautions, however, coverage of wartime surgery did focus on miracles, and the awestruck tone many writers adopted shaped popular perceptions about plastic surgery. In magazines ranging from *Coronet* to the *Ladies Home Journal,* and in newspapers across the country, titles like "New Faces for New Men," "Saving His Face," and "Giving the Boy a New Face" heralded the miracles of the "new" plastic surgery. "Saving His Face," for example, included photographs of five normal-to-handsome young men in uniform with this note: "The splendid-looking men pictured on this page would have faced hopeless disfigurement in the last war. They have been badly wounded. But in this war the miracle of modern plastic surgery has restored them as you see them here." On the whole, most of these articles were fairly balanced, and a thorough reading would yield a realistic picture of the trauma, and the limitations, of plastic surgery. Titles and captions, however, aimed at creating drama, and a reader who only skimmed would come away with the impression that plastic surgeons could work magic. Films like Bela Lugosi's *The Raven* (1935), *A Woman's Face* (with Joan Crawford, 1941), and particularly *Dark Passage* (1947), which starred Humphrey Bogart as an escaped prisoner and Lauren Bacall as the angel who takes care of him after plastic surgery, helped to buttress plastic surgery's magic aura.[2]

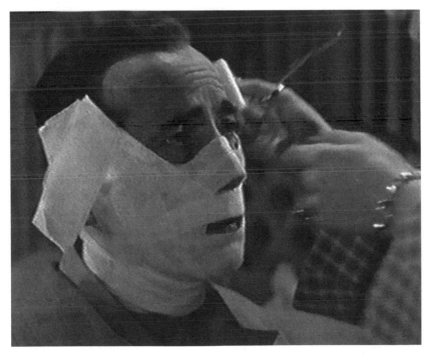

In 1947, Americans watched as Lauren Bacall cut the bandages to reveal Humphrey Bogart's "new" face in *Dark Passage* (video frame still).

As these wartime accomplishments were fanning public interest in plastic surgery, the specialty's new professionalism, heralded by the organization of the American Board of Plastic Surgery, seemed guaranteed to solve its old credibility problem. Beginning in 1942, all diplomates certified by the Board were listed in the American Board of Medical Specialties' annual *Directory of Medical Specialists*. To provide consumers with an easy means to identify those who were certified, the Board mailed out this list upon request. The specialty's professional image was further strengthened by the 1946 inauguration of its own journal, *Plastic and Reconstructive Surgery*, as well as by the continuing activity of its professional organizations. In the initial flush of postwar prosperity, plastic surgeons—better educated, better trained, and better organized than their predecessors—regarded with pride the profession they had created, believing its structure sound and its boundaries secure.

The specialty's new status soothed surgeons' fears that they would be regarded as quacks if it became known that they lifted faces, and the new antibiotics—the "wonder drugs"—and surgical techniques that came out of the war helped to break down their traditional reluctance to perform face-lifts. A more important factor, however, was the realization that the specialty's future was not nearly as certain as it seemed. During the war, some surgeons had expressed confidence that civilian casualties from accidents and burns would keep them busy in the postwar years, but not even large-scale industrial catastrophes would have generated enough patients to keep busy the increased number of surgeons the war produced. Plastic surgeons resolved this dilemma by going where no man—or at least, no reputable plastic surgeon—had gone before. In the years after World War II, plastic surgeons led what would become a widespread trend toward marketing medical techniques and technologies to particular groups. The first problem they targeted was aging, and the first audience they targeted was female—specifically, middle-aged, middle-class women.

This, it immediately became clear, was an astute strategy. The generation that came of age during World War II married and had children younger and lived longer than previous generations had. For the first time, at the age of fifty, a generation of Americans were healthy, affluent, largely finished with the tasks of day-to-day family life, and ready to enjoy themselves. They found, however, that the nation's attention was riveted on the generation they had created. Beauty, in America, meant youth: while aging gracefully continued to hold sway as a popular ideal, many Americans saw little grace in the reality, and no category comparable to the intriguing, attractive older woman the French so descriptively termed the "femme d'un certain âge" had developed in the United States. As the baby boomers bestowed cult status on Twiggy and the Beatles and vowed not to trust anyone over thirty, their mothers found that the transition to what some were beginning to call the "second half of life" was more difficult than they had anticipated. Postwar abundance enabled them to carry traditional notions of female responsibility for looking one's best to their logical, or perhaps illogical, conclusion, while the new emphasis on youth invested these notions with fresh significance.

The post–World War II medical and popular discussions of cosmetic surgery, in fact, suggest that thousands of middle-class women began thinking about aging at about the same time that hundreds of plastic surgeons began looking for new clients and realizing they would have to compete for those clients with the thousands of other doctors who were eyeing this growing market. For prospective patients, and for surgeons, the therapeutic ethos that came to dominate postwar American culture had significant implications. This ethos, which historian Elaine Tyler May describes as "geared toward helping people feel better about their place in the world rather than changing it," encouraged Americans to find private, personal solutions to social problems. For plastic surgeons, this ethos encouraged them to narrow their field of vision: rather than attempting to manage the practice of cosmetic surgery and shape its place in American culture, they directed their efforts to managing their own practices. Middle-aged women, in the years after World War II, were also pioneers in this process of individualizing social problems of inequality. They did not hesitate to criticize the culture that made them feel invisible, unnecessary. But, as so many Americans do, they concluded that it was easier to change themselves than to change the world around them, and no one—not their husbands, not their children, and certainly not their surgeons—disagreed.[3]

At this crucial juncture, plastic surgeons found that the social and psychological justification for cosmetic surgery they had developed before the war gave aging a whole new look, while many middle-class Americans, most of them women, found it easier to alter their own faces than to alter the cultural norms and expectations about aging that confronted them. Together, surgeons and their patients forged a new image of the face-lift as a sensible, practical, and relatively simple solution to the social problem of aging. In doing so, they became both producers and products of the modern "culture of narcissism" and created powerful incentives toward cosmetic surgery that are still in place today.

The Postwar World of Plastic Surgeons

After the Second World War, the United States, its physical plant untouched and its economy intact, emerged as the world's major economic and military power. In addition to producing a larger share of manufactured goods than ever before, the United States produced an increasingly large share of the world's science and medicine. New medical technologies and the expansion of scientific information accelerated the evolutionary process that had begun before the war; they were cause and consequence of an increase in both relative and absolute numbers of specialists. These changes were compounded by overall growth in the profession: in the years after World War II, the number of medical schools in the United States almost doubled, and the number of doctors more than doubled.[4]

Even against this backdrop, plastic surgery's growth was significant. By 1952, Chicago surgeon Paul W. Greeley reported, fifty-two of the seventy-two Class A medical schools in the United States offered training in plastic surgery. In 1960 the American Board of Plastic Surgery reported that the specialty had tripled in size since its founding two decades earlier. As of that year, the Board had certified 462 surgeons. Fifty-two had died and twenty had retired, but most were still practicing. The United States was widely acknowledged to be the leader in this field: of the eight hundred surgeons who attended the International Congress on Plastic Surgery in 1959, more than a quarter were from the United States. The specialty's journal also recorded progress. In 1957, American Society of Plastic and Reconstructive Surgeons president Frederick Figi reported that the number of paid subscriptions had topped two thousand, and a recent survey had identified the journal as one of the most widely read medical publications. Reliable statistics are difficult to come by, but it was generally agreed that the number of surgeries performed had also increased. According to one report, more than 130,000 Americans had plastic surgery in 1958, compared to just 15,000 a decade earlier, and the numbers were increasing annually. Plastic surgeons were not only more numerous, they were distributed more widely around the country. Starting from the east and west coasts where they had initially congregated, they were spreading out: by 1965 only five states—Idaho, Montana, Alaska, South Dakota, and Wyoming—had no plastic surgeons.[5]

Plastic surgeons generated support for the specialty's growth and expansion through a series of energetic promotional efforts. Decades of rumors, tragedies, and scandals had left the specialty with an image problem that was only partially offset by favorable wartime publicity. It was in part the residual effects of this image that turned plastic surgeons' sights toward the horizon of public relations. The article that would set the tone for much of the postwar media coverage appeared for three successive weeks in the spring of 1946 in the *American Weekly,* a widely read Hearst newspaper Sunday supplement. Penned by science editor Robert Potter and endorsed enthusiastically by Morris Fishbein, editor of the *Journal of the American Medical Association,* the series "Farewell to Ugliness" drew an explicit link between wartime experience and postwar possibilities: "In giving new features and new courage to battle-torn veterans . . . the army is training specialists who soon will turn their war-developed skill to making brighter futures for thousands of girls and women. . . . The matron with too many crows feet around the eyes will have new hope and faith because of plastic surgery on wounded veterans."[6]

Some surgeons found this article objectionable, but the enthusiastic public response to it and to other articles like it encouraged plastic surgeons to take public relations more seriously. In 1950 the American Society of Plastic and Reconstructive Surgeons for the first time engaged a full-time director of public relations and began to include the cost of public relations in its annual budget. The society actively fostered the preparation and publication of articles in popular magazines, at the same time attempting to discourage the sensational publicity with which the specialty had been plagued. According to surgeon Leon Sutton, who led these efforts, the key to the society's public relations strategy lay in two words: "*factual* and *unsensational* . . . we are not becoming publicity seekers . . . we are attempting to guide public information . . . so that the layman may understand our specialty, both its potentialities and its limitations."[7]

In 1955, in his outgoing presidential address to the ASPRS, William Milton Adams congratulated the society's members on their accomplishments but urged them to continue their efforts, as too few potential patients were having plastic surgery: "To be convinced of this fact," Adams noted, "one has only to walk a block down a busy city street; probably one of every five persons one meets will have some defect which could be improved or completely corrected by plastic surgery." Adams's colleagues apparently found overzealous his recommendation that the society sponsor a public relations campaign on the scale of those undertaken to vanquish tuberculosis and syphilis (and a campaign of this magnitude was never undertaken), but plastic surgeons continued to generate publicity. By 1962 the public relations committee, at the executive council's direction, had moved from "passive cooperation" with those seeking information to an "active educational and public relations program." This posture was unique to the United States. A journalist who attempted to begin her research on plastic surgery in Britain in the late 1960s was told in no uncertain terms, "A British plastic surgeon who is weak enough to talk to a journalist is automatically expelled from our society. His career, I daresay, is finished."[8]

Plastic surgeons were not alone in developing their public relations skills; the larger medical profession was moving in the same direction. The change was heralded by the American Medical Association's revision, in 1949, of its Principles of Medical Ethics. For the first time, doctors were encouraged to cooperate with the press in disseminating information to the public. The new attitude was reflected in an unprecedented article in the association's journal entitled "Dr., Meet the Press," which appeared in 1952. According to John L. Bach, the Chicago director of press relations, the increased number of news reports in papers, magazines, and on the radio was evidence of the public's desire for information, and physicians should respect that desire. "The facts about American medicine," he wrote, "have to be told by those who know the facts. If a reporter cannot get the facts from you, the doctor, he will go elsewhere and your chances and the chances of the medical profession, generally, of getting an accurate story before the public may be lost." C. Lincoln Williston, manager of the University of Illinois Office of Public Information, supported Bach's position. "No matter what physicians and scientists might accomplish, newspapers, magazines, radio and television are going to report on subjects currently within the realm of medicine," he counseled. "The choice then is not between publicity and no publicity. . . . It is . . . between authentic news reports prepared with the active cooperation of physicians on the one hand, and 'black market' publicity of questionable accuracy on the other."[9]

But plastic surgeons' promotional efforts were more energetic, and more successful, than those of other physicians. This was in part due to exactly the phenomenon surgeons were trying to combat: the aura of magic and mystery that had surrounded the field since its inception made for great copy. More important, however, was that surgeons were finally ready to talk about cosmetic surgery. This had not always been the case. In 1922, journalist Ethel Lloyd Patterson, a self-described "woman standing with reluctant feet where thirty-nine and forty meet," had attempted to interview a "conservative surgeon" about face-lifts for a magazine article and had been severely rebuked for her interest. "I would not touch any woman at any price who came to me and asked me to remove the legitimate trace of her years," the surgeon told her emphatically. "There are too many people afflicted by real suffering . . . for me to be willing to throw away my time. . . . And . . . quite aside from the ethics of my profession, I am opposed to so-called 'beauty surgery.' . . . The average woman who seeks to have a 'beauty operation' . . . well, I have no words for her. A woman of forty years of age, or more, ought to be ashamed to have a face without a wrinkle." In the postwar years, however, surgeons began to court rather than castigate women like Ethel Patterson. They did so by reconstructing plastic surgery's image. Rather than a long, arduous operation involving general anesthesia and great risk, surgeons explained, a face-lift—like the new "wonder drugs"—was simply one more way in which medicine was helping to improve modern life.[10]

The terminology of sewing, which during the war had proved so useful in persuading thousands of Rosies that they could rivet, provided the perfect metaphor for this new, domesticated image of cosmetic surgery. In 1957, surgeon Walter C. Alvarez told *Good Housekeeping* readers that surgeons lifted faces very much the way dressmakers fitted frocks that had stretched out. "After [the surgeon] has loosened the skin so that it can be moved," Alvarez explained, "he pulls it up and outward to straighten out the wrinkles, and he shapes it to the face, just as a seamstress might fit a dress over the shoulders of a woman. . . . He puts in a few 'basting' stitches to guide him later and cuts off the excess . . . skin. Then with a fine and almost invisible suture (stitching), he brings the two edges of the cut together." In her "Diary of a Face Lift," recorded for the *Ladies Home Journal* in 1962, the anonymous liftee wrote of her postoperative consultation: "He says my ears have been shortened over a centimeter. It seems they sort of eased the lower third into place, like putting in a sleeve when you make a dress."[11]

The new awareness of middle-class America as a growing market led some surgeons to reconsider the economics, as well as the image, of cosmetic surgery. New York surgeon E. Hoyt de Kleine, in 1955, urged his colleagues to acknowledge that the specialty's future lay with the middle class and thus with the cosmetic operations in which the members of that class were most interested. "In a competitive economy," de Kleine wrote, "prosperity can continue only if we render more and better service to our people. . . . The prime objective of our specialty should be an overall quantitative increase in high quality cosmetic work for people of all economic levels. . . . If we do not care for this need others will. Whether the control of cosmetic surgery remains with the ethical medical profession (and with plastic surgeons) depends on what we do with it in the immediate future. For the hours spent, there is no way in which so much human suffering can be relieved as through our cosmetic work." Plastic surgeons had erred, de Kleine continued, in refusing to acknowledge cosmetic surgery's importance. Securing a niche in American society meant finding a place in the competitive world of middle-class consumer culture. To do this, de Kleine asserted, surgeons would have to correct the "gross overpricing" that was rampant within the field. Specifically, "the total cost of standard cosmetic procedures must be brought down to prices not exceeding what the average man pays for his television."[12]

De Kleine's suggestion was not greeted with unanimous praise, and the cost of most cosmetic surgical procedures has remained well above the cost of the average television. But one of his key points could not have been lost on his colleagues. Although plastic surgeons began the postwar period confident that the establishment of the American Board of Plastic Surgery would finally put an end to the quack problem, they realized quickly that competition was heating up from unanticipated directions. The "wonder drugs," which allowed virtually any physician to treat a variety of infections simply by prescribing antibiotics, had sparked anxiety among the members of several medical specialties, notably otolaryngologists (or ear, nose, and throat specialists), who began eyeing cosmetic surgery as a potential direction for expansion. In warning his colleagues not to price themselves out of the market, de Kleine was acknowledging that the position Board-certified surgeons had only recently achieved was already tenuous.[13]

The issue of competition between practitioners allied to different specialties, which would boil over in 1960, had begun percolating

immediately following the organization of the American Board of
Plastic Surgery in 1937. Conscious of its late start in relation to other
specialty boards, of its diplomates' diverse experience and training, and
of the public's confusion about what plastic surgery was, the Board's
initial strategy was to publicize its existence and the meaning of the certification it provided. Much of the publicity came from articles in
magazines and newspapers, which began advising readers to contact the
Board for information. Initially, Board members viewed these queries
as opportunities to publicize the fledgling Board's existence and believed
that providing information was the best course to take. In December
1939, journalist Gretta Palmer (whose article about plastic surgery had
appeared in that month's *Ladies Home Journal*) asked John Staige Davis
for a list of Board-certified surgeons to aid her in responding to the many
letters her article had generated. Davis replied that the list was as yet
incomplete, but if the *Journal* would forward the inquiries, he would
refer them appropriately. "By return mail, I got a large batch of letters,"
Davis later told Vilray Blair. "Maybe this will be a good way of steering
some of these poor people out of the hands of our unscrupulous
friends." All inquirers received letters giving the names of several local,
Board-certified plastic surgeons.[14]

The amount of correspondence generated by articles like these testified to the level of public interest, and surgeons scrambled to respond.
More than four thousand people wrote asking for information and
referrals in response to the 1946 *American Weekly* series; *Look*'s 1948 cover
story ("The Face Plastic Surgery Can Build You" by writer Geri Trotta)
generated even more work; a series entitled "Why Grow Old?" by syndicated newspaper columnist Josephine Lowman generated more than
two thousand letters in the spring of 1953. Journalist Maxine Davis con-
tacted New York surgeon Jerome Webster about this problem in 1949.
In response to an article she had published, she had received a desperate letter from a woman in St. Augustine, Florida, pleading for help. Her
efforts to contact the Board had been fruitless, so Davis turned to Webster, asking, "I wonder if you could possibly suggest what I can write to
this woman." Webster apologized for the Board's inattention, explaining that the secretary had been swamped with requests sparked by the
six different articles that had appeared in lay publications in the preceding
few months.[15]

In the early 1950s, the Board began referring inquiries to the
American Medical Association, which agreed to handle correspondence

with lists supplied by the ABPS. The Board also began asking writers, editors, and publishers to refrain from publishing the Board's name and address, but requests kept coming in as many authors simply picked up the information from earlier articles, which themselves continued to circulate. In a June 1960 letter to Alice Lake, the public relations officer of the ASPRS, ABPS corresponding secretary Estelle Hillerich commented, "You are right, the Board's address given in the June issue of *Harper's Bazaar* is bringing in around twenty to thirty letters for lists daily.... It is really becoming quite a nuisance." A month later, Hillerich noted wonderingly that letters were still coming in from articles that had appeared in some newspaper or magazine as long as ten years previously. And new articles continued to appear. "Your Trouble May Be as Plain as the Nose on Your Face," which appeared in the Sunday supplement *Family Weekly* on August 13, 1961, generated more than five hundred letters in five days.[16]

Surgeons like James Barrett Brown, who in 1948 characterized the 1946 *American Weekly* articles as one of "two very distasteful episodes of popular articles on plastic surgery" (the second was Trotta's 1948 *Look* magazine cover story), continued to express concern about the way their specialty was portrayed in the press, about the unrealistic expectations such portrayals fostered, and about the Board's role in this process. They feared that consumers would take the list as a recommendation or endorsement and blame the Board if they were dissatisfied. In some cases, this fear was justified. In 1949, for example, a Dunsmuir, California, woman wrote that the surgeon she had chosen to lift her face, whose name she had received from the Board, "only took a little sag out of the front of the neck." "It took me a long time to save $1,000," she complained. "I think you shouldn't mislead people with your flowery prose and advertisements." For the most part, however, the surgeons' goal was to shape publicity rather than to stop it altogether; even the most conservative surgeons were aware of its benefits.[17]

When the June 1960 issue of *Harper's Bazaar* appeared on newsstands, however, even those surgeons who encouraged publicity realized that it was a double-edged sword. The episode surgeons later termed the "*Harper's Bazaar* Hassle" began with an article by veteran plastic surgery writer Geri Trotta entitled "The Wish to Be Beautiful." The article itself was tame enough; it contained the (by-then) standard descriptions of the types of surgery available to correct noses, faces, necks, eyes, ears, and chins. The warning with which she concluded, however, sparked a nasty turf battle: "Some ear, nose and throat men (otolaryngologists) feel qualified to perform the nasal plastics . . . and no law can stop them. For your own protection . . . be sure that your surgeon has had the added years of study and experience which the American Board of Plastic Surgery certification guarantees." Despite Trotta's assurances that she had acted independently, in addition to thousands of letters from potential patients, the article generated angry protests from otolaryngologists, who accused the Board of planting the story in an attempt to protect its territory, and from other physicians who objected to the warning's uncollegial tone. After much discussion, the American Board for Medical Specialties asked all boards to refrain from giving out lists of their diplomates to the public, although they might continue to provide them to physicians for use in making referrals. The American Board of Plastic Surgery began responding to requests for information with printed cards advising people to ask their family doctors or local hospitals for referrals and redoubled efforts to curb the publication of its name and address.[18]

The Board's public relations policy from 1960 to 1973, when the issue again became a major concern, was much less active, and many Board-certified plastic surgeons, their feathers dirtied by the mudslinging resulting from the *Harper's* incident, were reluctant to speak publicly about their work. By then, however, women had become accustomed to reading about plastic surgery, and magazines had come to rely on such stories as staples, guaranteed to maintain interest among committed readers and generate sales among new ones. As one plastic surgeon observed, "Cosmetic surgery is so apparent that everyone considers himself an expert in judging it, so perhaps untrained authors find it easier to sell articles about this field than some others." Board-certified plastic surgeons were not the only practitioners doing cosmetic surgery, and as many others were eager to cooperate, the number of articles about plastic surgery continued to increase. In 1972, when the public relations committee of the ASPRS subscribed to a clipping service, it received more than twelve hundred articles in just six months.[19]

Women Face the Postwar World

In a very real sense, then, plastic surgeons actively drove the specialty's growth in the postwar years, but as the following anecdote suggests, this is only part of the story. In June 1944, Senator Ralph O. Brewster of Maine received an anonymous letter containing an unusual suggestion for boosting wartime morale: a federally sponsored lend-lease program to provide cosmetic surgery for wives and families of men in the armed services. "What woman, wife or mother, among us wants that man to return to a wrinkled face, dried up, flabby neck; knowing men do not age as quickly as women?" the writer had asked. "We've suffered at home—many of us are still in our 30s, but our necks and eyes, faces, do not respond to cream and exercises. We need these skins made youthful again. That would help the morale of returning fighting men." The *New York Times* treated the suggestion as a joke, but the letter Senator Brewster had received was a harbinger of things to come.[20]

Historians have recently begun to reexamine women's experience in the United States after World War II. Some have argued that the war was a watershed for women, opening up new opportunities in everything from career paths to lifestyles, while others, their vision shaped by Betty Friedan's pioneering *The Feminine Mystique,* have seen women as victims of a postwar ideology that contained them in the home. In recent years, works by scholars like Elaine Tyler May and JoAnne Meyerowitz have offered more finely textured interpretations that take into account women's diverse experiences. Among other things, these works have highlighted the danger of making sweeping generalizations about women's experiences in this period.

That beauty remained important for women in the postwar world and that it was most often equated with youth is, however, a safe generalization. As historian Lois Banner has shown, the cosmetics industry posted exponential growth, as novel discoveries like lanolin and aerosol spawned a generation of new products, while fresh advertising campaigns like Revlon's suggestive "Are You Made for Fire and Ice?" and Clairol's sly "Does She or Doesn't She?" spurred sales of established ones. The increasingly visual nature of American society and culture, too, has acted to increase the importance and value attached to women's looks over the course of this century. Embodied by Hollywood stars and models and presented to Americans in films and in an ever-growing and ever more standardized series of "photographs and articles, advertisements, models, and pinup girls," the ideal, historian Beth Bailey argues, had by the postwar years become nationalized, "held up to and available to a much greater percentage of the population—both men and women—than ever before." Americans of the 1920s, who had found the beauty budgets of their times scandalous enough, would have shuddered at the figures reported in 1956. According to *Life* magazine, American women had spent almost \$2.5 billion, a sum equal to twice Italy's defense budget, on cosmetics, beauty products and treatments, and weight reduction aids.[21]

And, in the postwar years, beauty was clearly equated with youth. As Lily Daché put it in her 1956 *Glamour Book,* "Today, there is no excuse for a woman to grow old, unless she is ill. . . . If you want to keep up with this modern, wonderful world, you must be young in thought, feeling and appearance . . . and all you have to do is stretch out your hand to receive the magic bounty of glamour that modern science has prepared for you." While Daché did not specifically mention surgery, other commentators clearly saw it as part of modern science's bounty. "Farewell to Ugliness," the series of articles that bid good-bye to the war years, provides an obvious example. Author Robert Potter framed cosmetic surgery as the quintessential product of postwar prosperity: "When a plastic surgeon wields his scalpel—and he is wielding it today with a skill far greater than ever before—he can change a man's inner self, his

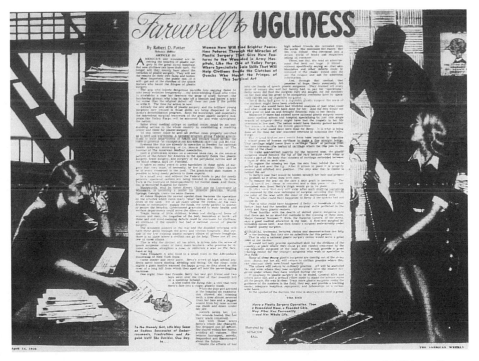

After World War II, magazines and newspapers encouraged Americans to bid "Farewell to Ugliness."

whole outlook upon the world, his attitude toward life." Suggesting that the psychological explanation surgeons had formulated before the war remained pertinent, Potter emphasized that the minor cosmetic surgeries "that mean so much to a patient's mental attitude" would be performed "far quicker than ever before." And costs would go down after the war, he prophesied, making such surgery accessible to the growing middle class. Most important, all of these benefits would be available to women, who "now [would] find brighter peacetime futures through the miracles of plastic surgery." The caption to a set of before-and-after pictures (a secretary, holding a handkerchief despondently to her large nose as her boss ignores her; the same secretary smiling as he looks attentively, and adoringly, into her altered face) made this point even more strongly: "To the homely girl, life may seem an endless succession of Embarrassments, Frustrations and anguish until she decides, one day, to . . . have a plastic surgery operation. Then a remodeled nose, a rounded chin, may alter her personality—and her whole life."[22]

The response generated by these articles—more than fifteen hundred letters in six weeks, four thousand total—suggests that women had an inexhaustible appetite for information about cosmetic surgery, even if they did not act on it. As writer Olga Kahler commented in a 1948 article about face-lifting: "Some think it's wonderful; some think it's silly; and a few think it's horrible. But all, including the horrified, are extremely interested and listen eagerly to the smallest detail." Kahler's article generated so much interest that it was picked up by another magazine a few months after its initial appearance with the notation that the "unusual number of requests for information about this particular branch of plastic surgery" had prompted the reprint.[23]

For women, beauty and youth were important determinants of economic security. Some limited their discussion to women "gainfully employed" in positions demanding contact with the public (secretaries and those in the fashion industry were usually cited as examples), while others granted a place on the surgeon's waiting list to "the woman whose social standing demands that she appear her best at all times." All, however, agreed that for at least some women, face-lifts were essential. As surgeon and psychiatry buff Adolph Abraham Apton noted in 1951, "Not vanity, not self-esteem alone, but tyrannical reality enforces the demand for surgical relief."[24]

Their words attest that reality did indeed seem tyrannical to women of this generation. Eugenia Harris commented in 1961 that "vanity, wealth, and leisure time aren't enough to persuade women to entrust their valued and only faces to the surgeon's cold knife. It takes an urgent reason, like the economic one of the need for a pay check." This assertion was supported by a woman who described the prevailing atmosphere in the fashion industry, emphasizing the clear divisions between generations and the surprising suddenness with which a woman crossed that line. "Up to a point, being an old hand gives us an advantage," she explained. "But then suddenly that point is passed. The very slim, very chic, but obviously mature women of last year suddenly remind you of the tall gaunt madwomen of Chaillot; their faces seem to *go* all at once. It's not quite decent that they're still working—to say nothing of looking for jobs." Suggesting that a youthful appearance had become as important in the pink collar world in which most women worked as in the higher echelons of the fashion industry, writer Ramona Leigh described a similar situation to *Popular Medicine* readers the following year. "To a business woman face lifting is almost as important in dollars and cents as it is to those on the stage," she asserted. "When a man has furnished an office with heavy carpets, colorful walls and draperies and the very latest in office fixtures it is only human to wish for a secretary to be not only proficient and experienced but as up to date looking as the rest of the office." *Science Digest*, in 1964, also warned its readers about the danger inherent in America's new emphasis on youth: "In a society that places a high value on youthful appearance, surgery for many older people is an economic necessity. An older widow or divorcee or an older man with sagging jowls and baggy eyelids meets rebuff in work applications."[25]

Jerome Webster saw many prospective patients in these years, almost all of them female, who believed cosmetic surgery was necessary to hold onto the jobs they already had. Nightclub singer Adela Captiva, age forty-seven and worried that her career would not last much longer, came to see Webster about a face-lift in 1937. The next year, the *New York Herald Tribune* told its readers that "no reputable surgeon attempts" to lift faces, but only weeks before, *Tribune* editor Jean Swenson, fifty, had told Webster that she had already dyed her hair but was afraid that she would lose her job within the next year if she could not manage to look younger. Virginia Walther wrote Webster in 1949, "I am a working lady and have to keep up my appearance to hold the position I now occupy and a sagging skin of the chin line is no asset." Daisy Benton, one of the most famous actresses of the century, secured a television contract in 1955 but believed a face-lift was necessary to retain the loyalty of her public. In 1956 Pauline Bertacci, a beautician, insisted that in her line of work it was "essential to keep young." These women had already achieved their desired positions but were worried about losing them; security, not mobility, was their goal. Cosmetic surgery, they believed, would alter the way others perceived them and allow them to maintain the power they had acquired through long years of hard work. Webster tried to discourage this belief. In 1949, for example, in response to Mrs. Theodore Collins's inquiry, he chided gently, "There is, of course, much to be said for a person's being her own age and not worrying about the effects that age brings." He turned down Captiva and Bertacci. But on occasion even he could be persuaded: he agreed to perform surgery on Swenson and Benton (Walther did not pursue the matter after this initial correspondence).[26]

As comments such as these suggest, women who worked outside the home—and more and more women did—described aging primarily as an economic problem and tended to see a face-lift as simply a practical step toward solving that problem. Surgeons encouraged this view. As one told *Cosmopolitan* in 1959, "Theatrical people are matter-of-fact. They regard their faces and figures as tools. They talk sensibly to the surgeon. I reject—among the general public—more than half of all patients who want face lifts or other operations . . . they need psychiatry more than surgery. But I cannot recall ever turning down a star. Stars expect no miracles from the surgery. Only a help in getting on with their careers—not a transformation in their whole lives." Or, as another surgeon told *McCalls* nearly a decade later, wanting to look better was a perfectly valid reason for having a face-lift. "What we mistrust is the romantic woman—or man—who presumes that a face-lift is going to guarantee a happy new future." Surgeons counseled women, in short, not to expect miracles. A face-lift, they insisted, would not save a marriage or make the world a significantly different place, and those who attached too much psychological importance to it were likely to end up disappointed.[27]

But even as they advised middle-class women to view a face-lift through the same lens as they might view a coat of paint on a house— as a practical, cost-effective step that would add value to an important commodity—surgeons' descriptions of the personal transformations that surgery brought about must have encouraged women to hope for miracles. Their faith was affirmed by a slew of popular magazine articles, most of them positive. And even articles that adopted a cautionary tone underscored surgery's transformative potential. In 1965, for example, a surgeon told *Esquire* that knowing how to judge which patients were likely to react badly was an important part of the surgeon's art: "Sometimes it's very hard to decide about the patient," he observed ruefully. "I had a woman patient recently; a very smart, chic, well-dressed woman. Middle-age. She wanted a face-lift. She was married to a very responsible man in an upper-income bracket, and she wanted to look better for her husband. It sounded okay. . . . Later on I heard she absolutely ran amok—divorced her husband, ran off to Mexico, took a twenty-five-year-old boy as a lover—the whole route. It was dreadful." It is hard to imagine that middle-class women read this anecdote as the apocryphal warning the surgeon evidently intended, and in any case most transformations were described in unswervingly positive tones. Syndicated newspaper columnist Josephine Lowman, in 1953, attributed remarkable transformations to face-lifts: "Over and over again," she noted, "women have won a husband, gone ahead in a job, or just plain felt more confident and happier after an operation."[28]

Indeed, commentators suggested repeatedly, a face-lift might well be the beginning of a brand new life. According to writer T. R. McCoy, its benefits included "a more relaxed attitude, a more vigorous step, a stronger feeling of security, sometimes economic, sometimes marital." Ramona Leigh's article made the same point: "If you wish the operation to hold a husband it might be well to remember that a youthful face alone will not do it. Still, it might so renew a right spirit within you that the same result would be obtained." The remarkable tale of "Mrs. B." illustrated this lesson for *San Francisco Chronicle* readers, in 1969, in concrete terms. Within two weeks of her face-lift, the sixty-two-year-old widow received three dinner invitations from men in their thirties and shortly thereafter married a forty-four-year-old man who thought her younger than he. And surgeons' accounts bore this out. As Robert Alan Franklyn, author of the autobiography *Beauty Surgeon* and for years one of Hollywood's most celebrated (and most controversial) plastic surgeons put it in 1972, a patient's surgical transformation "not only saved her job but it gave her a warmer personality and a brand new attractiveness to men who previously shunned her as a 'crotchety old bag.'"[29]

The "Youthquake," as fashion editors dubbed the craze that swept the country in the 1960s, gave new impetus to traditional fears: women searched for the words to describe the very basic questions about personal identity that the aging process raised. *Vogue,* in 1961, described it this way: "the *fading* of beauty is almost imperceptible . . . a beautiful woman just seems to have become plain; a desirable woman, unalluring for no reason that anyone can put a finger on. It's simply that an elusive something has vanished." Eugenia Harris described a similar feeling in *McCalls*: "Looking—and feeling—'old' tends to desex a woman, because men stop looking at her as if she is a woman," she wrote. Several years later, an anonymous liftee confessed to *Harper's Bazaar* readers, "For years I guess I hadn't thought of myself as attractive—not since I was young."[30]

The identification of beauty with youth was often implicit rather than explicit; it had to do with a "look" or a "feeling" rather than with a chronological age, but the widely held conviction that Americans held rigid ideas about what chronological age meant compounded the problem. Women's words suggest clearly that they thought about the problem of aging in terms of norms and deviation from those norms. Olga Kahler, author of the popular 1948 "I'm Glad" article, described the problem in this way. Over the years, she wrote, she had grown accustomed to looking, and feeling, younger than her chronological age. After she passed fifty, she continued to feel younger, but her appearance caught up with her. "I'm sure there are many women my age (fifty-one) who feel younger than they look," she observed. "And this lack of harmony between the inner woman and the outer is psychologically disturbing." In *Cosmopolitan* in 1958, writer Elizabeth Honor put it this way: "What about the woman who looks into the mirror one morning and realizes that, unlike her friends, she is not aging gracefully? She may even be so unfortunate as to age prematurely." Actress Edith Meiser, in 1959, cited the disjunction between her appearance and her attitude as the reason for her face-lift. "I have managed, without too much stress and strain, to retain a reasonably youthful figure and point of view," she explained. "My step is brisk, my eye is clear. What I resented bitterly was promenading down the street on a bright sunny day, feeling as brisk and debonair as I did when I was thirty, and unexpectedly seeing that droopy, dreary face mirrored back at me in a shopwindow. I resented it bitterly."[31]

As if the general problem of aging were not bad enough, women were widely believed to wrinkle earlier and more dramatically than men because they were more emotional and more expressive than men. Echoing Charles C. Miller, the visionary turn-of-the-century practitioner who advocated cutting facial muscles early in life as a preventive measure, self-appointed advisors cautioned women to take care lest they speed the wrinkling process by their own actions. New York surgeon Murray Berger, author of a 1951 book about the benefits of plastic surgery, asserted that women ruined their faces through "reckless expenditure of emotion" and "careless indulgence in tricks of unlovely expression." Surgeon John Conley, in his 1968 book on face-lifting, also charged women with being the instruments of their own destruction. "The constantly enforced and exaggerated smile in vogue today is a major offender in causing wrinkles about the commissures of the mouth, the nasolabial fold and the eyes," he scolded. "This habit is so deeply ingrained in some persons that it is not possible for them to order a dozen bananas at the local grocery store without staggering the clerk with a Hollywood smile. This is certainly conducive to the production of wrinkles at an early age." Beauty advisors echoed these pronouncements. In her 1977 consumer guide, Sylvia Rosenthal commented, "Those who learn to cope with [stress] will hold onto the freshness and vitality of youth a little longer. Profound, uncontrolled emotion leaves its imprint on our faces for the world to see." Ironically, women learned, it was femininity itself that caused aging.[32]

Some Americans continued to believe that the risks inherent in a face-lift outweighed the problems wrinkles caused. As late as 1948, *Hygeia* cautioned surgeons and other readers that a face-lift carried inherent dangers: "A person who has had the wrinkles erased may feel that she *is* as young as she *looks*. Dangerous strains may be put upon failing body resources as a result." In the postwar years, however, surgeons increasingly advocated face-lifts as the most practical, effective solution for the problems of aging. As one husband told *Vogue*, his wife's surgeon had altered his initial opposition: "I pointed out that what I most admired was a woman who could grow old gracefully. The doctor made me see that age per se hasn't a great deal of charm, that there is no particular virtue in putting up with unattractiveness, and that a drooping chinline, wrinkles and a sagging jaw are grace*less*, not grace*ful*." As they shared their perspectives with prospective patients and their spouses, families, and friends, surgeons helped turn the public's sights toward plastic surgery. As one surgeon explained, "The plastic surgeon cannot make time stand still, but he can certainly lessen its ravages on those who do not want to appear old before their time or who want to look as young as they feel." "Beauty surgeon" Robert Alan Franklyn put it even more succinctly: "Personally, I believe it's tragic when women who still feel youthful look tired and old," he noted. "It is so unnecessary."[33]

In the postwar years, middle-class women came increasingly to see face-lifts as the solution for the empty feeling that plagued so many of them as they approached middle age. In 1961, after describing this vague malaise, *Vogue* explained, "And just as indescribably, without anyone's knowing why or being able to *see* why—after expert artistic surgery—a woman seems to become a going concern again, out of the age limbo and back in competition as a woman." Eugenia Harris advised *McCalls* readers that, although many surgeons insisted otherwise, a face-lift could change their lives "because it gives you an inner lift that goes hand in hand with your newly youthful appearance and thus helps you move more confidently and happily and effectively among people who are important to you. . . . For the normal, not-too-neurotic woman, the beneficial changes a face-lift can make in her life are basic indeed. . . . After a face-lift, she responds to the stimulus of being regarded as desirable once again." The *Harper's* liftee, too, was elated: "But here it was—that 'you're attractive' feeling back again after how long!"[34]

The quotidian vocabularies of postwar domesticity—sewing, housecleaning, and cooking—supplied the vocabulary and frame of reference that allowed women to claim this solution as their own. As one patient put it, "It makes me mad and sad to think of the years and energy I wasted thinking up reasons why I shouldn't get my face neatened. . . . [Now, it's] on with the face-tidying." When Amy Vanderbilt went public with her face-lift in 1971, she employed carving and cooking as metaphors: "With a small scalpel the surgeon cuts along these lines, much as a whittler would. He reveals excess fat and tissue and then pulls it out with little pincers, much as you might remove the membrane from sweetbreads in preparing them." Words like "neatening," "tidying," and "fixing up" made cosmetic surgery seem less foreign and less threatening to middle-class women; at the same time, they expanded the limits of domesticity to include plastic surgery.[35]

Straightforward discussions of cost also demystified cosmetic surgery. In 1961, *Vogue* described the back-in-town-after-summer lunch meeting of two female friends. One had "taken a look at the Aswan temples and dipped down into Nigeria." The other, in what she described as "the best summer of her life," had stayed home and had a face-lift. For middle-class Americans, these vacations were comparable: "While the operation involves a respectable sum," *Vogue* acknowledged, "it is no more than, if as much as, the standard American luxury-necessities—a car, a boat, a European jaunt." *Esquire,* in 1965, quoted a woman who described face-lifts as "much better for your morale and your appearance than going around the world or to Europe. Heaven knows they're cheaper than those trips, and you get much more out of them in the long run." Two years later, another liftee urged *Harper's Bazaar* readers, "Don't feel guilty about spending the money it costs. It's no more than the cost of just one fabulous ball dress." And in 1969 a liftee told *Harper's Bazaar* simply, "We belong to a nice club, but we're not rich. I'm not at all the spoiled rich-woman type." These examples speak to upper- or upper-middle class social choices, but an article the following year in the *Ladies Home Journal* explained the economics of face-lifting for the more marginally middle-class: "For three years I had earned and saved money from the oddest assortment of jobs a housewife ever tackled. . . . I boarded pets, played the organ for funerals, raised puppies, became a vacation-time receptionist, pounded a typewriter, altered clothes, sold household accumulations . . . and stashed into the bank every gift of money I received—along with the dimes and quarters I won on the golf course and at the bridge table. At the end of three years I had saved $1,500. . . . A lot of money, but not out of reach for anyone who can budget a trip to Europe or a good fur coat. Any really determined woman can do it."[36]

As they laid claim to the therapeutic benefits of the face-lift, women redefined cosmetic surgery itself as simply one of the many products that postwar prosperity had made available to the growing middle class. But money was not the only issue. Over and over, in articles like these—perhaps in an attempt to counteract the stereotype of face-lift patients as vain, rich, and spoiled—women assured each other that face-lifts were not only affordable but appropriate for normal, suburban women. In 1961, *Vogue* reassured readers that the majority of face-lift patients were "neither narcissists nor hedonists." Rather, they were "serious, thoughtful women—often with good jobs or small businesses—whose working years are going to be lengthened by ten, fifteen, or even more; active women who intend to keep up with their busy lives attractively; women who have had children late in life and want to be on a pleasant par with other younger mothers; affirmative women with good lives who believe in keeping them that way as long as they can." The self-described "small-town, Midwestern housewife who was terribly concerned over her appearance" whose diary appeared in

Ladies Home Journal encouraged women to assert themselves and claim their rights. "I was not the plastic surgeons' preferred patient—a celebrity who needed their help for real economic reasons," she wrote. But she didn't give up: "Why, I asked myself, should a firm face and smooth neck be the exclusive prerogatives of 'past 45' celebrities? If they could rebuild their morale with restorative surgery, so could I!" Describing her three interviews with potential surgeons, a liftee told *Harper's Bazaar* readers simply that "waiting in the three anterooms was reassuring. You see that it's a nice normal-looking lot of people who've been having facial surgery done." By the end of the decade, even *Newsweek* had taken note of the new trend. "Cosmetic surgery has long been regarded as an indulgence sought only by aging actresses and rich and narcissistic matrons," the magazine commented in 1969, "but the pattern is changing rapidly."[37]

As it turned out, the specialty's new willingness to take seriously the problems of middle-class, middle-aged women was a wise move. As a 1958 study conducted by the Johns Hopkins University found, the typical face-lift patient was forty-eight, married, white, Protestant, upper middle-class, socially active, and employed or otherwise involved in the world outside her home. Plastic surgeons found these patients gratifying. As one surgeon noted, "They are enthusiastic and grateful patients. They do not tend to forget quickly their original condition, and, years after operation, they continue to express their satisfaction." The sources that shaped women's view of the postwar world—newspapers, films, and particularly popular magazines—heralded the new youth culture and offered few positive models of aging. One of the more than one hundred women who attended a seminar on plastic surgery offered by Gimbels department store in 1972 explained that fourteen of her friends had selected her to attend and report back to them, while a spokesman for the store, marveling at the audience's enthusiasm, noted, "The cooking or sewing classes were not as exciting as this. . . . We've never had such an interested audience."[38]

The picture of middle-class culture that emerges from these accounts is not a pretty one. "This is America in 1965," Dixie Dean Harris told *Esquire* readers: "Competitive, youth-oriented, money-conscious, affluent America." Some commentators framed the change in terms of the nation's historic emphasis on self-improvement. As a *McCalls* article lauding the face-lift put it, "We're living in a time when there is no stigma attached to improving yourself in any way." Many more decried the new trend and the superficiality in American society that fostered it, but, even among these, resignation was the most common response. In the years after the Second World War, the social and psychological limbo brought about by aging began to seem just as hellish as the purgatory to which halitosis had sentenced sufferers in the 1920s and 1930s, and the pervasive anxiety that had then driven Americans to the drugstore counter now drove them to the surgeon's office. By the mid-1960s, this message had become ubiquitous throughout a wide range of publications for both lay and medical audiences. As the editors of *Newsweek* put it in 1969, "The furrowed brow, the wrinkled cheek, the baggy eyelid and the sagging jowl have no place in a modern America, where the smooth, firm flesh of youth has become a cultural totem."[39]

Real Men Get Face-Lifts

As middle-class Americans became increasingly convinced that an aging face exacted significant social, economic, and psychological costs, men began to see their wrinkles in this new light. The more enthusiastic surgeons of the 1930s had waxed ecstatic about the benefits that cosmetic surgery might bestow on men, and a few more restrained surgeons had voiced their willingness to accept male clients. Men, of course, had been plastic surgeons' first patients. During World War I, they had spurred the specialty's organization, and during World War II they had provided surgeons with the training and experience that helped to fuel the postwar boom.[40]

But face-lifts were rare among men for several reasons. First, according to popular belief, where age made women ugly, it made men mature and distinguished. As a 1975 article in *LA Magazine* explained, "Men simply don't *need* plastic surgery as much; or when they do, it's never as radical or as all-encompassing as in females." Second, until after the war, surgical techniques were less than effective: in the standard prewar lift, the surgeon simply removed a crescent-shaped piece of skin and pulled up the slack; the resulting tension often caused scarring, and this was more of an issue with men because men could not style their hair to hide it, as women could. Third, and perhaps most important, was that the culture of masculinity, as it developed in the United States, was homophobic. Real men did not care about their looks; ergo men who did care were suspect. In 1957, surgeon Walter C. Alvarez noted that "a few men, some in the public eye, want to have a face lifting or really need it to hold their places in the theatre or on the concert stage. A few 'gay birds' may also want to be rejuvenated, as well as a few elderly men married to young women." As late as 1967, a study of 325 repeat plastic surgery patients asserted that "nearly all" were "mentally disturbed unmarried males between the ages of 20 and 35." These "latent schizophrenics" were characterized by "grandiose ambitions, low self-esteem, little heterosexual interest and high anxiety." Surgeons, in short, generally agreed that any man considering a face-lift was "effeminate" and "narcissistic"—in the words of Los Angeles surgeon Michael Curtin, "either an aging actor, a homosexual, or both."[41]

Beginning in the early 1960s, the cultural barriers that had kept men from the plastic surgeon's office began to crumble. *Coronet* broke ground in 1961 with a report of a study of fifty-three west coast men who had found face-lifts extremely beneficial. Most were commission salesmen and sales managers, all were middle-class and in their fifties and sixties, and all were heterosexual. One year later, their incomes had increased, on the average, by $1,300. Foreshadowing the hundreds of articles that would follow in publications ranging from *Forbes* to *Gentleman's Quarterly,* author Marilyn Mercer explained, "We put such a premium on youth today that a more youthful appearance may be necessary for survival"—an observation that has an oracular ring to it more than thirty years later.[42]

The economic justification provided the vocabulary and the frame of reference that enabled surgeons and their patients to reframe cosmetic surgery as masculine common sense rather than effeminate vanity. Addressing a science writers' seminar entitled "The Quest for Youth and Beauty" held at Philadelphia's Temple University in 1969, for example, one surgeon characterized the typical patient as a businessman who was either starting a new job or afraid of losing his current job to a younger man. Patrick McGrady Jr., in *Vogue,* acknowledged that men's new interest in cosmetic surgery was related to the new ethic of self-improvement and personal presentation that had them paying more attention to fashion and hairstyling as well. "But behind the facade of self-indulgence and 'let's see what they'll think when we try *that,*'" McGrady continued, "lie some rather cruel social and professional pressures. Although a face-lift may be a real-estate centi-millionaire's valentine to a sweet young thing, or the only way a fading actor can watch his TV re-runs without cringing, it may represent nothing less than survival itself to a psychologically murdered salesman." As employment counselor Harry Adams put it a few years later, "The sales executive is particularly vulnerable in these times of business recession and an abundance of sharp young go-getters who are out to get his job."[43]

The economic justification was important because cultural barriers do not fall all at once; the historic suspicion of male vanity continued to inform the way that many surgeons looked at their male patients. Two Miami plastic surgeons, for example, wrote that an increasing emphasis on youth in advertising and the media and a wider knowledge of plastic surgery's benefits had upped the number of men among their patients to between 15 and 20 percent. Most were successful businessmen, often in their early fifties, who were married and well adjusted and simply looked older than they felt; these men, the surgeons wrote, made fine patients. The others, however—described as widowers or divorcés who were dating younger women—might be unstable, the surgeons warned their colleagues.[44]

Although in previous years surgeons had characterized male patients as unpredictable and likely to initiate lawsuits, by the 1970s the *New York Times* was reporting that some surgeons, especially in southern California, where face-lifts were more common among males, had come to prefer them to women. San Diego surgeon Matthew Gleason, who by 1971 had lifted dozens of men, told the *Times* that men were easier to work with because their expectations were reasonable: "Unlike women, the men don't come back and complain about every wrinkle that's left," Gleason asserted. In comparison to "the stout and 60-ish woman who brought in a photograph of Mrs. Jacqueline Onassis to give the surgeon an idea of what she had in mind," the male patient "doesn't expect the impossible . . . doesn't ask us to make him handsome, only that we try and erase 10 or 15 years. . . . He's not trying to turn November back to May. He's satisfied with July or August."[45]

If Americans were more comfortable believing that it was economic reality that generally drove men to the surgeon's office, they were aware that a variety of benefits accompanied them home. Several male celebrities who openly admitted to having had cosmetic surgery in the 1970s helped to smooth the way for others. Hair emperor Vidal Sassoon, in 1973, had no qualms about discussing his eyelid surgery: "Why should I look like an old man when I feel young? I am in great physical shape. I am married to a young woman, am chairman of a young company, and all my staff is young. Only my eyes betray me." Senator William Proxmire, too, discussed his hair transplants and eyelid surgery with the press, explaining that it was not vanity but insecurity that inspired him. "If you're very vain, you wouldn't want to improve your appearance," he stated. "You'd feel, 'Well, I'm perfect; how could I be any better?'" Only a deep-seated insecurity and "feeling of ugliness" had led him to "submit to the pain and the cost and the difficulty and the ridicule, especially the ridicule." Surgeons and personnel executives agreed that the results were likely to change a man's "personality and his outlook on life," and other observers backed them up. One lawyer's secretary stated, "He had his face lifted last year. . . . He's much happier and far easier to get along with."[46]

Despite the pioneering examples of celebrities and the warm welcome surgeons had begun to offer, most men took up residence in this new world only uneasily. According to post office authorities, men were more likely than women to be victims of mail fraud, because they were embarrassed about pursuing beauty. The *New York Times* reported that men were more likely than women to go abroad for surgery, cloaking their real purpose in the disguise of a vacation (the percentage of male patients among those who went to Mexico for surgery tripled between 1972 and 1977). The anxiety and embarrassment men felt was probably compounded by the fact that many surgeons retained a lingering distrust of the men who consulted them. One Florida surgeon, in 1974, observed cynically that of the fifteen men who had consulted him recently, most cited business reasons, "although two were retired and four had younger wives." A Los Angeles plastic surgeon voiced similar sentiments the following year about the Washington, D.C., politicians who, in increasing numbers, were heading west in search of hair transplants: "These people are involved with literally controlling our destiny, yet they're willing to come out here and let me drill holes in their heads."[47]

Comments like these testify to the vague discomfort many felt as they watched increasing numbers of American men join the quest for youth and beauty. Perhaps the most frightening picture of middle-class men gone surgery mad was painted by writer David Lilienthal in his 1963 novel *Seconds* (later made into a movie starring Rock Hudson). The novel begins as the protagonist—a middle-aged, upper middle-class New York attorney identified only as "Mr. Wilson"—receives a late-night phone call from Charley, an old friend who had (Wilson believed) killed himself a year before. Intrigued, Wilson follows Charley's directions. First, his own "death" (more costly than Charley's "suicide,"

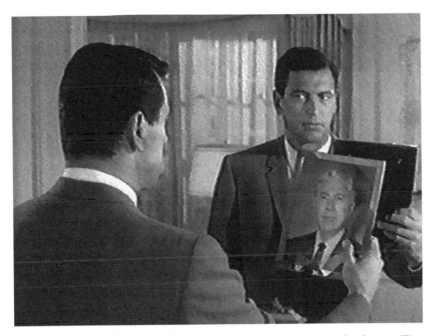

Rock Hudson contemplates his total transformation in *Seconds* (video frame still).

but easier on survivors, his guides tell him) is arranged. His face is then remodeled, with phenomenal results. Looking into the mirror, Wilson muses, "The surgeons had done an extraordinary job. They had taken a face that tended to be rounded, florid, and a bit jowly, and had somehow made it lean and long and hard, with prominent cheekbones and chin; and the weeks and weeks of dieting and exercise that had accompanied the surgical process had produced a physique to match. Only the eyes were the same." Wilson is then literally installed in a new, more romantic life commensurate with his transformed look: a painter, complete with landscapes to back him up, he lives beachside on the swinging coast. Initially thrilled at this second life, Wilson soon develops misgivings, which are compounded by the discovery that his new "friends" are not real but makeovers like himself: the world that has been given to him is entirely false. He escapes from the colony and heads for his old life but is captured and taken back to "headquarters," where he learns the truth about the pyramid scheme of which he has become a part. Wealthy men buy into the system, but those who can't make the transition are dealt with severely lest they topple the pyramid. Only by recruiting more men, as

Charley recruited him, can Wilson avoid the fate of becoming the corpse used to fake another man's death.[48]

With its futuristic vision of plastic surgery as (literally) the creator of life itself, available for purchase by the wealthy and privileged, *Seconds* may have inspired some second thoughts. In general, however, the boom in face-lifts for men was accepted with the same resignation that had characterized the nation's response to feminine face-lifting. Echoing the conventional wisdom surrounding the 1960 presidential debates, which held that John F. Kennedy's young, tan, and healthy appearance gave him a significant edge over his pale, pasty, and five-o'clock-shadowed opponent Richard Nixon, in 1971 Captain W. D. Latham, chief of plastic surgery at Bethesda Naval Hospital, forecast that plastic surgery was clearly "the thing of the future" for politicians. In 1977, several surgeons cited the "current emphasis on physical fitness and youthful appearance" as the reason for the recent increase in male patients, noting that "the economic pressure on a man, particularly in his middle years, to look as young and vigorous as possible is very real." Men's experiences tended to support such assertions. As a fifty-five-year-old man noted ruefully about the job he had gotten after his face-lift, "I'd have had to be 80 to have all the experience they wanted—but if I hadn't looked 40, they would never have hired me."[49]

New York Times columnist Russell Baker, in 1978, offered a lighter view: "The central question," he mused, "is whether the smooth mug is here to stay or just another fashion flash in the reorganized pan. . . . If I get an expensive new tight face it's a sure bet that the following week Jerry Brown will turn up in Malibu wearing the brand-new Miz Lillian Carter wrinkles and trying to pretend he knows John Dillinger from Henry Kissinger. This is the same reason I haven't bought pink eyeglasses." But to Dr. Norman Pastorek, inventor of the hair transplant, the trend was clear. In business, he observed, "A number of years ago, there was the elder who was the king. That's not true anymore." By 1980, no less respected a source than *Business Week* was suggesting, "The dawn of a new decade signals a time for fresh starts, and one of the things you might want to treat yourself to in the 1980s is a new—and younger—face." Estimates of the percentage and number of male face-lift patients vary widely, but most sources agree that increasing numbers of men are following the magazine's advice. According to the American Academy of Cosmetic Surgery, men accounted for 26 percent of cosmetic surgery patients in 1994, up from 10 percent in 1980. Women still constitute the overwhelming majority of those seeking face-lifts, which suggests that Americans still believe that aging exacts a higher cost from women than from men. But the frontiers have continued to expand for men as well as for women, with liposuction in the early 1980s, calf and pectoral implants a decade later, and most recently penile enhancement—procedures that are more difficult to justify on economic grounds. If men continue on the path they began to forge in the late 1960s, and there is no reason to expect they will not, the numbers may soon be even.[50]

Second Thoughts about Cosmetic Surgery

At its simplest, the story of the role cosmetic surgery has played in American society over the past half century is one of more surgeons, more dollars, and more surgeries on more parts of the body. Americans, who once classified such surgery as vanity and deemed vanity not a reasonable response to social conditions but a serious, if not always deadly, sin, have in general come to accept such surgery as a fact of life. *Psychology Today*, in a recent study, found that sixty million people do not like their chins, while another six million are dissatisfied with their eyes. *USA Today* similarly reports that of the eight thousand men and women who responded to a recent survey, 40 percent rated their bodies "C" and 14 percent would consider liposuction. Many of those who choose plastic surgery today are not rich. According to the ASPRS, only 23 percent of patients come from families earning more than $50,000 per year. Families with incomes under $25,000 account for 30 percent of patients, while those earning between $25,000 and $50,000 account for another 35 percent. And more and more people believe that cosmetic surgery is acceptable, for others if not for themselves.[51]

If the overall picture is one of continued expansion, however, it is important to note that Americans have had some misgivings about expanding the definition of self-improvement to encompass the surgical approach. These misgivings have not slowed the specialty's growth, nor have they dissuaded significant numbers of potential patients, but they have made some patients uneasy about their decisions. Olga Kahler, in her pioneering 1948 article, dealt with the issue of shame with a rhetorical question: "Is it any more false to lift your face than to recap your worn-out teeth, rouge your lips, or tint your nails and hair?" Two decades later, *W*, the bible of the fashion industry, proclaimed that for both women and men, "cosmetic surgery has come out from behind the bandages . . . as the BP [beautiful people] openly admit that a stitch in time can save a sagging ego." In 1971, no less a BP than Amy Vanderbilt went public. "Perhaps by writing frankly about my experience I can help dissolve the last traces of prejudice against cosmetic surgery," Vanderbilt explained. "It can be a blessing, a need, a delight." With characteristic humor, comedienne Phyllis Diller also directed attention toward her new face in 1972. "What a pity these operations are so shrouded in secrecy," she commented to *Life* magazine. "I think if a woman can afford it, she's inconsiderate to herself *not* to have this done, if only to *feel* younger."[52]

Despite this defensive rhetoric, cosmetic surgery remained for many a dirty little secret. Surgeon Walter Alvarez reassured women in 1957 that most surgeons were aware of, and would respect, patients' desires for secrecy. Dr. McCarthy DeMere of Memphis scheduled women under assumed names for a "bilateral operation on the face" to protect their privacy. Eugenia Harris, in her 1961 article, recounted an anecdote in which a woman entered the hospital with her daughter for a double nose-bob, having previously (and secretly) arranged for the surgeon to lift her face at the same time. "My daughter never caught on. Neither did my husband. Isn't that cute?" the woman exclaimed. "My friend is going to sneak in a face-lifting too, along with *her* nose." The author of the enthusiastic 1969 *Harper's Bazaar* article assured her readers, "Remember, if you decide to take The Step, the world is on your side." Nevertheless, she had gone to a great deal of trouble to avoid recognition, including scheduling her lift at an out-of-town hospital. "So you can see," she confided, "I couldn't possibly sign my name. You wouldn't, would you?"[53]

While cosmetic surgery's critics have themselves often been stigmatized as offering only "sour grapes"—old, ugly, inflexibly Puritan, or too lazy to enter the race, they instead sit back and shoot barbs at those brave, adventurous, committed, resigned, or rich enough to undertake surgical improvement—the continuing preoccupation with secrecy testifies to a haunting unease. As so much of the commentary seems to suggest that cosmetic surgery has been smoothly incorporated into a pre-existing moral framework, a brief look at several instances where controversy has arisen may help illuminate the process by which cosmetic surgery became part of American culture.

One of the most interesting discussions of cosmetic surgery took place among authorities of the world's leading religions in the early 1960s. The exchange was sparked by Pope Pius XII, who in 1958 cautioned plastic surgeons that although "numerous reasons" rendered plastic surgery legitimate, it was morally unlawful to operate on someone who wanted surgery to enhance the "power of seduction, thus leading others more easily into sin . . . to hide a criminal from justice, or if it damages the normal functions of the organs of the body, or if it is desired only to satisfy vanity or the caprice of fashion." The topic was taken up at the 1961 meeting of the American Society of Facial Plastic Surgeons, and this discussion was reprinted in installments in the December 1961 and January, February, and March 1962 issues of *Eye, Ear, Nose and Throat Monthly*. Noting that the scarcity of religious comment on plastic surgery precluded definitive statements, the Reverend Robert B. Reeves Jr., Father Charles G. O'Leary, and Rabbi Immanuel Jakobovitz volunteered to extrapolate from their faiths' general principles and explain their faiths' respective views.

Predictably, none had trouble with the question of reconstructive surgery. For Protestants, Reverend Reeves wrote, the two most relevant principles were that of personal honesty—"that a man should be as he is created to be; that David should not parade in Saul's armor"—and what might be termed wholeness: "that whatever contributes to a man's total effectiveness and happiness, in all his life's relationships, is good; that whatever deters, detracts or hinders him . . . would be bad." Reconstructive surgery, defined as "restorative, reparative and remedial," was clearly consistent with these two principles. "With this class of surgery," Reeves concluded, "I cannot see that there is any ethical issue involved." Father O'Leary similarly found reconstructive surgery consistent with the Catholic Principle of Totality, in that violation or destruction of parts, while not to be undertaken lightly, was acceptable when undertaken for the good of the whole. Likewise, Rabbi Jakobovitz concluded that while Jewish law prohibits endangering one's own life except for an overwhelming reason and objects to any mutilation of the body, these conflicts were clearly resolvable in reconstructive cases where healing was the central issue.[54]

The question of cosmetic surgery proved more complex. Jakobovitz began with the Hippocratic oath, only to discard it as irrelevant. Cosmetic surgery, he stated, was clearly in conflict with this fundamental principle, but so was much of current medical practice, including abortion and artificial insemination. Much of the modern physician's work, in fact, had nothing to do with healing the sick per se; in relation to these matters, the oath was outdated. Those who claimed that cosmetic surgery's psychological component defined it as healing, Jakobovitz continued, were either misguided or indulging in wishful thinking: "I very much doubt if, as a rule, the psychological stress, in merely pathological terms, resulting from the facial malformation to be corrected will outweigh and thus neutralize the health and other risks involved in the operation. In other words, the chief indication for such surgery, I suspect, is cosmetic pure and simple and not medical." After careful consideration, Jakobovitz concluded that the economic justification was the only one that might conceivably apply to men; cosmetic surgery was unacceptable for men unless it was necessary to enable them to support their families. Women might also seek such surgery out of economic necessity, he acknowledged, but other reasons might also be acceptable: a single woman who used it to enhance her chances of marriage or a married woman who undertook it to enhance her relationship with her husband would be in accord with Jewish law.[55]

O'Leary and Reeves also had trouble with the issue of cosmetic surgery. Noting that "physical beauty, even though it occupies a relatively modest place in the Christian scale of values, is a true value in itself," O'Leary concluded that Catholics should harbor "no moral objections to Facial Plastic Surgery in its current use," as long as such surgery had a psychological component, making it consistent with the Principle of Totality. Reeves was less sure. About "the kind of plastic surgery designed to give a different impression than an individual would give in his original state, with a motivation . . . to change the personal impact of that person in his other life relationship," Reeves mused, he would ask "very serious, probing questions" that were clearly designed to discourage the potential patient. Still, he acknowledged, there was no hard-and-fast rule; each case would have to be judged on its own merits. All three concluded that questions from congregation members had become common enough to merit further study.[56]

Surgeons, meanwhile, continued to insist not only that their work was perfectly consistent with a religious worldview but also that the psychological connection, which Jakobovitz had found so flimsy, provided a strong justification for cosmetic surgery. In 1965, physician Albert P. Seltzer asserted that while each case was different, "physical malformation is illness of a kind, for if it does not impair natural functions, it may nevertheless attack the complexities of the mental and emotional structure to create new maladies." In cases where an otherwise normal, law-abiding individual's chances for marriage or employment were being reduced by "a physical imperfection science can cure," Seltzer insisted, "cosmetic surgery becomes sanity, not vanity." When plastic surgery can "correct or relieve any detriment to human health and appearance," he concluded, "God endorses our skills." And as such surgery became more routine, religious objections decreased. By 1986, physician Reuven K. Snyderman could assure his colleagues that there was no conflict at all between cosmetic surgery and the Jewish faith. "The right of a woman to beautify herself is one that is honored in scripture and in the Talmud," he noted. "Since the cosmetic purpose is an honored and an important one, and since the operation is not likely to be a dangerous one, the ambiguous law against self-injury does not apply here and the woman is allowed by Jewish law to undergo cosmetic surgery."[57]

The revelation that military medical establishments were providing cosmetic surgery sparked another significant discussion in the early 1970s. This episode began when the *San Francisco Chronicle*, with the same glee with which it might have reported a public figure's exposure as a fraud, reported that face-lifts and other cosmetic surgical operations were being performed "with increasing frequency" at Bethesda Naval Hospital, the Walter Reed Army Medical Center, and Lackland Air Force Base Hospital. Columnist Jack Anderson quipped that he was amazed that the phenomenon had been kept so quiet, as it could have a significant impact on military recruiting, but the hospitals quickly marshaled their defenses (in order to maintain their accreditation as training centers, they had to provide complete training in plastic surgery, which meant providing the full range of plastic surgical services, they explained), and little more was said. In 1974, San Francisco newspapers reported that such practices were still going on. The previous year, readers learned, two plastic surgeons at San Diego's Balboa Naval Hospital, the world's largest military hospital, had performed twenty-seven face-lifts, seventy-six breast augmentations, and nineteen breast reductions. In explanation, Rear Admiral Willard P. Arentzen had said only, "It is care they are entitled to."[58]

At the time of the 1974 revelations, the Pentagon had promised to keep tabs on the plastic surgery it funded. But, as the *San Francisco Examiner* reported in a front-page article in October 1978, it had not. Under the banner headline, "Facelifts on the Taxpayer," the *Examiner* reported that surgeons at eight Public Health Service hospitals and a number of other military medical centers were busy providing approximately three thousand patients per year with "free facelifts, flab removals, breast implants, and other beauty operations unnecessary for health." A retired colonel defended the program on the grounds that it provided necessary services for veterans, explaining, "My jowls were beginning to sag. I needed a new image," but researchers revealed that veterans accounted for only a tiny minority of patients. Statistics from two hospitals indicated that 91 percent of the beneficiaries were female; at all hospitals, the majority were military wives. The cost? Between $1 million and $6 million annually, "but nobody keeps count."

As it had in 1974, the *Examiner* noted that "the beautification of military wives" was the price the nation paid for training military plastic surgeons, and the military defended its position. Colonel Robert Parsons, who had addressed the issue several years earlier in the journal *Military Medicine,* insisted, "this surgery is no more frivolous or wasteful than the use of live ammunition on artillery ranges." Taxpayers, however, were doubtful, and Health, Education, and Welfare (HEW) secretary Joseph Califano sided with them. On his decision to order an official investigation, Califano commented, "What we do question is whether the hard pressed American taxpayer ought to be paying the bill for a special group for plastic surgery that is purely cosmetic."[59]

The answer to this question, Califano announced definitively in March 1979, was no—at least, not at the eight Public Health Service hospitals over which he had jurisdiction—even if this decision required hospitals to break their residency contracts. The hospitals in question had been established by Congress in 1798 in response to epidemics among merchant seamen. Since then, the number of primary beneficiaries had been gradually shrinking in relation to the number of secondary beneficiaries. Of the 1,110 operations that had been performed between 1973 and 1977 at the hospital in San Francisco's Richmond District, only 185, or 17 percent, of the patients had been primary beneficiaries, such as members of the Coast Guard. In all, the report concluded, the eight hospitals had been spending $500,000 per year on five hundred "nontherapeutic cosmetic" operations—mostly face-lifts, but also breast augmentations and reductions, nose jobs, and neck and eye lifts, sought primarily by wives of retired or active military personnel who, according to HEW Inspector General Thomas D. Morris, often traveled great distances to obtain the free services.[60]

The "Facelifts on the Taxpayer" incident raised some of the same questions religious spokespeople had addressed a decade earlier and resolved them in the same uneasy way. Like Reverend Reeves, Father

O'Leary, and Rabbi Jakobovitz, Secretary Califano refrained from making sweeping pronouncements about the morality of cosmetic surgery. He simply stated his belief—which, coincidentally, many American taxpayers shared—that those who wanted it should pay for it themselves. Although the issue in this case clearly was not the morality of such surgery, but merely who should bear the cost, sly, snide phrases like "the beautification of military wives" implied that more was at stake than fairness to the taxpayers.

Women's personal accounts suggest a similar range of attitudes toward their own decisions. One of these, entitled "The Face Lift That Flopped," appeared anonymously in *Good Housekeeping* in 1978. The author confessed that her obsession with her aging appearance had been sparked by her children's departure and exacerbated by her husband's seeming inability to stop talking about his new graduate student: "How could I, a middle-aged housewife, my face marred with worry lines and crow's feet, compete with the freshness and sparkle of Meg?" she wrote. The face-lift she finally got—from a surgeon whose advertisement she had found in a newspaper—was a disaster: her face was uneven and one eye drooped noticeably, and she became increasingly upset and withdrawn. When she confronted her husband, he admitted that her obsession with Meg was partially justified: "I do look forward to seeing Meg," he confessed. "Her excitement about life, her sense of humor are a real pick-me-up after listening to your moaning about your face." Then he took her to meet Meg, who turned out to be a happily married woman in her mid fifties, with "salt-and-pepper hair [that] framed a soft, round face filled with wrinkles and creases." Like the author, Meg was an empty-nester, but her solution had been to return to school. "I can't say that a miracle occurred that afternoon," the author recalled. "But things did begin to fall into perspective. I began asking myself some important questions. Was I a piece of skin stretched over a facial bone structure? Or was I the woman underneath?" After finding another surgeon to repair her face and making up with her husband, she followed Meg's example and began looking for new interests.[61]

A similar account appeared in *Ms.* in 1986. Nineteen days after surgery, children's book author, magazine writer, and "card-carrying NOW member" Ann Scheiner wrote, she had had an epiphany. "Before the operation I rationalized how I wanted my face-lift so my exterior would match my interior. . . . I realize now I was lying to myself. I just wanted to look younger and prettier." At five weeks, she developed a serious corneal abrasion because her lids had been stretched too tightly. Six weeks after the lift, she tallied the score: "On the plus side: a smoother cheek and neckline. I have fewer lines. I know more truths about myself. On the minus side: serious eye problems. Fear of blindness. Hideous swelling and swollen eyes. Numb face and neck, which may last for months. A nasty fight with my husband. Loss of identity. Long-lasting scabbing. Loss of weeks of work. Lack of exercise for six weeks. The results last only four to eight years. After that, it's sags and bags again. Cost: $5,300 plus eye-doctor bills." Scheiner concluded ruefully that, although she had thought of publishing her article anonymously, "I decided it was important to admit in my own name how far I've had to travel to accept the natural process of my aging."[62]

The women in these last two accounts have much in common with Evelyn Ciardi, who was forty-eight in 1954 when she came to see Jerome Webster about a face-lift. Her husband, after teasing her about the new fullness under her chin, had left her for a younger woman. She was a writer but was currently working in Hollywood; her stories paid the rent, but she thought they were cheap. Ciardi and Webster talked for an hour, after which he made the notation, "To get herself straightened out, possibly with psychiatric help; to write something worthwhile." Several years later, Ciardi wrote to thank Webster for his encouragement; it had been a struggle, she wrote, but she had left Hollywood and was writing "real" stories again; she no longer had any desire for a face-lift.

Jerome Webster was a product of the interwar years; he prided himself on being a conservative surgeon, and he generally refused to perform face-lifts, believing—correctly, in Ciardi's case, at least—that Americans needed to deal with the deeper problems their discomfort with aging signaled. Ciardi was the quintessential middle-aged woman of the postwar, prefeminist generation; as did most women of this generation, when she looked for the power to direct and determine her life, she had instinctively seen her appearance as both the problem and the solution. The fact that it was a plastic surgeon who encouraged her to see this as the culturally determined reaction it was, and to consider the possibility that if appearance was not really the problem, a face-lift was not really the solution, suggests how much had (and had not) changed by the time Meg's rival and Ann Scheiner visited their surgeons. The question the *Good Housekeeping* writer raised—"Was I a piece of skin stretched over a facial bone structure? Or was I the woman underneath?"—reveals a worldview informed by feminism; as a "card-carrying

NOW member," Scheiner's allegiance is even clearer. But while feminism may have encouraged them to see aging as a social problem, it had not diminished the seductive allure of the individual solution—and by then, Jerome Webster's generation had retired and left the field to a new generation, who had given up any thought of trying to shape this unwieldy cultural phenomenon.

On one level, the second thoughts of women who went through the face-lift process, like the taxpayer incident and the religious discussion, suggest that Americans look at cosmetic surgery much as children regard being punished: they are sorry only that they got caught. But if, in the years following World War II, Americans appeared to subscribe to an ideal that proclaimed cosmetic surgery value free, in reality their notions and beliefs were more complex. Opinions about cosmetic surgery varied widely, but a significant number of Americans eyed the entire process with distrust, and its participants with pity or scorn. As a liftee noted matter-of-factly in her 1962 diary of a face-lift: "Day 8. Can't get over how painless this has been. It's a good thing too. This being elective surgery, you ask for no sympathy and get none. Glad there's so little to complain about." Almost twenty years later, women continued to feel guilty about having cosmetic surgery. A woman whose eye lift was unsuccessful wrote in 1981: "I had no right to feel sorry for myself, or expect anyone's sympathy. This misery was self-inflicted, all for the vainglory of looking good. You can't even pray. It's pathetic."[63]

The World As We Know It

In 1968 a group of vocal and visible young women gathered outside the Miss America beauty pageant. Jubilantly, they threw girdles, curlers, and other items they identified as "objects of female torture" into a giant Freedom Trash Can, and they crowned a sheep and led it through the streets of Atlantic City. With this very public protest, they heralded feminism's second wave. Like other social movements of the 1960s, feminism identified women's lack of power as a social problem, and feminists, like civil rights workers, labor organizers, and other reformers, proclaimed their faith that change, at the societal level, could be effected. Much can and has been said and written of the successes and failures of the 1960s. But whatever one thinks of the decade, it is clear that there existed then an optimism about the nation's ability to alter itself that has since dissipated.

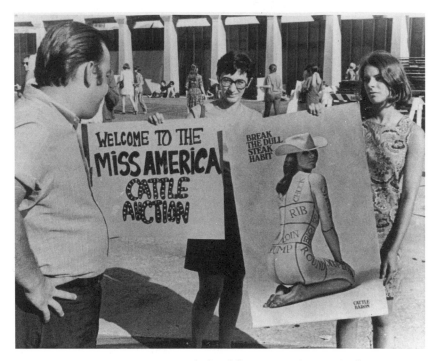

In 1968, young women declared, "No More Miss America."

Bumper stickers that read "Don't vote, it only encourages them" testify to voters' lack of faith in their government as an agent of social change. Shaken when U-2 pilot Francis Gary Powers was shot down over the USSR, this faith was fractured—perhaps irreparably—by Watergate. Today, when private, personal dramas like the trial of Orenthal James Simpson rate more media attention than constitutional scandals like Iran Contra, it is hard to remember that this faith once existed. But slogans like this are also indicative of a deeper malaise. The disaffection and alienation that once was (and is still) directed toward the federal government now extends to "society" itself, which—like the blob of science fiction fame or the enormous breast in Woody Allen's *Everything You Always Wanted to Know about Sex*—is presented as a discrete, independent entity that lurches across the landscape of its own mysterious volition. Those who once proclaimed their faith that American society could be shaped by its citizens now see their options in much more limited terms: duck and cover, or move to a walled and gated community.

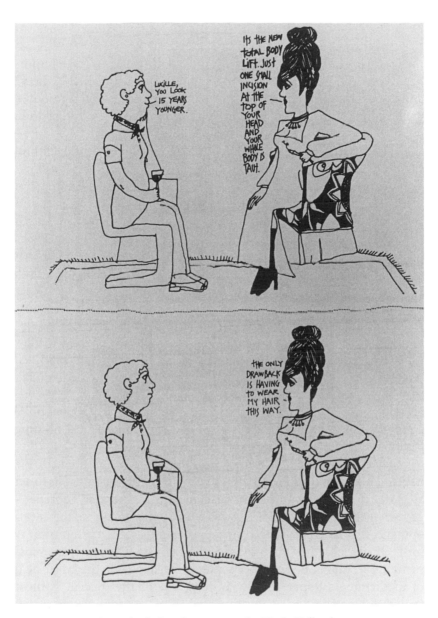

A novel solution, from cartoonist Nicole Hollander.

The rhetoric surrounding aging and cosmetic surgery suggests that this abdication of responsibility extends to this arena as well. Cosmetic surgery has remained a growth industry because, in greater numbers, American women gave up on shaping that entity called "society" and instead turned to the scalpel as the most sensible, effective response to the physical manifestations of age and because men, rather than question this course of action, blindly followed their lead.[64]

A few surgeons have attempted to address the social and cultural context in which surgery occurs, but consistent with their training as physicians, surgeons overwhelmingly limit their discussions to the arena of medicine, within which the "loose, sagging skin, jowls, creases, and wrinkles," the "wrinkles, pouches, bags, sags, and wattles" that are caused by the "inexorable process of aging" are defined simply as medical problems. As surgeons Richard Aronsohn and Richard Epstein put it, skin that is at first "pink, plump, smooth, soft, and translucent" takes on a "dull, yellowish, wrinkled, atonic, coriaceous stiffness" as its wearer ages. After three pages of such description, the authors concede, "even the words are ugly." Surgeons routinely use words like "deformity" and "pathology" to describe such conditions, further encouraging their patients to view aging as a medical problem. Informed by such convictions, surgeons often refer to the face-lift as something that is needed rather than desired, that may be delayed but not escaped. As New York surgeon Paula A. Moynihan put it in 1989, "If you start taking care of yourself when you're young, you may one day need cosmetic surgery, but instead of needing it at 40, it may be 50; or instead of 50, it may be 60."[65]

Given the specialty's history and the fierce competition in the field today, it is, of course, unreasonable to expect plastic surgeons to act as gatekeepers. As long as demand continues to increase, more surgeons will lift more faces. It is, however, instructive to look at the developments that have encouraged surgeons to abdicate the responsibility for their specialty they once guarded so jealously. The practice of cosmetic surgery has, of course, been altered by changes in the larger field of medicine. As Robert Goldwyn, long one of the specialty's most thoughtful members, has noted, hospital administrators, who in earlier years considered their staff plastic surgeons embarrassments, now push surgeons toward the lucrative field of cosmetic surgery: "Administrators now realize that more patients exist with sagging faces than with brain tumors. Catering in aesthetic surgery has several advantages: patients are healthy, turnover is quick, and payments are prompt and total." Malpractice insurance costs, which for plastic surgeons in 1988 ranged from $58,000 per year in Massachusetts to $100,000 per year in Miami, Florida, have contributed to this trend. "Under these conditions," Goldwyn notes, "most plastic surgeons, unless they have inherited wealth or married it, can keep financially afloat only through aesthetic surgery, even to the point of possibly having to advertise for patients."[66]

Competition for patients at the level of clinical practice has also had a significant effect on the way plastic surgeons regard their work. In the 1950s and 1960s, a few plastic surgeons tried to maintain some control over cosmetic surgery, but even then most gave up quickly. In 1981, Peter Fodor, a plastic surgeon at St. Luke's Hospital in New York, described to a *Harper's Bazaar* writer a situation that hearkened back to the days before the specialty's organization: "No other medical specialty includes so few doctors who are properly trained as in cosmetic surgery. Of the 40,000 who practice, only 2,000 are certified by the American Board of Plastic and Reconstructive Surgery."[67]

The proliferation of surgical options has promoted the "if I don't, someone else will" attitude. The "mini-lift," which enjoyed a brief renaissance in the 1960s, has been largely abandoned, but other techniques, such as the forehead lift, the eyebrow lift, and the eye lift, enjoy increasing popularity among those who quail at the thought of a full face-lift. The technique of chemical face peeling, popular among lay practitioners from the 1920s on, and adopted by surgeons and dermatologists in the 1960s, also continues to grow in popularity, as does the use of techniques such as collagen injection.[68]

The secrecy in which Americans generally shroud their surgery may be a holdover from an age in which people did not discuss their physical attributes, but it also offers a compelling reminder of the double burden the pursuit of beauty has historically placed on women and is now extending to men. We may someday become, in the words of historian Sarah Stage, "so fixated on the results that we are willing to accept, in face as well as in fur, the frankly fake." Yet for the most part women have been urged, and have urged each other, to maintain the illusion that a smooth, youthful appearance entails no effort. And just as they compliment women who manage to maintain this illusion, commentators ridicule those whose attempts are unsuccessful or too obvious. As surgeon Murray Berger put it in 1951, "The faded beauty who remains a coquette, who has herself painted, enameled and massaged, who resorts to electric treatment, rays and tissue-builders, and has her face half-baked, is a pathetic figure," as is her male counterpart, whether "aging lothario" or "gay bird."[69]

As long as grace and beauty are defined as external rather than internal qualities, the ideal to which Americans cleave—graceful, beautiful, aging—will be attainable only through cosmetic surgery. The husband of Olga Kahler, author of the 1948 "I'm Glad" article, evoked this "Stepford wife" situation when he wrote of her face-lift: "Without any loss of her priceless wisdom, my wife got back the same lovely face I took with me on my honeymoon!" *Vogue*, in 1961, described a similarly futuristic scenario. The growing popularity of face-lifts, the magazine suggested, "could, just possibly will, produce a distinctly new kind of charmer— the woman who borders on the ideal image—with all the raw edges of youth rubbed off, with a nice load of acquired wisdom and a face that's an extremely pleasant place for the eye to rest. She could be quite a combo." The end result of all this, as columnist Ellen Goodman notes, is the face Elizabeth Taylor presented to the world in the early 1990s, which reminds us that "it takes more confidence, more power, more nerve for a woman of a certain age to look that age, than to carry a condom in public." But before we, too, abdicate, let us speculate on the following scenario: if every magazine that denounces ageism made a point of using models with graying hair and crow's feet; if every personnel manager who complains of the prejudice against older men hired one; if every middle-aged man who ran a personals ad requested a woman his own age, rather than one a minimum of five years younger; if every woman took her cosmetic budget for the year and sent it to Emily's List, that alien entity called "society" might start to look more malleable.[70]

CHAPTER FIVE

The Michael Jackson Factor

RACE, ETHNICITY, AND COSMETIC SURGERY

Nowhere is the never-never land offered by plastic surgery more evident than in the face of musician Michael Jackson. Finely sculpted, with pale, almost transparent skin stretched over high cheekbones, tiny, chiseled, pointy nose, deeply cleft chin, and eyes always heavily lined, the face he unveiled in the late 1980s transcended all previously known categories of race and ethnicity (and, to some eyes, gender). As *Rolling Stone* writers Michael Goldberg and David Handelman described Jackson's "ever-evolving" features in 1987, his "pale, made-up face with its newly clefted chin looks anything but street; it barely seems of this world."[1]

Much of the favorable publicity that cosmetic surgery has received over the years has attempted to place it squarely within the American tradition of self-improvement, which sociologist Frances Cooke Macgregor has called the "American cultural tendency to change rather than to cope, to alter rather than to endure." Entertainers have been particularly enthusiastic about altering features that they believed would limit their careers or their chances for happiness. Jackson's reluctance to discuss his surgical transformation has only encouraged speculation about what motivated him to undertake it, but seen in this light, his surgeries—like those of Fanny Brice, Milton Berle, and a host of others—seem a practical response to the limelight's strict requirements.[2]

As even this brief list suggests, Jackson is only one among hundreds of thousands of Americans who have attempted, through plastic surgery, to minimize or eradicate physical signs of race or ethnicity that they believe mark them as "other" (which in this context has always meant "other" than white). These differentiating (and often contradictory) categories emerged from contemporaneous, and not unrelated, historical processes— for example, the impetus toward immigration restriction coincided with whites' increasing discomfort about a growing black presence in northern cities—and they shared the goal of defining "difference." From this perspective, Jackson's surgical choices are predictable. Race- and eth-nicity-based surgery has always focused on the most identifiable, and most caricatured, features: for Jews, noses; for Asians, eyes; for African Ameri-cans, noses and lips. Most of the operations with which this chapter is concerned, at least before mid-century, were performed on white Ameri-cans and European immigrants. Jews, Italians, and others of Mediter-ranean or eastern European heritage made the "nose job" a household word early in the century. Asians, in the years after World War II, began to pursue larger noses and folded eyelids. Their numbers are still small, but African Americans, too, have begun to alter their features through surgery in greater numbers than before. Unlike early-twentieth-century surgical pioneers, who were generally satisfied with altering one feature, Jackson has altered everything, but this may be simply a matter of tim-ing: since the end of World War II, surgeons have expanded their reper-toires to fulfill a wider range of requests, making transformations like Jackson's possible.

The extent, and expense, of Jackson's numerous surgeries probably account for at least some of the uneasiness and horror his efforts have generated. Advanced techniques, an adventurous surgeon, and lots of money have produced truly extraordinary results: Jackson looks less like his presurgery self and more like Elizabeth Taylor than either patients or surgeons in previous generations would have believed possible. As pediatrician Benjamin Spock put it in 1984, "He seems partly child, partly adult, partly masculine, partly feminine; he seems to be a person for all ages and all sexes. I don't see that he is doing any harm, but I'm not sure he's doing any good either." Jackson's status as one of the wealthiest entertainers in the world is common knowledge, and Ameri-cans have become accustomed to the phenomenon of celebrity surgery, but in this age of declining access to medical care, Jackson's repeated trans-formations seem like the most conspicuous kind of consumption.[3]

Fundamentally, however, what bothers Americans about Michael Jackson's face is the race issue. The results of his surgery suggest that if he is not trying to look white, he is at least trying to look less black, and a review of the coverage his surgery has received in the popular press suggests that the majority of Americans believe that Jackson's surgery is, at least in part, about race. The lighter color of Jackson's skin may well be due to a skin condition, as he explained to Oprah Winfrey in his 1993 television interview, but this, to most commentators, does not explain what has happened to his lips, nose, and chin. Jackson's haunting face signals not only that all is not well in never-never land; it suggests that something larger has gone awry in twentieth-century North America. Despite the longevity of the tradition described above, Americans of many colors apparently are not entirely comfortable with what is being changed, and why, and what is lost in the process.[4]

One of the most important questions raised by Michael Jackson's transformation concerns the role the medical profession has played in shaping standards of appearance. The frequency with which early-twentieth-century surgeons performed the classic nose job simply confirmed what most Americans already knew: a nose that called attention to itself and marked its bearer as "different" or "foreign" was a distinct disadvantage. Yet in their readiness to label certain nose shapes and types as deformities, surgeons helped to cement not just standards of beauty but standards of normality and acceptability in American minds. How plastic surgeons assumed the role of arbitrating between the issues of ethnicity, aesthetics, and "normal" or "standard" looks has remained unexamined. It seems clear, however, that as surgeons agreed with increasing numbers of prospective patients that, in fact, certain facial configurations were, if not unacceptable, at least undesirable, cultural standards of the range of acceptable deviation narrowed.[5]

Jackson's surgery also raises the larger issue of the role Americans have played in shaping these standards. Throughout the twentieth century, Americans have generally professed belief in the truism that norms of beauty are culturally determined; like fashions in clothes, fashions in faces change over time. On another level, however, Americans perceive at least some of these standards as basically unchanging and unchangeable: certain faces never come into fashion. From the early twentieth century on, the reigning cultural norms of beauty have been understood to demand an absence of what surgeons call racial or ethnic stigmata, and cosmetic surgery has consistently focused on altering features that differentiate patients from a norm that is always implicitly, and often explicitly, understood to be not just Caucasian but Anglo-Saxon or northern European.[6]

A brief review of American immigration and of the "science of race" that it inspired provides essential context for this discussion. Until about 1890, most immigrants to the United States hailed from northern and western Europe. Eighty percent of the fifteen million who arrived between 1890 and 1920, in contrast, were from eastern and southern European countries, including Russia, Poland, and Italy. Unlike the "first wave" of immigrants, many of whom took advantage of the federal government's commitment to facilitating white settlement of the plains and prairies by moving west, these new immigrants concentrated in the cities of the eastern seaboard. The widespread overcrowding, poverty, and poor living conditions among the new industrial working class combined to redefine immigration as a problem in the minds of native-born white citizens. In reality, the proportion of Americans who were born abroad increased only slightly during these years, but the prospect of submersion was no less threatening for being largely imaginary.[7]

The anxious atmosphere created by the new immigration inspired concern among individual nativist politicians and groups, including organized labor. Together, their efforts led, eventually, to the immigration restriction acts of the 1920s, which set quotas based on a nostalgic vision of how the country ought to look (after excluding first Chinese and then Japanese immigrants, legislators set strict quotas that privileged northern and western Europeans over those from the "less desirable" countries that had spawned the second wave). Such efforts also provided fertile ground for new scientific ideas about heredity, ethnicity, and race. In the late eighteenth century, comparative anatomist Johann Friedrich Blumenbach developed a widely accepted scheme for racial classification that depicted the European stock as the original racial type from which all others had degenerated. Swiss physiognomist Johann Lavater's theories similarly found their way across the Atlantic, and for a time the science of physiognomy—whose practitioners believed they could identify and classify facial and other features and from them divine personality traits—enjoyed wide publicity and popularity in the United States. In general, physiognomists believed that "small features indicated virtue and 'great delicacy of sentiment,' while large features indicated sensuality and slothfulness." Supporters of immigration restriction—such as nativist E. A. Ross, who in 1914 warned of "hirsute, low-browed, big-faced persons of obviously low mentality"—were clearly familiar with such theories.[8]

It is too simplistic to say that those who sponsored Jim Crow laws across the American South were likewise informed by ideas such as these, but it is true nonetheless. The Civil Rights movement of the 1950s and 1960s inspired an entire generation of scholars to explore and explain the historical construction of "blackness" and the mechanisms by which such constructions came to uphold a formidable legal structure that sheltered legalized racism in the southern United States and in the nation's growing empire and ignored the less-formalized racism that held sway elsewhere. A new generation of historians has turned this project on its head: in addition to demonstrating that what was constructed during these years was not just "other" than white but whiteness itself, these new studies of the construction of race remind us that, while their various incarnations may be place- and time-specific, the racial ideologies that permeated American culture in this period provided an all-encompassing framework through which Americans viewed the world and themselves.[9]

During the late nineteenth century, scientific schemes for racial classification and more vague (though no less powerful) ideas about racial definitions and boundaries met with great attention. They combined with Darwinian science, the rediscovery of Gregor Mendel's work on heredity, and fears of race suicide sparked by a declining birth rate among the white middle class of western Europe and the United States to produce yet another new and popular science. Eugenics was, essentially, the "science" of human improvement in which principles of plant and animal breeding were applied to humans. It taught that hereditary traits were dominant and could not be altered by environmental factors; breeding for the preservation of positive traits as well as for the elimination of negative ones was the only solution. On the American side of the Atlantic, not surprisingly, eugenicists were most often "old stock" Americans who were confused and dismayed by the changes they observed in their world. Geneticist Charles B. Davenport, whose New England Puritan father could trace his ancestry back to 1086, for example, was known to mourn publicly that "the best of that grand old New England stock is dying out through failure to reproduce." But the eugenics movement drew interest and support from a wide range of Americans, from social reformers concerned about the new industrial working class to politicians seeking to defend segregation. According to one tabulation, between 1910 and 1914, general-interest magazines carried more articles on eugenics than on the topics of slums, tenements, and living conditions combined.[10]

Eugenics provided a transition to more specific ideas about race that were taken up, in the early twentieth century, by men like William Z. Ripley, a Harvard economist, and Madison Grant. In the encyclopedic *The Races of Europe*, first published in 1899, Ripley went further than Blumenbach in applying the principles of scientific classification to humans; his system, for the first time, differentiated among white Europeans along "racial lines" (northern, Teutonic "tall, blond longheads," central, Alpine "stocky roundheads," and southern, Mediterranean "slender, dark longheads"). Ripley combined this racial typology with Mendelian theories and proposed, according to historian John Higham, "a thoroughly biological explanation of the foreign peril"—the suggestion that the racial intermixture in America represented an irreversible "reversion to a primitive type." In doing so, he set the stage for Madison Grant, whose alarmist jeremiad about racial purity (*The Passing of the Great Race*, first published in 1916) tapped broader currents of popular nativism and raised nativist thinking in the United States to an entirely different level. America, once populated solely by Nordics (in Grant's words, "the white man par excellence"), was being destroyed by Alpine, Mediterranean, and particularly Jewish immigrants, he warned darkly. Popular acceptance of the insidious parable of the American Melting Pot, Grant wrote, was facilitating this decline: contrary to popular belief, race mixing did not result in a blend; rather, it "gives us a race reverting to the more ancient, generalized and lower type." Thus, the Nordic stock could be destroyed by mixing with lower European races and particularly by mixing with Jews. In one of his most widely quoted phrases, Grant asserted grimly that "the cross between any of the three European races and a Jew is a Jew." Grant was not the first to employ science toward racist ends, but his work pioneered in offering a "systematic, comprehensive world view" based entirely on race.[11]

Historian Lois Banner notes that, despite the rampant nativism and prejudice in this period, American ideals of beauty remained surprisingly democratic. Commentators commonly heralded the ideal American female as "an amalgam of ethnic types . . . proof that the American melting pot could work." The original model for the Gibson girl was rumored to be Irish, or perhaps half-French and half-Cuban. In contrast to reversion theories, as far as beauty was concerned, the process of ethnic mixing was understood to produce a higher type than any of the individual ingredients: "truly unique, democratic, and American."[12]

But American ideas about beauty were not entirely unaffected by racist ideologies. Experimental psychologist Knight Dunlap is perhaps best remembered for placing the psychology department at the Johns Hopkins University (and later the departments of psychology, anthropology, and sociology at the University of California at Los Angeles) on firm ground, but early in his career, as did many respectable scientists, he toyed with eugenics. In 1920 he brought his combined scientific knowledge to bear on the topic of beauty; the resulting work, *Personal Beauty and Racial Betterment,* offers a compelling illustration of the way ideas about race and beauty might, and did, intersect. Dunlap identified beauty as a "positive condition" that could be said to be present only if "negative conditions" were absent. The first of these negative conditions— identifiable signs of race—was particularly visible in "negroid characters." "Here, where the suggestion or indication is of an inferior race," Dunlap asserted, "the negative condition is especially important." The second negative condition was signs of disease, deformity, or weakness. The third negative condition—significant deviation from the average—seems to imply relativity, but here, too, race was paramount. "The type which is highest in value tends to approximate the European type, wherever the European type becomes known," Dunlap explained. "All dark races prefer white skin," and both men and women tend to choose superior partners (meaning, in Dunlap's terms, a partner with skin lighter than one's own). Dunlap was unusually explicit, but his assumption that "white" features constituted the standard against which all were judged was not uncommon.[13]

For those whose features fell short of this standard, cosmetic surgery offered hope. In general, prospective patients viewed surgery as an option according to the amount of prejudice they encountered, the identifiability as ethnic of particular features, the availability of surgical techniques to eradicate the offending features, and money. In the early decades of the twentieth century, Jews and Italians most often met these criteria. They were (or were thought to be) identifiable to American eyes; they encountered prejudice; the feature that most troubled them was the nose, against which surgical techniques had already proved effective; and they were upwardly mobile. Not all who met these criteria, of course, sought cosmetic surgery: those who spent most of their time in ethnic enclaves probably did not realize the extent to which they were perceived as different; some simply tried harder to surpass the barriers they faced, confident that their success would help to destroy existing stereotypes; still others relied on white Americans' legendary inability to identify ethnicity to claim membership in a less-stigmatized group (according to one account, Italian immigrants seeking clerical jobs often claimed to be French, Spanish, or Turkish). Many new immigrants and members of less-favored ethnic groups, however, came to see cosmetic surgery as the most effective solution to the problems created by features that identified them as something "other" than the Anglo-Saxon American standard.[14]

The human costs of this long and often sordid history are visible in Michael Jackson's face. Jackson's injured air and defensive demeanor may arise from his conviction that he has altered everything about his face that might conceivably give offense: Why, then, don't we like him? The answer to this question, of course, has as much to do with Jackson himself as with his face. But the fact that the image of America his face reflects is so unflattering accounts for much of our discomfort.[15]

From Fanny Brice to Barbra Streisand

Throughout her life, comedienne and actress Fanny Brice insisted that looking Jewish had played no part in her decision to alter her nose, which she did (to great fanfare) in 1923. She had, she claimed, always been proud of being Jewish, and as she had met with "very little" anti-Semitism, she had no reason to want to look less Jewish. Late in life she recalled, "Nothing ever made me angrier than the gossip that I had my nose operated on so I'd look less Jewish. I wanted to look prettier and my nose was a sight in any language, but I wasn't trying to hide my origin." The explanation Brice offered most often was that she had done it to make herself eligible for a wider variety of roles; she had especially hoped to play Nora in Ibsen's *A Doll's House*.[16]

Despite Brice's denial, most of her contemporaries believed that the desire to look less identifiably Jewish played a role in her decision, and biographer Barbara Grossman concurs: "She must have hoped that the operation would make her look less Jewish. . . . Ethnicity was definitely not fashionable in the 1920s." On a personal level, Brice may in fact have been comfortable with her looks. She publicly proclaimed her pride in her religion and her heritage and indeed built her career on playing

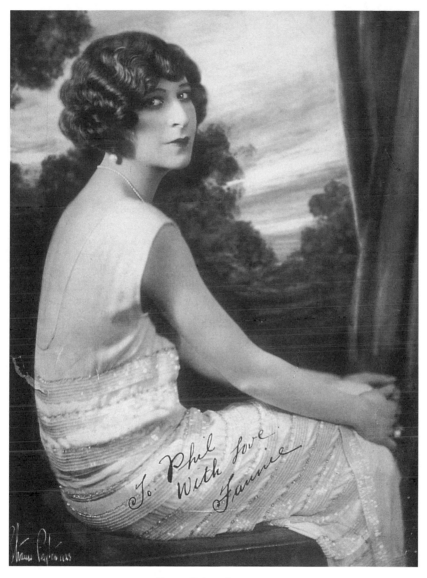

Fanny Brice, circa 1930.

Jewish characters to Jewish audiences. On a professional level, however, Brice evidently realized that a successful career depended on beauty, and that beauty meant the absence of the clear signs of race or ethnicity that could be damaging, if not fatal, to an entertainment career.[17]

The first group of Americans to undertake surgical alteration of ethnic features in any numbers were, like Brice, Jews who did not like their noses. Inspired by the work of New York's John Orlando Roe and Berlin's Jacques Joseph, American surgeons had begun to experiment with nasal plastic surgery in the late nineteenth century. While most early reports of nasal operations employed general terms like "overlarge," "humped," or "too-prominent" when describing the kinds of noses that were desirable of improvement, Dr. John B. Roberts's 1892 reference to "the Roman nose, the Jewish nose, and the nose with an angular prominence on its dorsum" suggests that, even before the turn of the century, the "Jewish nose" required no further description. Certainly by the 1920s most Americans were aware that noses that fit these categories most often hailed originally from southern or eastern Europe and that many of their bearers were Jewish. Thus, when Brice's nose job became public, Americans were already familiar, in general terms, with the "sciences" of race and ethnicity, as well as with the negative connotations that attached specifically to the "Jewish nose."[18]

Some Americans fought against the growing surgical trend. In her popular 1927 advice book, Girl Scout advisor Hazel Rawson Cades endorsed the camouflage that clever hat and hair arrangements might provide, but warned young women, "noses may not be cut off, either to satisfy or spite one's type." Surgeons, however, had already recognized that Jews and other ethnic Americans represented a large potential market for nasal plastic surgery and were making a move to claim it. In 1930 William Wesley Carter noted that the "modification of accentuated family or racial characteristics, such as are sometimes observable especially in semitic subjects, is not only a legitimate procedure, but it is frequently of great importance to the individual. . . . In the moving picture field . . . the possession of a shapely nose is frequently the deciding factor." While he had originally opposed such surgery, by 1936 Vilray Blair had come to believe that a Jewish nose was as deserving of correction as any other type of nasal deformity. "Change in the shape of the pronounced Jewish nose may be sought for either social or business reasons," he noted.[19]

Surgeons and Americans who by the 1930s had defined the Semitic or Mediterranean nose as undesirable had probably become acquainted with the scientific theories that had influenced American ideas about beauty in the previous decades, as well as with the new disciplines of psychology and psychiatry. As we have seen, in the years between the two world wars, the conviction that plastic surgery could be of particular benefit in helping to heal an inferiority complex was widely held. Family members, potential employers, and the general public who revealed their distaste for a physical feature might, surgeons believed, engender an inferiority complex. From this understanding, it was natural that they should begin to believe that a feature commonly defined as ugly—for example, a Jewish nose—might be just as likely to cause an inferiority complex as a congenital abnormality or a traumatically induced defect.

World War II gave new impetus to the link surgeons had forged between outer appearance and inner peace or lack of it. The war was crucial to the growth of the psychiatric profession: for the first time, the U.S. Army officially recognized psychiatry as an important branch of military medicine, and the military endorsement meant that psychiatry and psychology continued to receive wide coverage in the popular press. At the same time, the extent of American anti-Semitism was revealed in sharp relief. Laura Delano's response to the Wagner-Rogers bill, which would have relaxed quotas to allow the entrance of twenty thousand German refugee children—that "20,000 charming children would all too soon grow into 20,000 ugly adults"—was in many ways typical of American opinion in 1939. Even watching the 933 refugee passengers on the *St. Louis* head back to Europe in despair after being refused entrance did not significantly alter the widely shared conviction that Jews were the least desirable addition to the melting pot. After the war, as mental health practitioners joined surgeons in exploring the psychological indications for and implications of cosmetic surgery, a spate of articles that tied the inferiority complex to ethnicity appeared in a variety of medical journals. For prospective patients who carried the facial "stigmata" that identified them as members of minority groups and had inferiority complexes because of this, surgeons asserted, surgery was a positive step. By altering the feature or aspect of a feature that gave offense, surgery could eliminate the reaction it inspired in others and the inferiority complex this interaction had caused. A nose job, in other words, could mitigate the damaging psychological effects of prejudice.[20]

The image of hundreds of ethnic Americans undergoing cosmetic surgery to mask their ethnicity recalls the stereotype of people of mixed race "passing" as white, which has been well established in literature and film. Plastic surgeons and their patients, however, often explicitly disavowed any connection with this tradition. Surgeons justified their work in medical terms: as responsible and responsive practitioners, they insisted, they were trying to fulfill their patients' requests for a more attractive appearance, as well as a healthier mental outlook. In general, patients too claimed to have limited goals. They had no desire to deny their religion or their ethnic heritage, they asserted; they merely hoped to blend in better, to become indistinguishable and thus to reap the benefits that were generally available to those not perceived as different.

This oft-expressed desire for ethnic anonymity suggests the extent to which the stereotypes evoked by the nineteenth-century "sciences" of race—which, by the 1930s, had been largely discredited—continued to permeate popular culture and consciousness. This desire was sparked by the knowledge that in the United States the face, or particular features, often led others to attribute to the bearer particular personality or character traits. Facial features that might lead to the attribution of criminality, drug addiction, or disease were and continue to be of concern. A high forehead was often taken as a sign of superior intelligence, while a low forehead or receding chin (immortalized in the popular cartoon figure Andy Gump) was taken to indicate poor intelligence, weak character, and, in men, lack of strength, masculinity, and resolve. Racial and ethnic stereotypes, too, were widely recognized. In her path-breaking studies of plastic surgery patients, sociologist Frances Cooke Macgregor found that the so-called Jewish nose—"characterized by considerable length and height, convexity of profile, a depressed tip with a downward sloping septum, and thick, flared alae or wings"—was of primary concern to Italians, Armenians, Greeks, Iranians, and Lebanese (who feared being mistaken as Jewish) as well as to Jews. Individuals in all of these groups, she wrote, wanted to alter the noses that they believed offered "visible clues to an ethnic or religious group that they perceived as having unfavorable or stigmatic connotations." "In a milieu where racial or religious prejudice prevails," Macgregor commented, "a large convex nose, the Jewish stereotype, may automatically assign to its possessor all the physical, mental, emotional, and moral characteristics with which that group is supposedly endowed."[21]

The process of Americanization through surgery is difficult to decipher because no statistics were kept. Generally, patients did not discuss their motivations publicly; when they did, as in the pages of women's magazines, they seldom discussed issues of race and ethnicity openly. Several studies that were completed in New York using data collected between 1946 and 1954 provide clues. One of these found that of seventeen potential patients, fourteen were children of immigrant parents and most of these were from Mediterranean or eastern European countries: six were eastern European Jews, five were Italian, one was Armenian, and one Greek; only one was Irish. Individual surgeons often published their own conclusions, drawn from anecdotal evidence collected in their practices. A unique window onto this world is offered by the patient records kept by New York plastic surgeon Jerome Pierce Webster. Covering primarily the years from 1930 to 1950, these records allow us access to the motivations and desires of patients who came in requesting surgery during these years.[22]

Of almost 400 patients who came to see Jerome Webster about their noses in these years, almost three-quarters were female. Most of the women (204) were single; 73 were married, 12 widowed, 7 divorced or separated; the marital status of the rest was not given. Of the men, 56 were single, 33 married, 2 divorced or separated. The greatest number of patients (128 women, 32 men) came between the ages of fifteen and twenty-four, although many came later (82 women and 14 men from twenty-five to thirty-four; 37 women and 18 men from thirty-five to forty-four). Given the fact that a nose job is a cosmetic operation—by definition, elective and expensive—the socioeconomic status of these patients is surprisingly broad. For both men and women, student was the occupation most commonly given (54 women, 23 men). Many in this group were already self-supporting (in general, those in college or postgraduate programs such as law school); for minors, parental occupation (not recorded consistently) generally identified the family as middle class (a few, clearly, were wealthy; more often, the family was poor). The two next largest occupational categories for women were clerical (45, ranging from bookkeeper to receptionist to telephone operator) and "at home" (38, mostly housewives). Performing arts came next (23), then beauty and fashion (19). The men, in general, described themselves as white collar (15) or professional (12). A surprising number of men and women named occupations that were clearly either blue collar or working class in nature and in income: Webster's patients included florists, laundry managers, farmers, produce and dairy workers, piano teachers, firemen and policemen, laboratory technicians, electricians, and factory workers as well as aspiring movie stars.[23]

The nature of their complaints varied considerably: disease, trauma, sinus problems, and infections brought some patients in. By far the largest number, however—251 of 376, or two-thirds—were motivated solely by cosmetic concerns. Of these, 17 specifically cited career reasons; an additional 26 cited cosmetic concerns as one of two or more factors.

Only a few prospective patients specifically cited ethnic concerns. But the terms they used to describe their noses suggest that many of these patients were aware of racial and ethnic stereotypes and reveal the extent to which "normative" standards had permeated their consciousness. Thus, while only 14 described their noses as "Jewish" (and only 1 said "Italian"), the terms prospective patients used to justify seeking cosmetic correction clearly describe noses that were stereotypically un-American. In descending order: 84 described their noses simply as "bad"; 58 used the word "deformed"; 23 complained of a bump, hump, or lump; 12 thought their noses "large"; the same number complained that the nose tip was unattractive; 7 said "long"; 4 said long with a hump; 2 said "crooked"; 1 used the term "broad"; another, long and thick. Those with what they considered abnormally small noses used similarly coded terms: only one said "negroid," but seven more said "saddle-nose"; two said "flat"; one, "broad."

Anecdotal evidence from these patient records allows us to take a closer look at the complex ways in which ethnic and racial stereotypes, self-image, and aesthetic standards intertwined with the perceived demands of consumer culture. First, let us consider those patients whose primary stated concern was to advance their careers. Their stories are predictable, their words generally innocuous. In 1939 Alicia Martin was promised a screen test, contingent on a nose job. Stage actress Audrey Banks came in two years later because she wanted to make the jump to screen; she had passed the screen test, but her nose needed "touching up." In 1943 one of singer Alice Hansen's agents suggested that an improved nose might enable her to cross over to film. In 1957 secretary Christina Skouras and model Janet Cameron saw new profiles as stepping stones: Skouras had been invited to Hollywood but cautioned to change her nose before going west; Cameron had enjoyed some success making commercials but "T.V. experts said she is held back by [her] nose, especially profile."[24]

As these cases suggest, many Americans believed that occupational mobility and opportunity were contingent on a particular facial configuration. Unemployed or underemployed at the time they sought Webster's help, they believed that surgery would enable them to move up within their chosen field or make the jump to a more lucrative and more interesting occupation. Clearly, all of them aspired to careers that would place them (if in some cases peripherally) in the "public eye." But as the next group of cases demonstrates, many other Americans subscribed to these same standards.

Robin Shapiro, Hope Steinberg, Cindy Ross, Rachel Frank, and Marcy Goldberg—all young, single, and Jewish—came to see Webster between 1933 and 1953. Over a two-decade span, their concerns were remarkably similar. Shapiro had inherited her father's nose; it had not bothered her until friends started referring to her "beak" and asking why she didn't have something done. Steinberg—whose mother, Webster noted, had a "racial" nose—was "absolutely determined" to have hers altered. Ross was "extremely self-conscious" about her "Jewish nose" and was particularly distressed by the "bulbous tip." Frank, too, had been unlucky: her sister had inherited their father's straight nose, but she had inherited the nose her mother had altered years ago. Goldberg, Webster observed, came by her large nose "honestly" as "father has large nose and mother's is definitely racial."

Americans of other ethnicities shared these young women's perception that less noticeable noses were desirable. Ida Davis, born in Lithuania and employed as a maid when she saw Webster in 1941, complained of the "prominent tip" of her nose. Reza Hakim, an Iraqi immigrant, had begun to feel while living in Chicago "that the normal hump of the near East people's nose was not satisfactory." Susan Harjanian's schoolmates teased her about the large nose she had inherited from her Armenian parents, while Michael Baglione and Rita Cacciotti were both dissatisfied with large Italian noses.

Many of these patients cited the explicit or implicit goal of ethnic anonymity. They did not want to become something other than what they were: none cited a desire to pass, none changed their names, none planned to move away. But they did not want others to be able to identify them on sight as something other than generic American. They wanted to be seen as individuals rather than as members of a group and to be able to control what they revealed about themselves to others. The fact that so many prospective patients from a wide range of ethnic backgrounds cited the issue of "difference" suggests that this concept clearly had as its reference point a standard of appearance that derived from a particular definition of "whiteness"—not just Caucasian, but Anglo-Saxon. Americans, as Italians and others told sociologist Frances Cooke Macgregor, were quick to categorize people they met, and they often

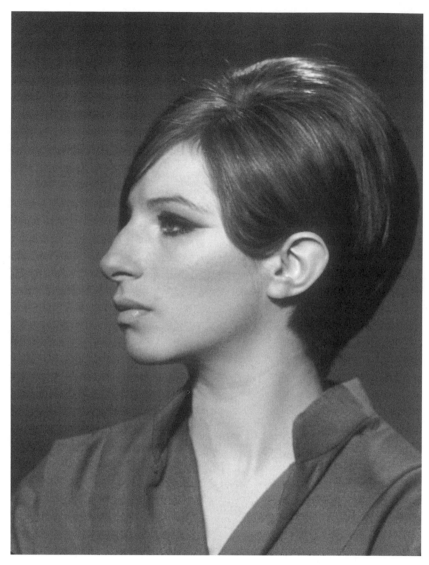

Barbra Streisand, 1971.

mistook Italians for Jews, or Greeks for Italians, but rarely, if ever, did they mistake "ethnics" for WASPs.[25]

Potential plastic surgery patients often claimed to hold no prejudices themselves: rather, they asserted, they were simply responding to twentieth-century American social conditions. Rita Cacciotti, for example, told Webster that while she had always disliked her nose, reading magazine articles had increased her dissatisfaction. On this point, however, no words are more revealing than those of non-Jews who feared and resented being mistaken for Jews.

Eleven prospective patients—seven women, four men—came to see Webster with this specific complaint between 1929 and 1957; the following stories are representative. Gretchen Algren, a thirty-five-year-old housewife, was married to an army officer stationed at Fort Leavenworth, Kansas. She had always been teased about her large nose, she explained, and had learned not to mind; recently, however, several people had revealed in chance remarks that they had [mistakenly] assumed she was Jewish, and she feared that she was holding her husband's career back. Webster's notes on Vivian Wolf's 1938 appointment read, "She is frequently mistaken for a person of Jewish heritage, although she is Catholic. At the New Haven Hospital the Jewish interns ask her to make dates." The twenty-six-year-old medical technician had been engaged to an Irish medical student, but he broke it off—in large part, she suspected, because his friends kept asking him why he was marrying a Jewess. Jane Hatch arrived from England in 1941 to find that her nose—which in England was acceptably British—was, in the United States, assumed to be Jewish. She believed an operation would enable her to find a job that would better support her two children.

William Gordon was the most plainspoken of this group. In 1957 he was twenty-four; he had recently moved from New York's West Side because "every Jewish rabbi would talk to him in Yiddish." Gordon had been horrified by being "taken for a Jew," because (Webster recorded) "his great hero is Hitler." Gordon's attitude was extreme among this group, but the sentiment was not unusual. Several complained that they had developed inferiority complexes because of these experiences. In all cases, patients were insulted that others had mistaken them for Jewish and were convinced that a nose job would eliminate the "social handicap" under which they labored.[26]

Like their fellow immigrants who made a point of losing their accents, learning English, and wearing typically American clothes, most of those who sought the more drastic solution of surgery wanted to blend in with people around them; they wanted to look "American." This desire was complicated by the fact that the face of America differed from region to region and had changed considerably due to successive waves of immigration and migration. But many Semitic and Mediterranean patients were not at all confused about what constituted the American face. The nose that looked most American, they believed, was the one that a few generations earlier had been widely caricatured as decidedly foreign. It was Irish.[27]

The story of twenty-eight-year-old "Arthur Steelman," née "Arthur Schulberger," who participated in one of the studies documented by sociologist Frances Cooke Macgregor, is illustrative. Steelman had been conscious of anti-Semitism throughout much of his life. He was particularly sensitive to Jewish stereotypes and resented the extent to which Americans subscribed to them. "They try to put me in a category," he explained, "and Lord help me if I did anything vulgar or loud, or if I cheated. . . . Socially and economically I could be strangulated by this [his nose]." In the army, Steelman's ideal had been "any good-looking Irishman with a turned-up nose," and he had "a burning desire to be accepted" by gentiles. He did not want to "pass," however, but to subvert the stereotype he was sure others held: "If my nose is changed, then I can show [gentiles] by my behavior that there are nice Jews. I'll be a goodwill ambassador. I can prove to people that I'm not only a 'white man' but a 'white Jew.' "[28]

Like many Jews of his generation, Steelman left the operating room with the turned-up nose he had requested. Adjusting to a new self-image was, at least initially, more difficult than he had anticipated: he was badly shaken by his first look in the mirror. "It's like . . . having someone else look back at you," he recalled. "A Jew has tremendous pride. That's why it's so difficult to get other Jews to admit their reasons for wanting a nasal plastic. . . . I wanted a Jew to know I was a Jew. . . . At the same time I didn't want others to know I was a Jew. At first I was horrified when I looked like an Irishman. I was a man without a country. Now I'm beginning to get used to it." Once accustomed, however, Steelman claimed that not looking identifiably Jewish had enabled him to accept—even to enjoy—being Jewish, in his own way. "I think I'd prefer to marry a Jewish girl . . . we'd be the kind of Jews they'd like," he noted. "I can afford to be generous and accept Jews now because I know I don't look like one. Before, I identified myself with them and resisted them." Steelman's family also had to adjust. In front of Steelman, his brother told the interviewer that he had no problem with the surgery. Alone, however, he revealed the complexity of his own feelings about the operation. "Now I'll tell you how I really feel," he confided. "You see, I'm a Jew and I'm not ashamed of it, but it's a shock to have your brother look like an Irishman—not that I have anything against the Irish."[29]

Some were more analytical and thoughtful about their motives than others, but most patients were aware that their desire for surgery had to do with what they perceived as the social realities of the United States. In other words, they were responding to standards of appearance and beauty peculiar to their adopted culture rather than to objective "aesthetic" norms. As surgeon Adolph Abraham Apton put it in his 1951 book on the psychological importance of plastic surgery, "I have operated on many persons of different ethnic groups who doubtless would never have considered surgical correction . . . if they had remained within their native borders. A nurse, of Lithuanian origin, confessed as much. She was anxious to be rid of her broad 'Slavic' nose and to have one in conformity . . . to that of the average American. A similar expression was that of an Armenian whose dominating desire was . . . [for] a nose along what he considered American citizen lines—a nose that would not be 'too different.'" In their belief that a clear norm existed, that deviation from it had costs, and that surgery was the best solution, patients were encouraged by the surgeons who offered correction. "What is considered a shapely nose in one culture might be considered a handicap in another," Oklahoma City surgeon Gilbert L. Hyroop observed in 1965. "There are certain persons who feel their racial characteristics are a hindrance to them, that they set them somewhat apart." In America, Hyroop contended, the outcome was obvious: big noses—even classical Greek or Roman noses, long considered the height of artistic beauty—were simply no longer fashionable.[30]

Again, Jerome Webster's case files offer an illuminating view of how the aesthetic standards and ethnic prejudices to which surgeons and patients subscribed intertwined with the propensity of medical practitioners to view requests as purely medical challenges to create powerful incentives toward homogenization. Audrey Scott came to see Webster in 1941. She was twenty-nine and single; she worked at the Metropolitan Museum of Art. She had been "conscious of her nose all her life," but this consciousness did not keep her from accepting invitations, and (Webster noted with relief) she was not neurotic. She was "occasionally told that she is Jewish, or asked if." Webster then described the complaint in clinical terms. "Nose is fairly long, has a very slight hump, is somewhat broad near the tip and the tip bends down, giving somewhat the appearance of a Jewish nose." In words that reveal his own aesthetic prejudices, he concluded, "I think there is sufficient deformity to warrant changing the nose."

While nose jobs could facilitate adjustment to American society for white ethnics, they might create unanticipated problems for patients, particularly if they had children, surgeons noted. In 1949, Drs. Lewis Linn and Irving B. Goldman described one such case. The woman in question was Jewish but had been raised in a gentile community and had had a nose job at nineteen. She had never told her husband about her nose job (it is unclear from the article whether or not he too was Jewish); now, at thirty-five, she had become obsessed with the fear "that her secret would be exposed in the noses of her [three] children." The doctors expressed their concern that this patient was deeply neurotic, but concluded that, in her case, surgery had been appropriate. "Where antisemitism and xenophobia are widespread," they noted, "specific nasal configurations add to feelings of loneliness and rejection. . . . Alteration of their features in the direction of greater conformity to the social average helps overcome this sense of 'not belonging.' In addition it facilitates identification with certain culturally determined aesthetic norms."[31]

Several studies in the next few years corroborated the hypothesis that the desire to avoid discrimination inspired many cosmetic surgery patients. One group of physicians noted that nine of eleven girls in their study group were Jewish, but none was anti-Semitic. Instead, the girls expressed "the wish not to be looked at in a stereotyped way . . . to be looked at as an individual rather than as a member of a class." A larger study that compared the requests of Jewish women and Italian men for nasal plastic surgery revealed that "wishes not to be stereotyped as alien contribute to desires for physical conformity . . . we suggest that conscious motivation concerns itself with the patient's desire to be viewed as an individual rather than as a member of an alien group." None of the Italian men, the physicians reported, wished to change religions or to deny Italian nativity, but "they did find unacceptable those class attributes of poverty, crudeness, alcoholism and brutality." Another study, completed in 1961, came to similar conclusions. "Nearly all of our patients under 20 years of age were Jewish and many attended the same high school," the study's authors noted. None desired to abandon or disassociate themselves from their religion, but "there seemed to be a wish not to be socially stereotyped as 'alien,' 'strange,' or 'foreign.'" Another surgeon recounted a similar case of a young Jewish girl who wanted her nose changed "not with the idea of obliterating her racial features, but so she could be considered as an individual personality rather than a stereotype."[32]

Doctors focused increasing analytical attention on rhinoplasty operations in the postwar years in part because of the rapid and significant increase in requests for them. Psychiatrist Joost A. M. Meerloo, in 1956, noted that he became interested in plastic surgery when he realized that "an epidemic of plastic surgery is going on among teen-agers wanting to correct prominent 'semitic' (Armenoid) noses." The postwar expansion of the middle class made this increase possible. In the years before the war, patients were often in their mid-twenties to mid-thirties by the time they had saved enough money for surgery. After the war, young people who wanted plastic surgery could have it—courtesy of their parents—before college or even in high school.[33]

Postwar publicity also fueled the increase in requests for plastic surgery. After World War II, advertisements for appliances such as the Anita genuine nose adjuster and M. Trilety's nose shaper, which appeared in *Photoplay* during the 1920s, were supplanted by articles heralding the wonders of nasal plastic surgery, but the significance of the nose as a focal point of beauty remained undisputed. In 1954, journalist Geri Trotta brought this point home to *Harper's Bazaar* readers. Describing the accompanying photograph of a lovely model, the copy read, "By any standard, this is a pretty face. . . . But what if the nose were a horrid shape or an awkward size? How inconsequential the large eyes would seem then, how irrelevant the apricot-gold skin, the nicely curved lips. For, while an imperfection can be a delightful distraction . . . a malproportioned feature is downright ugly; a defect no amount of make-up artistry can ever quite deny. It calls for more than camouflage. It calls for alteration. Frankly, it calls for surgery." *Cosmopolitan* similarly encouraged readers to change noses they did not like. Writer Elizabeth Honor noted in 1956 that the "most dramatic and popular of corrective operations is the nose operation to correct a humped, hooked, or over-long nose." Newspaper supplements spread the news to an even wider audience. "First of all, let's face the fact that there are few naturally pretty noses," began one article published in the mid-1950s. Another reassured its readers that nose surgery was safe and more common than ever: "More than 50% of plastic surgery is performed on the nose."[34]

Like surgeons, authors of popular magazine articles attempted to normalize the nose job; they stressed that patients were not neurotic but simply motivated by the healthy desire to fit in. In 1959 an *American Weekly* article noted, "Where plastic surgery is concerned, doctors are increasingly aware that it is not a desire for beauty, but a healthy minded wish to 'look as good as' everybody else, that this year will swell their waiting lists." In *Family Weekly,* another supplement, author Terry Morris quoted "a leading plastic surgeon," who told readers, "It is not empty vanity that drives them to the decision. . . . The majority of our patients seek the contrary effect. They want to be inconspicuous." Such comments confirmed the normative nature of beauty. A 1960 *Life* magazine photo essay about a young couple and their infant daughter made the point even more plainly. Inspired by her husband's new nose, Mom had hers done as well: "Everything's the same, yet it all seems different. . . . It's like being born all over again," she gushed. Everything was so much better with a small nose that baby, too, would be taken to the surgeon's office when the time came. "I'm not going to let her go through life with the kind of nose I had," the mother vowed.[35]

Popular magazines that carried news about plastic surgery to the public continued to speak of "large" or "humped" noses rather than to identify the ethnicity of such features. The ease with which popular magazines referred to these noses, however, suggests that they simply saw no need to define their terms. Writers and publishers believed that Americans shared a common cultural definition of the limits of the acceptable nose. It was assumed that readers would understand exactly what was meant by "over-large," "oversized," "excessively large," "humped," or "hooked" and that they would be able to judge their own (and others') features accordingly.

This was the world that greeted Barbra Streisand, the woman who would cement her reputation and her career by playing Fanny Brice, just forty years after Brice's celebrated nose job. In the early 1960s, everything about Barbra Streisand seemed to amaze the media. She was young, and she had made the move from Brooklyn to Broadway, which Brice and others of her generation had found so difficult, with ease. She emphasized her status as the first star of the youth generation and of the 1960s by wearing her hair long and straight, dressing in unusual combinations of thrift store clothes, and ignoring the conventions according to which entertainment personalities had traditionally dealt with the press. And, of course, there was her voice.[36]

But, above all, there was her nose. The *New Yorker* described it as "aquiline." *Newsweek,* less kindly, termed it "absurd." The *Saturday Evening Post* called it "the nose of an eagle," but to *Life,* Streisand had a "nose like a witch." Almost all of the many articles about her in these early years (more than twenty ran in national magazines in 1963 and 1964 alone) mention her nose. As if to forestall anticipated questions, many specifically informed readers that Streisand not only had a big nose but planned to keep it. The *Saturday Evening Post,* for example, told its readers that Streisand "has firmly decided against doing anything to her prominent proboscis."[37]

The national preoccupation with Barbra Streisand's nose is easier to understand if one recalls the context. By the middle of the twentieth century, the American ideal of beauty was understood to require a small nose, and the nose job had become a routine operation. After World War II, plastic surgeons spread out across the country, making nose jobs available almost everywhere, and Americans became accustomed to thinking of them as an option for many and a rite of passage for some. Chief among this latter group were girls like Barbra Streisand: as one article described them, "Jewish and Italian teenage girls" from urban centers "who get nose jobs for their high school graduation presents" or for their birthdays. In "rarefied, sophisticated" circles like New York and Los Angeles, a nose job before college was "as routine as the SAT," and for some people "fell almost into the same category as having teeth straightened." In 1961 a major Sunday supplement told hundreds of thousands of Americans that between thirty thousand and sixty thousand rhinoplasties were performed each year; sixteen- to nineteen-year-old girls constituted the largest group of patients.[38]

Streisand's nose was so surprising because it was so different from the nose then in fashion. In the early 1960s, when Streisand entered the scene, the Jackie Kennedy nose—"a small, slightly turned up nose on the short side" reminiscent of the Irish nose that had so enthralled Jewish immigrants decades earlier—reigned supreme. This style was so common that "in some circles . . . an upturned nose had practically become a middle-class status symbol, and hundreds of teenage girls in New York seemed to be wearing the same design. The bone was narrowed, the tip pinched into a triangle, and there were two distinct bumps above the nostrils." To the American people, the most amazing thing about Barbra Streisand was that she had not bobbed her nose.[39]

Some commentators theorized that by her courage Streisand might break the mold not only for herself but for others as well. In 1964, less than a year after it had likened her to a witch, *Life* noted simply that her nose was "big" and forecast, "it may be only a matter of time before plastic surgeons begin getting requests for the Streisand nose (long, Semitic and—most of all—like Everest, There)." James Spada, one of Streisand's many unauthorized biographers, credits her with ending, once and for all, restrictive standards of beauty that emphasized a white, Anglo-Saxon norm: she was a symbol to millions of hopeful girls who "could realistically feel it wasn't necessary to be beautiful to succeed." But as *Newsweek* noted in 1966, Spada and the millions of hopefuls for whom he claimed to speak were due for a disappointment. For a short time, nose jobs had seemed to be on the decline: "First there was the Mediterranean look, personified by Melina Mercouri, whose long classic nose was thought to be 'more sensual' than the Hollywood bob. Then Barbra Streisand became a coast-to-coast sensation, a fashion beauty and glamour queen." Now, however, "bobbsy girls" were back in town, participating in a new "teen-age frenzy for physical perfection," which involved looking less Jewish, less Italian, or perhaps achieving the ultimate, "a profile like Grace Kelly." Even Streisand, according to *Newsweek,* was only the exception that proved the rule. She was popular among teenagers, but her success "had little effect on the way they wanted to make themselves look." As one fifteen-year-old at New York's Lenox School asked the reporter incredulously, "Streisand? . . . That's her look. Would you believe it on anyone else?"[40]

Streisand's reception suggests that Americans in the 1960s had not adopted significantly broader standards of beauty than those that had inspired Fanny Brice to bob her nose. Although they were willing to make an exception in the case of Streisand's significant talent, most Americans continued to see her as just that—an exception. As eminent New York surgeon Clarence Straatsma told *Newsweek* in 1966, "Nothing changes. Today I'm doing the daughters of mothers I did before they were married." Several years later, nineteen-year-old Barbara Wagner of Flushing, New York, told *Seventeen* magazine readers a similar story. Wagner, whose mother claimed that her first thought in the delivery room had been, "Oh no. We'd better start saving money for a nose job!" had recently gotten a new nose from the same surgeon who had operated on her mother twenty-three years earlier. "It won't solve all your problems and it didn't solve all mine," she told her readers, "but yes, yes, it's worth it!"[41]

That Barbra Streisand, despite the star power she pulled in the early 1960s, could not singlehandedly change the standards by which American beauty was judged is not surprising. Americans continue to voice

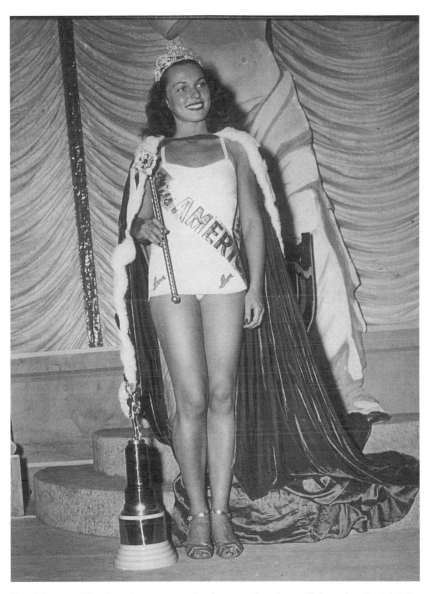

Bess Myerson, Miss America 1945, was the first—and to date, still the only—Jewish Miss America.

admiration for those who resist the pressure to conform. At the same time, however, the belief that large noses are identifiably ethnic and therefore something "other" than American, and that possession of such a nose is likely to limit its bearer's social and economic options, remains common. By the time Streisand emerged on the scene, the nose job was so well established that Americans had come to expect that those with large noses would have them reduced. That journalists and other commentators publicly voiced their surprise at Streisand's refusal suggests the extent of the change that had occurred in the forty years since Fanny Brice was called upon to explain why she had given up part of *her* nose.

From Shima Kito to William White

In 1926, with the headline, "Changes Racial Features: Young Japanese Wins American Bride by Resort to Plastic Surgery," the *New York Times* reported what was perhaps the first plastic surgery in the United States to westernize Asian features. Shima Kito of Boston and Mildred Ross of Dubuque, Iowa, first met in Detroit in 1925. Kito eventually proposed, but Ross felt she could not accept his offer: although she "preferred him to other young men of her own race whom she had met . . . she loved her parents and would do nothing that would hurt them" (especially, the article implied, marry a man of a visibly different race). The situation seemed hopeless, but love—and news of "the wonders accomplished by plastic surgery"—ensured a happy ending. Kito "consulted Miss Ross and then put himself into the hands of a surgeon," who "cut the eye corners so that the slant eye so characteristic of the Japanese race was gone. He lowered the skin and flesh of the nose so that the upturned trait disappeared, and he tightened the pendulous lower lip." Evidently, Ross—and perhaps more important, her parents—judged Kito's surgery to be successful, and the couple became engaged. Kito told the *Times* that he intended to complete his transformation by changing his name to William White, "which is nearly an English equivalent to his native name."[42]

William White's story may have suggested to some Asian Americans that the road to happily ever after led through the plastic surgeon's office, but despite widespread racism and prejudice, particularly on the west coast, Asians did not seek plastic surgery in significant numbers until after World War II. After the war, however, surgery to westernize Asian eyes became increasingly popular, first in Asia and then in the United

States. With the American occupation of Japan and the conflict in Korea, American films, magazines, and soldiers familiarized Asians with western models of beauty, and surgeons began to explore what they called "revision" of the "Oriental eye."[43]

Some surgeons were troubled by this trend. In his autobiography, surgeon Donald Moynihan recalled his experience with Mrs. Muncie, a Korean war bride who came to him in the early 1950s requesting double-fold eyelids and a new, more American nose. Her husband had fallen in love with her in Korea, she explained, but now that they had returned to the States he was ashamed of her. Moynihan was outraged, but after discussing the situation at length he decided that "Mrs. Muncie's problem wasn't all that different from a prominently hooked nose. . . . If it was making her unhappy, she had a right to have it altered." Moynihan performed the surgery to the satisfaction of Mrs. Muncie and her husband but continued to ponder the case. "With all my rationalizing," he recalled, "I still wasn't too happy with the outcome. Had I been writing the script, her husband would have materialized with the assurance that he loved her exactly the way she was. But I guess that's not the way the world turns."[44]

Moynihan was clearly troubled not only by Mr. Muncie's boorish behavior but by the larger implications of such surgery. The reaction of Miami surgeon D. Ralph Millard, however, was more typical. In early 1954, Millard was stationed in Korea. In response to requests to change oriental eyes to occidental eyes, he began to research the process and found that little had been published, so he devised an original solution and in 1955 published a report of his work in *Plastic and Reconstructive Surgery.* Millard was surprised and offended when a "communist magazine" picked up the story and "devoted a two-page spread . . . stating that 'Herr' Millard had taken it upon himself to improve, by westernizing, the races of the population of the entire Orient." He commented, "By neglecting to mention that this surgery had been carried out at the request of the patients, facts and motives were twisted out of all proportion."[45]

Millard's indignation may have been due in part to the fact that Asian surgeons were also performing such surgery. When he traveled through Asia, he found that different techniques prevailed in different places, but already in Seoul, Hong Kong, Tokyo, and the Philippines, surgeons were daily westernizing hundreds of Asian eyes. Millard's contention that he was only performing such surgery in response to patient requests, however, reveals more about why the story troubled him. To Millard, as to most plastic surgeons, features that patients identified as sources of distress were surgical challenges. Medicine, in general, trains its practitioners to meet such challenges rather than inquire into the cultural and philosophical issues surrounding them. For Millard and many of his colleagues, then, Asian eyes were, in technical terms, merely eyes in which the superior palpebral fold was absent or indistinct. In responding to requests to create this fold surgically, Millard believed he was fulfilling his responsibility as a physician and surgeon.

Like Millard, most surgeons—Asian and American—defended eyelid surgery. Leabert R. Fernandez, reporting in 1960 on the popularity of such surgery in Hawaii, noted that although the single eyelid fold is genetically dominant, the request for such surgery "should not be considered abnormal because, in one-half of the Orientals, this fold is normally present." In addition, Fernandez noted, "Those desiring [the operation] . . . usually have a strong complex about the lack of the folds and derive a psychologic lift from the procedure." When they did criticize such surgery, surgeons tended to make their objections on technical grounds. In 1963, surgeon George V. Webster noted that "the urge to Westernization of the Japanese people has created a demand for cosmetic improvement of the essentially small breasted Japanese women, and the excessively flat nose and heavily padded Oriental eyelids." Webster was highly critical of the methods some practitioners were employing: "Correction of hypogenetic defects, such as small breasts and flat nose by the use of implant materials has led to the employment of a great variety of foreign bodies, some of which are unquestionably poorly tolerated by the human host. A reversion to the injection of paraffin-containing materials is especially to be condemned." Significantly, however, he voiced no misgivings about the goals.[46]

Like American surgeons, Asian surgeons had few qualms about performing eyelid surgery and were matter-of-fact about the reasons such requests were increasing. Khoo Boo-Chai, who practiced in Singapore and published extensively on this topic, acknowledged in 1963 that westernization was sweeping the East: "Our Eastern sisters put on western apparel, use western make-up, see western movies and read western literature. Nowadays, there even exists a demand for the face and especially the eyes to be Westernized." Boo-Chai asserted that such a demand had existed for decades in both China and Japan, but that English-language medical journals had only recently begun to document the phenomenon. According to Boo-Chai, Asians wanted surgery for several reasons. One was socioeconomic: western eyes could be a status symbol and might aid in finding a job. A second was "domestic": double-fold eyelids might ensure personal happiness and domestic tranquillity. Finally, local beliefs and superstitions also played a part. Boo-Chai explained that, for example, the trait known as the "mouse-like eye" was particularly unpopular in China, and girls who possessed it "find it rather difficult to acquire a husband."[47]

By the early 1960s, Tokyo, with 108 clinics serving two hundred thousand women each year, was the destination of choice for Asian women who wanted plastic surgery. Dr. Fumio Umezawa, director of Tokyo's Jujin Hospital of Cosmetic Surgery, told the *New York Times* that he often operated on as many as forty patients each day and that the hospital's one-day record for all cases was 1,380 operations, performed on a wide range of Asian women who shared "a general desire to look like Elizabeth Taylor." At Jujin in 1957, the double-eyelid operation cost $8.33. By 1965 the cost had increased substantially to about $56, but Umezawa believed it was still underpriced. Suggesting that Americans had succeeded in exporting not just the practice of cosmetic surgery but the philosophical basis for it as well, Umezawa asserted that a price of a million yen (about $2,800) would be reasonable, because the operation would "release a woman from neuroses to enter a life of happiness." "The women treated here become happier and more joyful as they discard their inferiority complexes," Umezawa explained. "When women are confident of themselves they look prettier. To beautify women by measures endorsed by science also benefits men and therefore society itself." As in America, performing such surgery was gratifying for the surgeon as well. "The thing I like best," Umezawa noted, "is to stand at the door and watch the faces of the patients as they leave. The happiness they feel enhances the work we have done for them. They look beautiful!"[48]

The escalation of American involvement in Vietnam extended Americanized visual culture farther around the globe. As well as internalized standards of female beauty, American GIs brought with them external representations in the form of *Playboy* magazines and pin-up posters. In what observers insisted was not a coincidence, more and more Vietnamese women began to seek plastic surgery. Some of these women were famous: Madame Nguyen Cao Ky, wife of the premier of South Vietnam, registering at Jujin in 1966, commented only, "I want to be more charming to my husband." Most Vietnamese women who sought cosmetic surgery were less socially prominent and less wealthy; they could not afford to travel to Tokyo for surgery, but, as the war progressed, surgery came to them.[49]

Saigon surgeons had no doubts about what inspired plastic surgery's popularity in Vietnam. "Vietnamese girls have beautiful, classic faces, but remove their clothing, and they look like boys with long hair," one surgeon told *Time* magazine in 1966. Surgeons Pham Huu Luong and Pham Ba Vien offered a similar explanation for the marked increase in plastic surgery since the American buildup in 1965. "A bargirl's capacity to earn is based on her ability to attract American males," Dr. Luong told the journalist. "Many desire operations to make themselves more beautiful to them. Others just prefer larger noses and breasts. Some are giving into the fad of the time." Vietnamese surgeon Vu Ban also cited the American buildup. "The bargirls said the GIs preferred them with rounded eyes and big breasts and hips. . . . It became part of their livelihood. Then they found it helped them get jobs and American husbands," Dr. Ban told the *New York Times* in 1973. Mrs. Ngo Van Hieu, owner of a well-known Saigon clinic, told another reporter that bargirls who were influenced by magazines like *Playboy* made up 40 percent of her customers: "Vietnamese see pictures of the girls in the magazines and this becomes a standard of beauty," she explained.[50]

Some Vietnamese physicians found the increase troubling. Although cheaper in Vietnam than in the West, surgery was still costly, and, according to several surgeons, amateur clinics offering cut-rate procedures were springing up to meet the growing number of requests. Dr. Thai Minh Bach thought the phenomenon had gone too far: "They're just pumping in silicone everywhere," he complained. Years later, Jerome Webster saw evidence of such practices. Linda Wong told him that in Hong Kong in 1942 she had gone to a doctor who had injected both her breasts with paraffin; her condition necessitated multiple operations and resulted in severe disfigurement. Like their American colleagues, however, Vietnamese surgeons were more likely to voice concerns about the practical problems of bringing cosmetic surgery to the public than about the underlying cultural implications. They were concerned about untrained practitioners and dangerous procedures, but they were proud of the operations they had pioneered. Dr. Ban claimed to have given thirty-four-year-old Tham Thuy Hang, South Vietnam's top film star, new eyes, nose, breasts, hips, thighs, and even fingers: "She has even had dimples put in her cheeks and a cleft in her chin. You might say she was an entirely different woman." Like other plastic surgeons, Ban believed his surgical skill offered more than just "superficial beauty." "By removing a woman's complexes we give her confidence and transform her psychology," he asserted. "It's a lot of fun. And it's an art form in itself." Dr. Ban particularly prided himself on his ability to remove "natural Asian defects" in an hour.[51]

The surgical craze that swept through Asia in the years after World War II influenced Asians living in the United States as well. Jerome Webster saw his first case in 1946. Mrs. Anna Lee, then twenty-four, told him she believed "reduction of the upper lids" was essential to her plan for an acting career. Webster was unsympathetic, noting, "Patient has typical Chinese eyes, somewhat full on upper edge but I feel that operation is not indicated." In Hawaii, where the phenomenon was particularly evident because of the large Asian population, teenagers who could not afford such surgery (or whose parents would not allow it) often used cellophane tape, which—left on the eyelid overnight—created the desired effect, at least for a day. According to one Honolulu surgeon, Chinese Hawaiians were more conservative than other ethnic groups and did not seek surgery in large numbers. "Percentagewise, Koreans and Southeast Asians probably avail themselves more than the others," he noted, "but numerically, the largest group is still Japanese."[52]

Coming of age in a country that had historically described them and their communities as "Oriental"—in scholar Elaine Kim's words, "east of and peripheral to an unnamed center"—and that had recently defined as alien and incarcerated more than a hundred thousand Japanese Americans, posed particular problems for young Asian Americans. Attempting to make a place for themselves in the affluent consumer culture of post–World War II America, young men and women of Asian origin were as aware as their Caucasian peers of the reigning economy of appearance. As historian Beth Bailey suggests, in this "culture of consumption," dating "afforded public validation of popularity, of belonging, of success. . . . In this system, men and women often defined themselves and each other as commodities, the woman valued by the level of consumption she could demand (how much she was 'worth'), and the man by the level of consumption he could provide." Repeated reminders from magazines, movies, and their peers that this culture ranked blonde above dark, buxom above flat, wide-eyed over narrow, and pale above all could not help but have some effect on the way young Asian Americans saw themselves.[53]

In his 1971 autobiography *American in Disguise,* Daniel Okimoto recalled how awareness of these values complicated his dating years: "In this white dominated society, it was perhaps natural that white girls seemed attractive personally as well as physically. They were in a sense symbols of the social success I was conditioned to seek. . . . In the inner recesses of my heart I resisted the seductive attraction of white girls because I feared I was being drawn to them for the wrong reasons. I was afraid that my tastes had been conditioned by white standards. Behind the magnetism there may have been an unhealthy ambition to prove my self-worth by competing with the best of the white bucks and winning the fair hand of some beautiful, blue-eyed blonde—crowning evidence of having made it." In *Farewell to Manzanar,* her memoir of internment, Jeanne Wakatsuki Houston described a recurring dream that haunted her when she was young: "I see a young, beautifully blond and blue-eyed high school girl moving through a room full of others her own age, much admired by everyone, men and women both, myself included . . . watching, I am simply emptied, and in the dream I want to cry out, because she is something I can never be, some possibility in my life that can never be fulfilled." As Houston's account makes clear, familiarity with the standards held up by the majority culture did not necessarily engender a desire to capitulate to them but, rather, a desire for the benefits and privileges that seemed contingent on them. "I never wanted to change my face or be someone other than myself," Houston wrote. "What I wanted was the kind of acceptance that came so easily to [my friend] Radine."[54]

As writer Kesaya E. Noda observes in her essay "Growing Up Asian in America," in this country, those whose "difference" is visible know that choosing an ethnic identity is not an option for them, as it has been for most whites: "A third-generation German American is an American. A third-generation Japanese American is a Japanese American. Being Japanese means being a danger to the country during the war and knowing how to use chopsticks. I wear this history on my face." Out of such realizations came a new sense of identity and pride, which, given impetus by larger societal developments of the late 1960s and 1970s, resulted in increased opportunity and visibility for Asian Americans. Documentary filmmaker and former television reporter Felicia Lowe recalls, "*Change* was the key word in those days, and in some convoluted amalgamation of what was happening then, the Federal Communications Commission ordered television stations across the country to begin hiring women and minorities." But even the most vociferous supporters of "natural" (and, thus, more inclusive) standards of beauty find that images and ideals long held and deeply engrained cannot be easily or quickly altered by reason and logic.[55]

According to scholar Judy Wu, the Miss Chinatown U.S.A. Beauty Pageant drew on all of these traditions when it was founded in San Francisco in the 1950s. Chinese American businessmen organized the pageant both to foster pride within the community and to raise the community's stature in relation to the larger city—in other words, to draw tourists to Chinatown. The winner—described in the evocative phrase, "loveliest daughter of our ancient Cathay"—would, pageant sponsors proclaimed, represent the best of both worlds, combining the grace, modesty, and beauty of traditional Chinese women with the ambition and talent (including the ability to walk in high heels and wear a bathing suit onstage) necessary to succeed in America's modern consumer culture.[56]

Despite the pageant's name and proclaimed purpose, however, some contestants charged that the standards on which pageant judges relied reflected preferences shaped by the standards of beauty valued in the dominant Caucasian culture. Some contestants believed that taller candidates were preferred. To others, it was clear that larger eyes with double-fold eyelids and longer lashes offered an advantage. A 1973 contestant, asked if she had any special attributes, cited her eyes, which were "larger than some of the girls'." The souvenir book from the 1970 pageant carried an advertisement for a surgeon who claimed a special technique for converting "Oriental eyelids" to "Caucasian eyelids" and a clientele of "movie actresses, singing stars and participants in beauty contests." Today the "double eyelid" operation is the top choice among Asian American patients. According to the American Society of Plastic and Reconstructive Surgeons, surgeons certified by the ABPS operated on 39,000 Asian patients in 1990; since many Asian Americans go overseas or to other practitioners, the real number is likely much higher.[57]

Commenting on an increase in nose augmentations among Asian Americans, several San Francisco plastic surgeons, in 1970, expressed surprise and resignation that a desire to appear more "western," or more Caucasian, had inspired many of their patients: "In a time of social upheaval, with emphasis on self-determination and ethnic pride, it seems paradoxical that the number of non-caucasians undergoing cosmetic surgery is increasing. It appears that attainment of a caucasian aspect is desirable to these patients." Other surgeons, however, insist that race has nothing to do with such surgery. Double-fold eyelids, a Chinese surgeon insisted in 1987, were not "western" but "pretty." Two years later a group of surgeons from Seoul, Korea, Fukuoka, Japan, and Los Angeles similarly insisted that the objective of the eyelid operation was not "caucasianization of the Oriental eye" but, rather, the creation of subtle, "aesthetically pleasing supratarsal folds" that were naturally present in 30 to 60 percent of Asians. Such surgery often resulted in a more western appearance, but this, the surgeons asserted, was not patients' primary goal. The "overwhelming majority of patients" who request such surgery, they explained, "are merely trying to look more attractive within the current aesthetic norms of their own culture. It is believed that the 'double fold' makes the eyes look bigger and hence more attractive." Nor was the question of how norms are produced, reproduced, and disseminated surgeons' concern. The San Francisco surgeons concluded, "Nature inexorably mixes the races of man, while legislatures ponderously seek to equalize them. And plastic surgery, committed to the goal of helping each patient achieve social maturity, adds a measure of 'instant homogeneity.' ... The socioeconomic and psychological impact of the final results has been visibly significant ... and highly gratifying to the surgeons."[58]

As anthropologist Eugenia Kaw noted in a recent article, despite surgeons' and patients' protestations to the contrary, cosmetic surgery among Asian Americans is about more than objective aesthetic standards. Just as decoding the terminology used to discuss Jewish noses suggests that many nose jobs are about erasing visible signs of ethnicity, decoding the terminology used to discuss eyelid surgery among Asians suggests that here race (and the meanings attributed to it) is also the central issue. For Asians—as for Jews, who feared that their noses would be taken to indicate undesirable character traits—the long tradition of the "sciences of race" looms large. Asians who seek cosmetic surgery often do so because they believe that, in the United States, negative characteristics attach to Asian features. As one of Kaw's informants explained, single-fold eyelids evoke "the stereotype of the 'Oriental bookworm' ... who is *dull* and doesn't know how to have fun." Surgeons, in general, have confirmed these readings; as one surgeon explained to Kaw, "the upper eyelid without a fold tends to give a sleepy appearance and therefore a more dull look to the patient. Likewise, the flat nasal bridge and lack of nasal projection can signify weakness in one's personality and by lack of extension, a lack of force in one's character." The centuries-old practice of divining character traits from facial configuration continues to shape the perspectives of surgeons and patients alike. The generally unspoken standard to which surgeons hold patients and patients hold themselves is, just as clearly, Caucasian, as the comments of two Beverly Hills plastic surgeons suggest. In 1989 Ronald Matsunaga said of his patients: "They get the magazines, the movies, they see all the models. They're looking at the Western world"; of himself, Toby Mayer said, "I realize my judgments are by Western standards."[59]

Surgeons and patients, in short, are confident that, by altering individual facial configurations, cosmetic surgery can confer a wide range of benefits that together add up to the American dream—and they are right. But as prospective patients hurry to stake these individual claims, all the while congratulating themselves on their perspicacity in dealing with the world as it is, they sanction, if unintentionally, the belief that social problems can be ameliorated only by individual solutions. There are, still, other voices—voices that call for pride and acceptance and confidence and hope, voices that proffer a vision of the world as it might be— but the chorus singing the praises of individual self-improvement gets louder and more relentless every day.

Ebony and Ivory

Michael Jackson's transformation has allegedly inspired an increase in requests for plastic surgery among young African Americans, including members of his own family, but until recently blacks have been less likely than members of other racial or ethnic groups to seek plastic surgery. That dark skin is particularly likely to develop keloid scars probably accounts for some of this lag: the formation of large, hypertrophic scars may be judged inevitable when surgery must be undertaken for reasons of health, but the possibility that they might result from an elective operation designed to improve appearance has meant that many surgeons and patients have judged the risk too great. The melanin that gives skin color also affords protection against ultraviolet rays, which means that black skin is less prone to sun damage and generally shows age less quickly than white skin. Until late in the twentieth century, many African Americans were unable to afford the high cost of elective surgery, which must be paid for in advance. Finally, as Lawrence Otis Graham points out so eloquently in his memoir, black skin is a marker that no amount of plastic surgery can hide.[60]

The fact that black Americans have not, in large numbers, had plastic surgery, however, does not mean that black features have been considered attractive. Facial characteristics such as wide noses and thick lips have been featured prominently in caricatures ranging from political cartoons to salt-and-pepper shakers to films like D. W. Griffith's epic *Birth of a Nation.* Images like these—and the character traits such representations were intended to evoke—were often explicitly cited as the basis for anti-miscegenation laws and for the widespread adoption of Jim Crow laws at the turn of the century; they offer convincing documentation of the distaste with which whites viewed black features.[61]

The questions of how African Americans have defined beauty in their own communities and what effect white standards have had upon those definitions continue to generate debate. Historian Jacqueline Jones notes that "in some slave quarters mulatto children were scorned as the master's offspring," while other accounts hold that even under slavery lighter skin and smaller features were prized, taken as evidence of higher class status (deriving from indoor work rather than agricultural labor), income, and education. Whatever their genesis, standards of appearance that helped enforce the color bar between blacks and whites—and that created a hierarchy of color among blacks—were clearly in place by the turn of the century. The significance attached to the "Black Is Beautiful" movement of the 1960s suggests just how oppressive American standards of beauty seemed to many African Americans, and that movement's evaporation suggests just how tenacious such standards have been.[62]

That fear of being thought black could drive white Americans to plastic surgeons suggests the power with which Americans invested these standards. The number of cases is apparently small, but over the course of the twentieth century surgeons have reported cases in which whites requested surgery to forestall accusations or suspicions of having black blood. Surgeon Adalbert G. Bettman recounted such a case in 1929. "A young woman," he told his colleagues, "had protruding lips which raised the question as to Ethiopian origin. When the deformity was removed without leaving tell-tale scars, no more questions were asked and she went among her friends, freed of her psychologic as well as her physical impairment." Surgeon Jacques Maliniak noted that "a negroid nose is a distinct social and economic handicap to a dark-skinned Caucasian," as was the "negroid lip": "Except in certain primitive races," Maliniak explained, "a heavy mouth is not considered a social asset. The negroid lip does not satisfy the artistic canons of the present day."[63]

Henry Junius Schireson's veracity is questionable, but his tales are revealing nonetheless. "Miss M," a forty-year-old nurse, was heavily freckled; she wanted Schireson to remove the freckles because in dim light she looked to her patients "like a Mulatto." In a more problematic instance, a young man was brought to Schireson by the woman who had adopted him as an infant; she was disturbed because now that he was grown he showed "unmistakeable signs of black blood." These signs, Schireson wrote, included a distinct negroid upper and lower lip, dilated flaring nostrils, extreme length of legs, absence of calf, and an extraordinarily forceful thumb. Schireson explained to the disappointed woman that surgery had not advanced to the point where all of this could be changed; in 1938 "the youth could not escape his race." In other instances, however, he noted, "it is a simple matter to make the necessary corrections to lips and nostrils."[64]

Surgeons did not always respond positively to such requests for surgery, even from Caucasians. Several New York surgeons jointly reported an instance in which they had refused a patient's request. A thirty-seven-year-old woman, married but childless, requested a third nose job. "She was born in the South, to a family of fading aristocracy," the surgeons recounted, and had not known her father. "Early in life the patient developed the fantasy that her conception occurred in an assault, and that her father was a Negro. The 'flatness' of her nose was a constant reminder of her past; unconsciously, she wished to remove this hated stigma." The surgeons advised the patient to pursue psychiatric treatment rather than additional surgery. In this case, the surgeons involved were curious enough about the patient's motives—and probably tipped off to what they termed a psychological disturbance by the patient's previous surgery, which she judged unsuccessful—to ask more questions and eventually to refuse surgery. Jerome Webster's files contain two similar cases. In one, he noted that the patient had told another doctor that "she thought she had negro blood but didn't say so to me"; he suspected a "complex" and refused the request. In another instance, he received a letter from Elizabeth Cole, who explained, "The trouble is that my nose is absolutely flat, just like a negro's. In fact I have been afraid since I was a child that people would think I was part negro on account of it." His response has not survived.[65]

Other surgeons, however, took such requests at face value as surgical challenges and did not ask too many questions. Spokane surgeon Charles M. MacKenzie, in 1944, noted that maxillary protraction (protruding jaw) cases sometimes involved "abnormally thick lips, in some instances approximating the negroid type," which were simple to revise. Charles Firestone of Seattle regarded this challenge in a similar light. The "full, everted lower lip," Firestone noted in 1946, was exclusively a cosmetic problem of "unesthetic anatomy." The medical literature contained reports of lips everted because of scarring, Firestone continued, but not the "congenitally unesthetic" lip that was the subject of his paper.[66]

New York surgeon Milton Tuerk stated explicitly his belief that no explanation was required of a patient who desired lip reduction surgery. "If the end result produces patient gratification," Tuerk asserted, "the procedure is self-justified." The operation Tuerk recommended for what he called this "ubiquitous deformity" was not original, but he considered it worth describing because as of 1960 it had not been discussed extensively in the medical literature. Tuerk had begun to perform the operation because of requests from women who were distressed by the "moist and quite pallid" appearance of the everted portion of the lower lip. The "wetness and texture" of this part of the lip meant that it would not take a lipstick; "to many girls this is especially discomforting and objectionable," Tuerk explained.[67]

Articles and comments like these recall those Italians and Greeks who suffered what they perceived as the "undeserved" penalties of anti-Semitism earlier in the century, as well as the reactions of Jews themselves. The rhetoric here is clearly about race; the goal, just as clearly, about what it means to look "American" (with "whiteness" the implicit frame of reference).

Although surgeons were generally willing to fulfill requests from African American patients, some did so only to the extent that such requests were consistent with their own ideas about what constituted improvement in appearance. Surgeon Donald Moynihan, in his autobiography, recounted an example of a case he had refused. The prospective patient was a young black woman whose cornrowed hair and black studies major in college suggested to Moynihan that she was "really into the heritage thing," as did her request that he put a bone through her nose. "I respected the deep pride she had in her race," Moynihan recalled, "but the way I see it, no matter what, a bone through the nose is an unreasonable request. I turned her down."[68]

Reports from African Americans who have pursued the option of plastic surgery are few, but those that exist suggest that it was not the belief that their features were "congenitally unesthetic" that drove them to have surgery. Rather, they were responding to the limitations on their lives and careers that their identifiably black features imposed. As a nineteen-year-old model explained to sociologist Frances Cooke Macgregor about the time of the Montgomery bus boycott, "I don't find it advantageous to have decisive Negro features. The less you look like a Negro, the less you have to fight. I would pass for anything so long as I'm not taken for a Negro. With a straight nose I could do costume work and pose as an Indian, Egyptian, or even a Balinese." Sometimes, black patients were open about their desire not only to look less black but to look more white. In 1971 a Miami plastic surgeon reported that in a case involving a "young Negro female school teacher. . . . There was full knowledge that her basic desire was to resemble the caucasian; she thought this might enhance her future teaching ability in the public school system. Her husband was tolerant of this desire."[69]

Many African Americans, however, dispute the contention that race has anything to do with plastic surgery. Ouida Lindsey, a Chicago journalist, told *Ebony* magazine in 1977 that after her nose job a friend had accused her of trying to "be Caucasian." Lindsey, pointing to others in the room, asked: " 'Why couldn't you feel that I wanted my nose to be like a sister's whose nose was straighter than mine?' People tend to think there is a stereotyped look that all black people have. That is ridiculous." Lawrence Graham, similarly, protests that the very fact of his curly black hair and dark skin prove his nose job cannot be about whiteness and reminds us that black Americans have the same rights to determine their appearance as white Americans.[70]

Coverage of plastic surgery in black magazines has not been extensive, but it has generally been positive, contending that self-improvement is just as laudable a goal for black Americans as for white. That African Americans generally use words like "prettier" rather than "Caucasian" or "white" to describe the look they want is not surprising. Such usage is consistent with the way members of other ethnic and racial minority groups have framed their desires, as well as with the terminology surgeons have employed. Words like "prettier" and "better," however, are explicitly comparative in nature; they beg the question, "than what?", as well as the more complex question of how definitions and standards of appearance came to be. Once that historical question has been raised, accepting such terms at face value becomes more problematic. On the one hand, "the 'denial of heritage' accusation that is leveled at Black women" would seem to deny them the right to "have fun" with their appearance that white women claim so casually. On the other hand, as *Essence* editor Elsie B. Washington noted in 1988: "The wish to acquire what we were not born with, to adopt the coloring that has for centuries been touted as prettier, finer, better, carries with it the old baggage of racial inferiority and/or superiority based simply, and simplistically, on physical traits."[71]

Until recently, most surgeons have been as reluctant to confront the implications of cosmetic surgery in African American patients as they have to discuss similar implications in relation to Asian patients. In 1969 surgeon Thomas D. Rees commented on the increasing numbers of African Americans who were requesting nasal surgery. "It is sometimes thought that the Negro who seeks rhinoplasty is attempting, symbolically at least, to deny his heritage," he noted, but—like those who insisted that Asian patients were inspired by aesthetic, rather than ethnic, concerns—Rees expressed his belief that African Americans were seeking improvement according to objective, aesthetic standards: "Most Negroes who desire this operation simply wish to obtain a measure of improvement in personal appearance. They want a nose that is smaller, more symmetrical, and pleasing in three-dimensional contour." The complaints voiced by the increasing numbers of young African Americans seeking nasal surgery, surgeon Ferdinand Ofodile noted in 1984, encompass any or all of the following conditions: a wide bridge, a depressed or "low" bridge, a prominent or bulbous tip, and flared nostrils. Many request "the same type of procedure done on Michael Jackson," and they often bring photographs. Usually, Ofodile asserted, prospective patients are "attractive . . . with slender features in whom parts of the nose are disproportionately large. What they are seeking, therefore, are finer nasal features to match the face. There is no desire . . . to 'Caucasianize' their noses." In 1983 two Israeli surgeons concurred. Although they cautioned against extrapolating from the small sample of 289 patients they had questioned, the surgeons concluded, "In our experience, certain ethnic groups are blessed more bountifully in the area of their olfactory organs. Individuals so blessed are often not pleased with their noses and turn to the cosmetic surgeon to help alleviate their problem. We feel it is simply a matter of aesthetics and not stereotypes."[72]

Still, the issue of "Caucasianization" remains troubling. Thomas D. Rees, who in 1969 claimed that the issue was purely aesthetic had, by 1986, revised his interpretation. "In my 1969 paper," Rees wrote, "I made the point that most non-Caucasians seek rhinoplasty without a conscious desire to achieve Caucasian features. I am now not so sure of this interpretation, since Asian plastic surgeons assure me that it is the influence of Western movies and television that has increased the requests for such surgery among Asians. It seems to me that many, if not most, Negro prospective rhinoplasty patients are mightily impressed with the Caucasian-like transformation of the previously Negroid features of Michael Jackson, the noted entertainer." Compared to statements made by other plastic surgeons, Rees's comment is unusually prescient—or unusually candid. Like most Americans, plastic surgeons have found it difficult to discuss openly issues of race and ethnicity. But while Rees's interpretation of the meaning of such surgery had changed, his attitude about the role surgeons should play in it had not. The homogenization of world cultures, Rees noted, meant that more of these requests were inevitable, hence surgeons "should be aware of safe and reliable techniques for effecting these changes." Like generations of plastic surgeons who preceded him, Rees defined the field of plastic surgery as driven by public demand, in other words, by patients and their requests. This position is very much in line with past and current trends in the field of plastic surgery, but it leaves unexamined the role that surgeons' attitudes and actions have played in shaping American standards of beauty.[73]

A review of medical literature on non-Caucasian plastic surgery suggests that "Negro prospective rhinoplasty patients" are not the only ones who are "mightily impressed" with Caucasian features. In the same way that "over-large" came to be used to describe Jewish noses, which were understood to be excessively large in the implied comparison to the Anglo-Saxon norm, words such as "too-wide" and "flattened" are commonly employed to describe typical noses of nonwhite patients. With the goal of educating their colleagues about the anatomical differences between Caucasian and non-Caucasian noses, thus enabling them to operate more effectively, two San Francisco plastic surgeons, in a 1987 article, described some of the differences: "the non-caucasian nasal tip is usually flattened, bulbous, and lacks the subtleties of lights and shadows of definition," the surgeons wrote. "The base of the bony pyramid appears widened in non-Caucasians. The dorsal bridge seems depressed or saddle-like, and is broad. A deepened nasofrontal angle exaggerates the flattened look." Nowhere in the article is it stated that either the patient's or the surgeon's goal is to achieve a more Caucasian nose, yet the message is clear. All of the above-described conditions of the non-Caucasian nose are defined in relation to the appearance of the nose in Anglo-Saxon Caucasians. The postoperative photographs—which show narrower, pointier, higher-bridged noses in black, Asian, and Chicano patients—make this point explicit.[74]

The Caucasian orientation of plastic surgery is, of course, most clearly evident in Michael Jackson's face. Exactly what Jackson has done, and has had done, remains in dispute. In *Moonwalk,* his 1978 autobiography, he admitted to two rhinoplasties and an artificial cleft in his chin, but has consistently denied having additional surgery. At a September 1984 news conference, Frank Dileo (then Jackson's personal manager) read a statement that included the assertions, "No! I've never had my cheekbones altered in any way. No! I've never had cosmetic surgery on my eyes." Most observers, however, doubt these claims. According to biographer J. Randy Taraborrelli, by 1991 Jackson had had four primary rhinoplasties and two "touch-ups." Surgeons and others who have observed his transformation believe the number of procedures is higher—that cheekbone implants, permanent eyeliner, and surgical reduction of the lower lip may have played a role in Jackson's transformation.[75]

Although Jackson's motivations remain opaque, accounts of his life suggest that the question of self-hate—which most of the rhetoric concerned with cosmetic surgery and race emphatically denies—is worth considering. Jackson became aware early in his career that, in the world of American entertainment, being too black was a disadvantage. Motown president Berry Gordy reportedly warned the group that they could not afford to appear to be too black or too militant lest they alienate their white audience. "Listen, Diana Ross didn't become a star by being black. She became one by being popular," Gordy explained to one publicist. "As far as I'm concerned, The Jackson 5 aren't black either. So let's have none of that black stuff." In June 1971, when MGM records released Donny Osmond's first single, most entertainment world observers agreed that The Jackson 5 could not hope for similar teen idol status, because the teen magazines that created and awarded such status were predominantly white. On a more personal level, too, identifiably black features troubled Jackson; family nicknames like "Big Nose" and "Liver Lips" caused much pain. Jackson's personal history, as well as his current appearance, suggests that at the very least he is in pursuit of the same "ethnic neutrality" so many Americans have desired.[76]

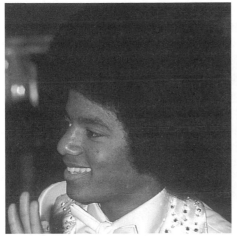

Michael Jackson, 1977.

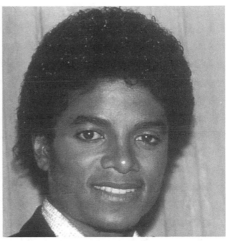

Michael Jackson in 1980, mid-transformation.

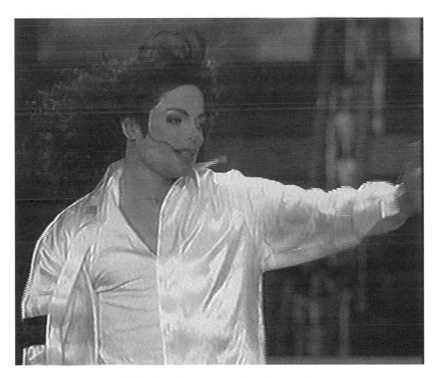

Michael Jackson, 1997 (video frame still).

It is the tension between politics and play that makes cosmetic surgery so problematic in this context. Tired of talking about oppression, which they relegate to the same cellar as the other "dreary and moralizing generalizations about gender, race, and so forth that have so preoccupied liberal and left humanism," those who insist that cosmetic surgery is simply one more way we amuse ourselves tend to affect what philosopher Susan Bordo describes as a uniquely postmodern sensibility, in which "all sense of history and all ability (or inclination) to sustain cultural criticism, to make the distinctions and discriminations that would permit such criticism, have disappeared." The postmodern conversation, Bordo writes, exhibits "intoxication with individual choice and creative *jouissance*, delight with the piquancy of particularity and mistrust of pattern and seeming coherence, celebration of 'difference' along with an absence of critical perspective differentiating and weighing

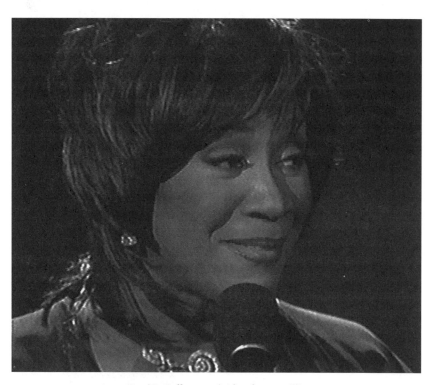

Patti LaBelle, 1997 (video frame still).

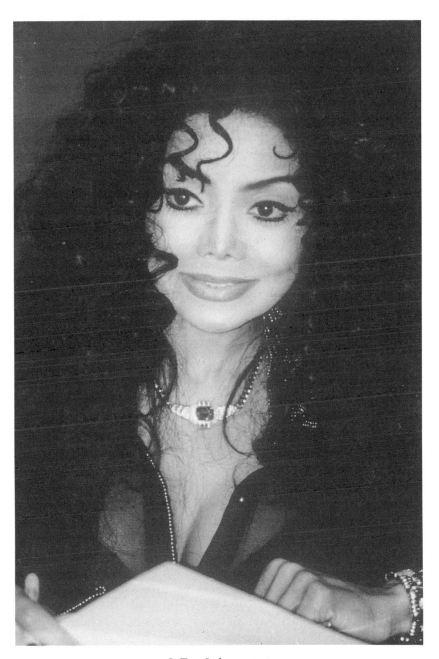

LaToya Jackson, 1994.

'differences,' suspicion of the totalitarian nature of generalization along with a rush to protect difference from its homogenizing abuses"—in brief, it flattens the "terrain of power relations." Its effect is destabilizing much as television is: its endless "pastiche of differences" prevents us from making any positioned social critique, formulating any critical generalizations, discerning any patterns. What is effaced is the "arduous and frequently frustrated historical struggle that is required for the subordinated to articulate and assert the value of their 'difference' in the face of dominant meanings—meanings which offer a pedagogy directed at the reinforcement of feelings of inferiority, marginality, ugliness."[77]

What is effaced, in other words, is history itself—in this case, the long history of racism and oppression that makes us wonder if the efforts of some Americans to remake themselves in the image of other Americans is not by definition a politically charged act. The difficulty, here as elsewhere, is that the kinds of transformations that are being effected are unquantifiable, even though there are visible differences among them. Consider the face of singer Patti LaBelle, who recently told talk-show host Oprah Winfrey that she once had a nose that "went from here to here" and is thrilled at her surgeon's work. Juxtapose her face with that of LaToya Jackson (whose surgery was obviously much more extensive): the contrast is noticeable—but that does not necessarily make it easier to talk about. The question of what is effaced raises the related question of what it is that cannot be effaced. What is, in fact, lost in Michael Jackson's face? Jackson's case tells us not only about a general disquietude respecting alteration but about the impossibility of actually losing racial identity. After all, how improbable, for black Americans, is the idea of looking into the mirror and seeing "a man without a country"—and yet how often has it happened (think of Paul Robeson, W. E. B. DuBois, Josephine Baker) that white racism has inspired precisely this emotion?[78]

Just as they mourn the blurring of once-distinct regional accents that has attended the proliferation of national media, some cultural critics have lamented the homogenization of appearance that has resulted from the acceptance of plastic surgery. In 1945, *Time* magazine interviewed Manhattan plastic surgeon Jacob Daley, who prided himself on trying to talk prospective patients out of having nose jobs. "Art takes the high road and seeks to create the unusual . . . rhinoplasty takes the low road and seeks to remove all traces of it," Daley told *Time*. To support his point, Daley showed *Time* the tracings he had had an artist make of the *Mona Lisa*, Titian's *Man in a Red Cap*, and Holbein's *Erasmus*, altered to demonstrate how "dull and uninteresting" the paintings' subjects looked with noses reduced to suit modern [1945] standards. "As further evidence," *Time* noted, Daley had "kept his own magnificently large, arched, craggy and overhanging neb." The New York Academy of Art's Xavier de Callatay visited a plastic surgeon's convention in 1984 to urge surgeons to preserve patients' individuality. "I can admire their desire for harmonious proportions," Callatay told a reporter, "but the artist I am worries about the uniformity this model implies. I was taken aback by the book cosmetic surgeons published for themselves, showing all those cute, bland faces. What happened to mortal beauty *and* divine beauty?"[79]

Almost unanimously, plastic surgeons counter that they are inspired by an abstract, artistic ideal of beauty rather than one that is culturally defined. Throughout the twentieth century, surgeons have claimed that they are artists, veritable sculptors in human flesh. Where once they relied on geometric measurements, they now claim to carve and mold according to their own highly developed aesthetic sensibilities. In a statement representative of such claims, which are legion throughout surgeons' writings, surgeon Murray Berger, in 1951, described the process of surgical artistry: "The well-informed plastic surgeon—essentially a sculptor—studies the proportions of his patient's facial features. . . . He has a sculptor's concept of the features that form the particular face under study and consequently can obtain a gratifying surgical result—gratifying to himself and patient alike." Some Americans have found this explanation persuasive. Repeating a message that hundreds of other publications had passed along to their readers over the previous decades, writer Jane Fort told *Teen* magazine readers in 1980, "The goal of cosmetic surgery is to normalize appearances so that your nose enhances the rest of your features."[80]

The mantle of artistry has allowed surgeons to claim a disinterested position—a position outside of culture. Their standards, their values, and their artistic sensibility, they say, derive from the same timeless canon of craft, skill, and beauty that produced David and the Mona Lisa. Always suspect, this claim is simply no longer supportable: their own history demonstrates that American plastic surgeons are both products and producers not only of a culture of medicine but of a culture that is unique to modern America. And an enormous, and impressive, number of recent historical and literary works have demonstrated that no canon is timeless. In a poignant piece that appeared in *Mademoiselle* in 1978, Diana Stephens recounted how her own thinking about this issue had

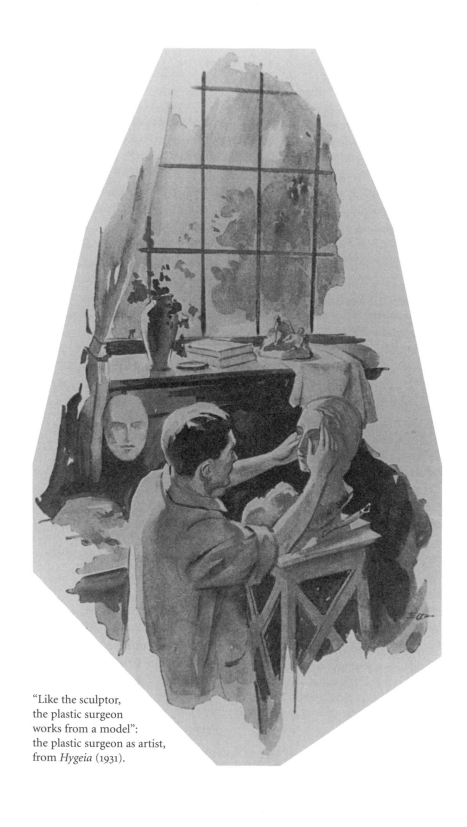

"Like the sculptor,
the plastic surgeon
works from a model":
the plastic surgeon as artist,
from *Hygeia* (1931).

changed. Stephens wrote that while she had never liked her nose, it was surgeons' claims to artistry that had persuaded her to alter it: "As the doctors said, there was a nose other than the one I possessed which belonged with my face. It was a nose determined not by genetics, but by an abstract, artistic idea of what nose was aesthetically most suitable for my eyes, my mouth, my chin, my face shape, my size. And this aesthetic quality, like art itself, seemed to extend beyond culture and be independent of it." After surgery, Stephens reevaluated her decision, and her surgeon's words; eventually, she decided that she did not believe in pure art, at least when it involved changing the human face. "One cannot separate the aesthetic norm from cultural conditioning," she wrote. "Aesthetic values can and do change from culture to culture, from century to century.... I went to my surgeon to have my nose bobbed because my society and culture prefer small noses to larger ones. As if it makes any difference."[81]

There has been some evidence in recent years that the voices that have decried the homogenization of appearance are now falling on more receptive ears. Some Americans believe that the standard of American beauty—and with it, the goal of cosmetic surgery—is beginning to change. Surgeon Samuel Bloom, in 1970, cautioned his colleagues against making women's noses too small: "Although a 'cute' nose may be acceptable to a woman in her 20's," he noted, "in later years it becomes inappropriate." In response to the requests of modern American women, who had concluded that the pert, turned-up style popular in earlier decades was no longer appropriate, New York's Dr. Norman J. Pastorek began to create noses for women that are "slightly assertive, longer and straighter, closer to handsome." Paraphrasing the explanations women gave him, Pastorek explained that women say, "I don't want to look too sweet.... When I'm toe to toe with those guys on the stock exchange, I don't want to look ineffective and vulnerable." Minnesota surgeon William J. Carter agreed. "The executive woman is in," he told *Newsweek* in 1985. "The Debbie Reynolds look with the cute turned-up nose is out the window." In 1987, *Health* similarly told readers, "These days, more assertive noses with stronger, straighter lines are in; cute little turned-up noses are out."[82]

By the mid-1980s, many commentators asserted, American ideals of beauty emphasized a more natural, and more ethnic, image. "More plastic surgeons now strive to preserve a person's ethnic look, rather than making everyone into the same Anglo Saxon mold," *Health* writer Paula Dranov told readers in 1987. According to New York plastic surgeon Henry

Sackin, the "squashed-tip-nose variety of the '40s" and the "scooped-out-bridge-pug-nose one of the '60s" were side effects of surgeons' emphasis on uniformity. Dr. Thomas J. Krizek of Chicago similarly noted that "the scooped-out nose, which used to be popular, just didn't occur in nature very often, and that bothers people today." New York surgeon Blair O. Rogers credited the sixties' generation with changing the bland standards that had held sway in previous decades. "A Mediterranean, Italian, Greek, near-Eastern look is coming in. . . . A lot of young patients today don't want to lose their ethnicity," Rogers noted.[83]

Stars like Cher, Dustin Hoffman, Al Pacino, and Ali McGraw, whose looks do not fit the typical movie-star mold, have been credited with fomenting a veritable revolution in America's attitude toward ethnicity. As Dr. Alvin Mancusi, a New Jersey surgeon, asserted in 1974, "People . . . are increasingly proud of their ethnic backgrounds." They want to "enhance, rather than change, their existing features." In the late 1970s, Susan Taylor, beauty and fashion editor of *Essence,* was similarly optimistic that standards of beauty would broaden still further in the years to come. And as M. G. Lord documents in her fascinating study of Barbie, there is considerable evidence that this "broadening" is occurring in a number of different arenas. In 1980, Black Barbie and Hispanic Barbie were introduced as the sole representatives of their respective cultures; today consumers select from a variety of Barbie dolls with complexions ranging from beige to mahogany (although most still come only with long, straight hair). The recent demise of the Crayola "flesh tone" crayon was heralded by many commentators as evidence of this trend, as was the 1993 *Time* magazine cover that carried a computer-generated portrait of the "new Eve"—a hybrid of every conceivable heritage heralded as the "new face of America."[84]

Indeed, widespread admiration for those who have chosen to keep unusual features suggests that conformity is not as enticing as it once was. Barbra Streisand continues to top this list. Physician Kurt J. Wagner, an outspoken critic of plastic surgery, has cited both Streisand and Sophia Loren as "true originals" and "non-conformists." In 1980, *Seventeen* magazine relayed a surgeon's message to its readers: "There are times when some girls must realize what Barbra Streisand knew years ago: that some noses—though not your standard, turned-up button—are beautiful." Four years later, *Seventeen* again cited Streisand as an example some teens might want to emulate: "Certainly we're not suggesting that a less-than-perfect nose or anything else *has* to be changed.

Many people are content with their distinctive features. They know that an unusual nose—or any other feature—can be special. Consider Barbra Streisand: Throughout her life, she has resisted suggestions to have a nose job, and it hasn't affected her career in the least." In their 1996 book *Divided Sisters: Bridging the Gap between Black Women and White Women,* psychologist Midge Wilson and poet Kathy Russell expanded the list but continued the tradition: "Certainly Barbra Streisand and Whoopi Goldberg are not traditionally beautiful," they wrote, "yet each has successfully managed, through her inner beauty and personality, to enlarge ideas of attractiveness in ways previously not thought possible."[85]

But if Americans continue to admire Barbra Streisand's character, most still do not want to look like her. In 1976, Julie Smith, a Florida student who had a nose job at seventeen, recounted the glee she felt when people who used to tell her she resembled Streisand began to say, "You look just like Barbra Streisand—except for your nose." In 1990, Streisand's profile was still haunting America's young (white) women. "They tormented me, first with Jimmy Durante and later with Barbra Streisand," Kathleen Rockwell Lawrence told *Glamour* readers about her childhood. A nose job later, the teasing had stopped. Philadelphia surgeon Julius Newman found Streisand's profile equally distressing and told an interviewer of his desire to work on her. " 'She'd be beautiful,' he predicted, 'I don't think I'd charge her.' "[86]

While moderate ethnicity may have become more acceptable, as *New York Times* personal health columnist Jane Brody cautioned readers in 1989, too much ethnicity is still considered undesirable. Her assertion that "a good surgeon will not try to erase ethnic features but merely modify those that are considered too extreme" suggests that when it comes to standards of beauty, changes have been less significant than constants. To eyes that in the 1970s saw actress Bo Derek's cornrowed hair as a positive comment on African American styles, Barbara Hershey's newly plumped lips signal a like acceptance. Yet to others, white women's indulgence in such experimentation seems to signal not genuine plurality but an unthinking display of privilege. "Cherry-picking" the best of all cultures, they enjoy the benefits of "exotic" looks without the oppression. The appeal of the "exotic" has its own long tradition in western culture, and the contemporary shift to exoticism may signal nothing more significant than advertisers' need to create ever new products and palettes that demand acquisition.[87]

What has indisputably changed, in the field of ethnic plastic surgery, is the number and range of available remedies. In her introduction to Frances Cooke Macgregor's 1974 study of plastic surgery patients, anthropologist Margaret Mead foresaw this trend. "Once there is a possibility that the defect can be reduced or minimized or compensated for," Mead noted, "our attitude changes from one of painful inattention to active concern. Something should be done. . . . Whatever is wrong that can be fixed, should be fixed." Popular knowledge about plastic surgery encouraged this process, as "those who know that something can be done are freer to say that something ought to be done." On one level, such predictions spark unlikely futuristic images straight out of science fiction. On another level, however, they contain more than the proverbial grain of truth. Dental surgeon Ronald P. Strauss, in 1983, offered the "relative maxillary protrusion, the class II malocclusion" as a compelling example of how this process works on a practical level to alter the way patients and surgeons define medical categories and allocate medical care. "The ability to alter appearance," Strauss asserted, "has affected how we respond aesthetically to differences." "A child who may have been acceptably 'bucktoothed' in the 1940s and who may have been a candidate for orthodontic braces in the 1950s and 1960s, now often has a dentofacial deformity, the treatment for which is maxillofacial surgery. The expansion of medical attention toward this non-life-threatening condition serves to increase its unacceptability as normal. As a result, a minor variant of normal becomes a deformity." As Strauss noted, "there does not appear to be a broad understanding of how medicine became involved in decisions about integrating or altering individual appearances differing from cultural norms."[88]

The project of redefining normal to encompass a broader range would require such an understanding, but if surgeons have been reluctant to dig too deeply into their own motives, so too have their patients. Strauss suggested that surgeons move from their patient-demand orientation toward a more active "surgical gatekeeping" role, but it is unrealistic to expect that they will pioneer in formulating standards of beauty that will diminish their incomes and decrease their social significance; nor is it likely that the ideals to which surgeons adhere will differ significantly from those admired by their culture. As M. G. Lord observes, the common thread in Mattel's Dolls of the World collection "involves Mattel's coding of an 'American' identity"; the original, "American," Barbie remains the standard against which these "aliens" are compared. Certainly, pluralism—however limited, however conditional—is better than no pluralism. But as yet Americans have only begun to chip away at the standards of beauty that were constructed early in this century.[89]

Ironically, what hope there is for change is embedded in reactions to Michael Jackson's masklike countenance, which suggest that the pursuit of sameness elicits a level of discomfort comparable to that once evoked by difference. Americans have made remarkably little progress in the past century when it comes to talking about race and racism, and in some sense this failure is understandable. As writer Marita Golden notes in her introduction to *Skin Deep*, a 1995 anthology on this topic, there is truth in the truism that "race is the tar baby in our midst; touch it and you get stuck, hold it and you get dirty." But if it offers nothing else, the haunting face of Michael Jackson provides a none-too-gentle reminder that the tar baby, like the proverbial elephant in the living room, does not vanish just because it is ignored.[90]

CHAPTER SIX

Beauty and the Breast

In November 1991, a Food and Drug Administration panel voted almost unanimously to reject the data provided by Dow Corning Wright Company, then the nation's leading manufacturer of silicone gel breast implants, on the grounds that they were insufficient to prove that the implants were safe. This decision seemed to foreshadow a ban on implants, and the country's newspapers that day carried headlines like "breast implants imperiled." As it turned out, this initial alarm was premature: panel members, after hearing hundreds of women testify to their need for implants, could not agree on whether, and where, to draw the line. As Dr. Rita Freedman told the *New York Times,* some women were terrified of receiving unsafe implants, while others panicked at the thought that implants would no longer be available; panel members found "the idea that we would decide which group should suffer . . . unconscionable." The very next day, the panel proclaimed implants a "public health necessity" and recommended that they remain on the market. FDA commissioner David A. Kessler, however, was more cautious. Early the following January, he declared a voluntary temporary moratorium on the manufacture, distribution, sale, and implantation of silicone gel-filled prostheses and scheduled public hearings for February.[1]

The FDA's fall decision reflected a broad cultural consensus, developed over decades, which held that what people choose to do with their time and money and bodies is their own business. Kessler's subsequent announcement signaled a sharp divergence from it. These events set in motion a drama that for months dominated the evening news and the pages of newspapers and magazines all over the country. At a press conference in Washington, D.C., later in January 1992, Dr. Norman Cole, president of the American Society of Plastic and Reconstructive Surgeons, told journalists that Kessler's failure to make available to doctors the medical and scientific data on which his decision was based was "unconscionable—an outrage" and accused the agency of creating "hysteria, anxiety and panic." As they began to explore the history of silicone, however, journalists asked whether the FDA's previous inaction was not more "unconscionable" than its recent decision. Dow Corning came off worst of all in the growing number of muckraking stories the controversy inspired. As medical writers and cultural commentators drew historical parallels between the silicone gel breast implant, the synthetic estrogen DES, and the tranquilizer thalidomide, business writers compared Dow Corning's crisis management strategy to others commonly regarded as woefully inadequate and unprofessional: Exxon's response to the Valdez oil spill, Johns Manville's to the asbestos episode, and of course that of A. H. Robins to the Dalkon Shield scandal. The company continued to insist that it had acted responsibly, but its swift move to replace chief executive Lawrence Reed was widely interpreted as a damage control measure.[2]

On February 20, following the hearings, the FDA advisory panel concluded that the information presented, which included more than thirty thousand pages submitted by Dow Corning, was insufficient, and recommended that implants be reevaluated. Although many commentators greeted this recommendation with relief, the various versions of the breast implant story that were being offered in the press suggested that the issue had already become too complicated for a simple regulatory solution. According to some commentators, the breast implant story was yet another chapter in a long history of national inattention to issues of women's health. Others held that breast implants represented one of many instances in which potential regulators had bowed to the powerful lobby of organized medicine. A more dramatic version held that Porsche-driving plastic surgeons, in collusion with the soulless capitalists at Dow Corning, had conspired for personal profit to suppress information that called the safety of implants into question. Still more far-reaching was the accusation that these same parties had deliberately conspired to undermine the personal and political gains promised by feminism's second wave by redirecting women's time and attention toward attempting to fulfill unrealistic expectations created by the advertising and fashion industries. These readings had in common an implication that some kind of restrictive or protective legislation was long overdue.[3]

Alternative perceptions, however—informed, variously, by the Vietnam generation's distrust of experts and by the neoconservative suspicion of government—equated the call to restrict the availability of implants with a threat to individual freedom. Perhaps most significant were the voices that argued that while implants may have originated as objects of oppression, women had utilized them toward their own, sometimes subversive ends: cancer patients' demands for breast implants had forced the male medical establishment to reevaluate its cavalier attitude toward the loss of a breast; implants enabled small-breasted women to turn the tables and triumph over cultural standards largely determined by male tastes. Recalling recurrent debates over protective labor legislation, these versions held that any attempt to restrict the availability of implants amounted to an attempt to restrict women's freedom of choice; such attempts were thus paternalistic at best and antifeminist at worst.[4]

Even those who opposed regulation, however, acknowledged that the FDA had been guilty of inconsistency: it had not cared sufficiently about the health of American women to require that breast implants be routed through the testing and approval system it had set up to oversee the health-care industry. To many commentators, the traditional belief that female vanity deserves what it gets seemed to explain why it was this particular case the FDA had chosen to ignore. As *New York Times* columnist Anna Quindlen noted, breast implants had been held to a negative standard—"not unsafe"—rather than to the affirmative standard that women deserved. This criticism, the validity of which was implicitly and explicitly acknowledged by the FDA, was met by the FDA's final decision, made public on April 16, 1992. Beginning immediately, the agency declared, the availability of silicone gel-filled breast implants would be severely restricted. Women who needed immediate replacement of leaking or ruptured implants could get them, as could those whose reconstruction was currently in progress. A woman who desired breast reconstruction after cancer or injuries or for congenital deformities could still opt for silicone implants, provided her surgeon certified that saline implants were not suitable in her particular case. Those who desired augmentation with silicone implants for cosmetic purposes, however, would have to review other options. Silicone implants would be available for cosmetic purposes only to approximately two thousand women who would agree to participate in, and were accepted into, a strictly controlled, long-term experimental study.[5]

The FDA's stated commitment to unraveling the intertwined, interconnected issues of health and illness, beauty and deformity, went against a long-established trend. Over the course of the twentieth century, lay and medical opinion in the United States gradually converged around a neutral definition of cosmetic surgery. According to this definition, cosmetic surgery had no larger moral, ethical, or cultural implications; rather, it was simply one of a number of reasonable paths Americans might choose to tread in their quest for self-improvement. Neither lay nor medical opinion was unanimous, of course: many Americans continue to feel ambivalent about a practice that defines vanity as a positive good, and many physicians continue to disdain it or at least its more aggressive proponents. Even those who are most critical, however, have generally adopted the "live and let live" attitude that informed the FDA advisory panel's recommendation that implants remain on the market. Commissioner David Kessler came to a very different conclusion, but his decision to withdraw implants from the market would prove to be a nostalgic attempt to return to an idealized and imagined world in which distinctions between medical necessity and vanity, and between reconstructive and cosmetic surgery, could be clearly drawn.

It is ironic, although not particularly surprising, that the solution at which the agency finally arrived provided something for all but satisfied none. Surgeons, current and potential patients, and commentators alike found the moral distinction between reconstruction and augmentation troubling for the same reason earlier generations had: such distinctions had proven impossible to maintain. While some women who had had or were considering reconstructive surgery after cancer, for example, were grateful that their concerns had been privileged over the "less serious" concerns of augmentation patients, others were insulted by the perceived implication that their illness made them expendable, appropriate for potentially dangerous experimentation. Those who defined the problem as a lack of information were angry that the FDA's decision seemed to ignore this point and to imply that if the government did not step in, women would choose breasts—or bigger breasts—over their good health. Some pointed out that the decision was inconsistent, leaving testicle, calf, and pectoral implants unregulated.

Despite approval of the largest product liability settlement in this country's history, the breast implant controversy remains a story without an ending. So many women registered for the class-action suit that the settlement was already in jeopardy when Dow Corning filed for bankruptcy protection (a standard Chapter 11 claim) in May 1995. A settlement involving three other manufacturers (Bristol-Myers Squibb, Baxter Healthcare, and Minnesota Mining and Manufacturing) seems at this writing fragile at best, as does the future of Dow Chemical (which, according to a 1995 ruling, may be held liable for claims against its subsidiary). The first epidemiological studies have found no cause-and-effect relationship between breast implants and known connective tissue diseases. But the thousands of women who, empowered by the movement to secure funding and attention for women's health issues, complain of a variety of health problems and are sure their silicone implants are to blame call our attention to the question of which women's voices get listened to and which ignored. Millions of women still have silicone implants whose long-term effects are unknown, and many others are looking to new and untested alternatives, such as implants filled with soybean or peanut oil. Still, if it did not provide an ending to the story, the FDA's decision suggested that its long and complicated beginning and middle are worth examination—and that the balance that Americans and their surgeons struck over the course of the twentieth century between vanity and self-improvement, mental and physical health, beauty and ugliness, was tenuous indeed.[6]

The First Breast Operation: Reduction

Breast augmentation is a fairly recent phenomenon, dating in its modern form only to the early 1960s. Breast reduction, however, was carried out much earlier as a solution to the problem variously termed macromastia or gigantomastia (literally, overlarge or gigantic breasts). Although it has been refined in recent years, the operation has not changed significantly since the 1920s. The surgeon makes two C-shaped horizontal incisions, underneath the breast and the areola, and two vertical incisions running between the horizontal ones. He removes a "wedge" of fat, tissue, and skin, reshapes the breast, and repositions the nipple and areola before closing the incision. The standard scar, after recovery, is anchor-shaped, running vertically from the nipple to the curved, horizontal scar, which is normally hidden underneath the breast. Side effects may include loss of sensation in the nipple and breast skin and an inability to breast-feed. As many women with extremely large breasts lack both sensation and breast-feeding ability, however, they often consider these consequences minimal, and for many more they are a fair trade-off. Because of the physical discomfort large-breasted women often experience, breast reduction has with few exceptions been considered reconstructive rather than cosmetic surgery.[7]

By the 1930s, as surgeons came to agree that huge breasts were a mental and physical handicap to their bearers, breast reduction surgery became fairly well accepted in medical circles, and books and magazines began to inform their readers about its benefits. As Maxwell Maltz put it in *New Faces, New Futures,* "Not only is there considerable physical discomfort in continually carrying enlarged breasts . . . but this over-development also causes psychological disturbance in the growing girl who feels physically abnormal and, therefore, at a distinct disadvantage socially or economically. From this come maladjustment, discontent, unhappiness and misery." Writer Maxine Davis carried a similar message to *Pictorial Review* readers the following year. Although body sculpture was for the most part out of the question, Davis asserted, breast reduction was "the one type of remodeling of the figure" that works: "Oversized, pendulous, or asymmetrical breasts are sometimes a tragic psychological handicap to young girls. In professions where appearance is important, they constitute a serious economic liability, as in the case of actresses, or women in the fashion industries." Davis assured her readers of the operation's safety and stressed that it was not cosmetic: "The reputable surgeon makes sure the operation is a psychological or a social or an economic necessity."[8]

Not all Americans were comfortable categorizing breast reduction as reconstructive. Some, in the 1930s, still thought it smacked of vanity, and criticized patients who desired it and surgeons who performed it. Philadelphia surgeon Hans May met this critique head on in a 1939 article. Breast reduction, he wrote, "is not merely a cosmetic operation due to vanity of the fair sex . . . the trend of modern times [is] influenced by active sports and styles. . . . Thus pendulous breasts are apt to be a physical and psychic handicap, resulting in inferiority complexes. When it is possible to correct a breast deformity safely and satisfactorily and thus restore the happiness of the patient, plastic reconstruction of the breast is a justifiable operation." In an article in *Independent Woman* that same year, writer Lois Mattox Miller made the same point. Many requests for breast reduction, she noted, "are motivated by vanity and the desire for a more fashionable figure; but most physicians and psychiatrists now admit that there are innumerable cases in which it is not only advisable but essential to a woman's mental and emotional well-being." As evidence, Miller offered the story of a young girl who in her teens developed "abnormally large breasts. At first, she tried all sorts of brassieres, never wore a swim suit, and avoided all occasions that called for evening dress." The girl's father, a physician, viewed surgery as vanity, but when he "noticed alarming changes in her personality, a tendency toward solitude and melancholy," he consented to the operation, with good results. "According to this doctor, the psychological change in his daughter . . . was amazing. She blossomed out, renewed old acquaintances, and married a few years later."[9]

Breast reduction's defenders often stressed its transformative potential. The story of the doctor's daughter provided a perfect example of these benefits, and it found its way into quite a few articles for lay readers. In 1943, for example, *Parents Magazine* used the same story to encourage parents to take their children's problems seriously. "Young girls often suffer untold embarrassment because of overdeveloped, pendulous breasts," the article noted, but adults too often minimized their concerns. One doctor who did not believe in it changed his mind when the patient was his daughter: "He had a chance to observe intimately in his own home environment the psychological effects of this handicap on the girl's personality. She was becoming morose, withdrawn, and anxious to avoid normal social contacts. He consented to an operation and the results in terms of her new poise and better adjustment to life made him an enthusiastic convert." *McCalls,* too, stressed transfiguring effects. In a 1948 article, writer Marguerite Clark narrated the story of twenty-two-year-old Ruth. Ruth was pretty and slender, but her huge breasts were making her "bitterly unhappy." Clark checked in with Ruth three months after surgery and found that "her whole body had undergone a miraculous change. Her posture was correct, her carriage proud. Her small, well-proportioned breasts matched the lines of her slender, 22-year-old body. She wore a trim tailored suit and a bright sweater—a combination that she had always longed to wear." Even more striking, to Clark, was the alteration in Ruth's outlook. "The change was not in the girl's body alone," she wrote. "The confident look in her brown eyes showed new poise and healthy self-assurance. *Plastic surgery at its modern best had reconstructed her abnormally large, prolapsed breasts into youthful, normal contours, and in so doing, had lifted the burden of a painfully unhappy and neurotic girlhood."* [10]

Mothers who read such stories with one eye on their adolescent daughters learned that they, too, could benefit from breast reduction surgery. As writer Elizabeth Honor explained in *Cosmopolitan* in 1956, "One housewife endured for years the physical discomfort of shoulder-straps cutting cruelly into her flesh . . . perspiration rashes in hot weather, and the backaches and stoopshoulders which had developed because of the excessive weight of her breasts; she had endured embarrassment that caused her to bind her breasts painfully tight in an attempt to look 'normal,'" but only upon noticing her daughter's discomfort did she consult a plastic surgeon. "So gratified were the woman and her husband with their daughter's new mental and physical health that two months later the mother underwent the same operation. Because she waited so long, she will always remain stoop-shouldered, and some of her psychological scars, too, will remain, but she is free of discomfort and embarrassment." Twenty years later, Ginny Evans told her own story to *Good Housekeeping*. At 5'2" and 117 pounds, Evans was a 34D. She had a hard time growing up, but until her mid-thirties had remained committed to accepting herself the way she was. At thirty-six, after ten years of marriage, increased pain and discomfort led her to change her mind. "For the first time in my life I feel good about my body," Evans exclaimed; she hoped her story would inspire other women to follow her example. [11]

Some Americans voiced misgivings about tampering with what, in this culture, is accepted as the most obvious marker of femininity. The explanations Americans formulated to cover other forms of cosmetic surgery, most notably the inferiority complex, clearly applied to breast reduction, but in most cases the observable, documented physical problems caused by huge breasts obviated the need for more involved explanations. The number of such surgeries increases yearly. In 1984, for example, 38,000 women opted for breast reduction, an increase of 18 percent since 1981; in 1992, 2,500 teenagers were among surgeons' clients. [12]

Early Attempts at Augmentation

Most surgeons did not begin to address the problem of small breasts until after World War II. Dr. Robert Gersuny of Vienna pioneered the use of paraffin injections for breast augmentation in the 1890s, but paraffin in the breast was found to cause as many, if not more, problems than paraffin anywhere else, and by World War I the practice had been largely abandoned. In the 1920s and 1930s, some surgeons experimented with a technique known as autologous fat transplantation, in which fatty tissue was transferred surgically from the abdomen and buttocks to the breast, but they found that the body tended to reabsorb fat quickly, sometimes in unshapely ways, and that the lumps that resulted from this process made the early detection of cancer difficult (proponents of the penile enhancement technique that became popular in the early 1990s would have done well to take note of this). The inevitable scarring of the donor sites was also deemed an unsatisfactory trade-off. The solution of the 1940s—transplants that included most of the dermis, in an effort to ensure that the grafts would not die—had similar results. As late as 1944, the *Archives of Surgery* recommended simply that surgeons learn how to construct "external prostheses of sponge rubber" for those women suffering from "congenital atrophy or absence of the breasts." Some physicians were reportedly prescribing estrogen injections for breast growth, but most simply did not define small breasts as a medical problem. As Marguerite Clark admonished *McCalls* readers in 1948, surgeons did not often agree to operate on small breasts "because women with small, infantile breasts do not suffer so much physical and psychological discomfort. These conscientious surgeons have neither time nor sympathy for vanity and vague longing for a beautiful body."[13]

Surgeons began the postwar years with a distinct lack of sympathy for the problems of small-breasted women, but this attitude changed quickly as women—encouraged by fashion magazines and inspired by movie stars such as Jane Russell and Marilyn Monroe to fill out Dior's "new look"—clamored for new solutions. Perhaps inevitably, Los Angeles surgeons were among the pioneers. In an article published in *Plastic and Reconstructive Surgery* in 1950, cosmetic surgery champion H. O. Bames identified three types of breast deformity: hypomastia, hypermastia, and gigantomastia. Surgeons had learned how to deal with the second two, Bames wrote, but were only beginning to realize that the first was just as deserving of attention: "Hypomastia causes psychological rather than physical distress. Its correction has been receiving increased attention only since our 'cult of the body beautiful' has revealed its existence in rather large numbers." Manufacture of "falsies" had become a multimillion dollar industry, but surgery offered a better solution. In this article, Bames proposed "reshaping" the breast to create "firmness, conical contour and fullness of bosom directly above the breast," which, while it did not alter "geometric measurements," would result in lifted morale and increased happiness. Just three years later, he introduced a new technique designed to address the geometry problem. "Free fat grafts with gluteal fat," he proposed, which, if accompanied by the fascia, provided rich tissue for vascularization (blood flow) on both sides of the graft, could solve the problems earlier fat transplantation techniques had had. The technique Bames pioneered did seem to ensure that grafts would not die, and it apparently became common for a time, but other problems remained. Over time, surgeons and patients found, the unpredictable tendency of the body to absorb these grafts led to asymmetry, and, as with earlier techniques, donor areas were left severely scarred.[14]

As Bames attempted to balance buttocks and breasts, another Hollywood surgeon stepped into the limelight. In August 1953, an issue of *Pageant,* a popular Sunday newspaper supplement, was distributed in a white paper wrapper bearing the legend, in boldface type, "The Operation That Remolds Flat-Chested Women." The article did not specify how the remolding was achieved, but it did inform readers that Los Angeles plastic surgeon Robert Alan Franklyn had invented a new and unique method for helping the more than four million women in the United States who suffered from the serious disease of "micromastia."[15]

In *Beauty Surgeon,* an as-told-to autobiography published in 1960, Franklyn recounted the background of his discovery. His idols, Berlin's Jacques Joseph and New York's J. Eastman Sheehan, had lived in a time when small breasts were not regarded as problems. By the 1940s, however, "the mores of our times had glorified the bountiful breast and a new beauty problem had been created," and Franklyn resolved to solve it. Franklyn's interest was piqued toward the end of World War II when he observed imitation foam rubber (later called polyurethane), which German chemists had invented during the war. After several years he succeeded in importing a sample of the raw material and found a fabricator in the United States. "Endless hours, endless weeks" of tests later, "Surgifoam"—which, according to Franklyn, was lightweight, durable, resistant to bacteria and fungi, nonallergenic, easily sterilized, and easily shaped—was born.[16]

Franklyn's colleagues in the medical world reacted to his discovery—and the manner in which he chose to publicize it—with anger and disdain. A November 1953 column in the *Journal of the American*

"The Story of Linda Lee—A triumph of beauty surgery over misery," which illustrated Dr. Robert Alan Franklyn's 1960 book *Beauty Surgeon,* put the inferiority complex in a new context.

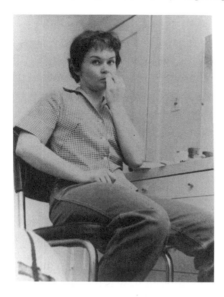

"Let's call her Linda Lee because that is not her name. Let me sketch her as she was [in] those uncertain days before she visited my office. She wore clothes she hoped would hide the fact that she was flat-chested. When she talked of her problem, she could not face it. She used such indirect words as, 'My bosom is very small.' She did not, she could not, say, 'I have no bosom at all.'"

"She was a lonely girl. She rarely had a date. She would go to the corner drugstore or the high school cafeteria and try to become part of the crowd, but the fact that she was under-endowed as a woman had already left a strong imprint on her personality. She was withdrawn, shy, insecure. She had an inferiority complex that made her manner abrupt and discourteous."

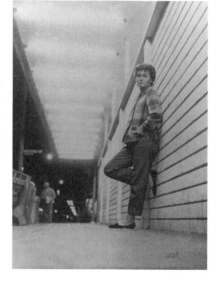

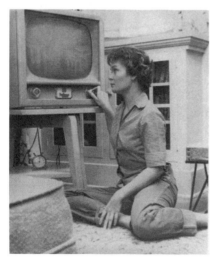

"As a child, she told me later, she had been full of confidence—a bright, light-hearted, warm-hearted girl. She had been pretty, and the problem of a flat chest had not yet colored her personality. Later she had wanted to retire from life. I privately wondered if she had made any attempt at suicide as some of my patients, in desperation, had done."

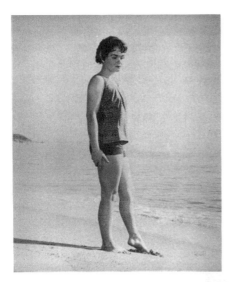

"She hated to be seen on a beach, and never removed the loose blouse she wore to hide her flat chest or joined other young people in their fun in the water."

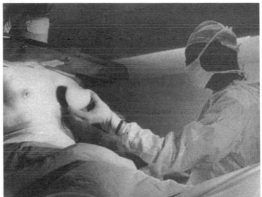

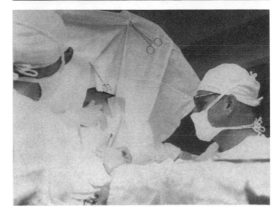

"The day of the operation, she was not nervous. She gave me a shy little smile, almost afraid her dream would not come true."

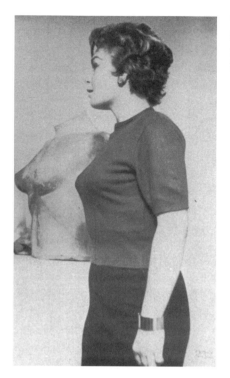

"When she came out of surgery, she looked down at her bosom. Although heavily bandaged, she could see she had a new figure. She started to cry. Rarely have I been so moved."

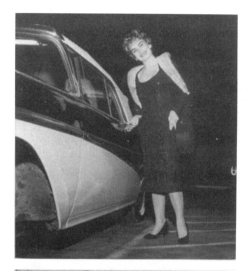

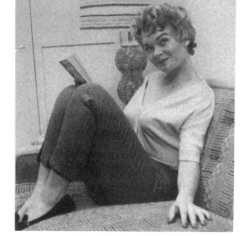

"When she went out into life a few weeks later, she was a changed girl. She was wearing figure-revealing clothes. She had a new self-confidence that warmed my heart."

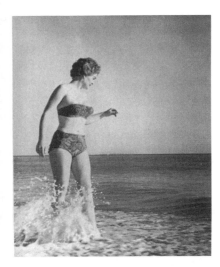

"She began having dates, going to the beach—something, incidentally, that she had avoided since she was fifteen."

"In time, she dropped by to see me with that special young man. You can always tell it's *the* special young man by the stars in a young girl's eyes. You could see his admiration for her voluptuous figure in his eyes. You could also see his depth of character as he explained to me that Linda Lee had told him about her before and after operation. He told me, quite earnestly, that he would have fallen in love with her if she had been as flat as the desert."

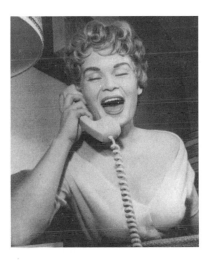

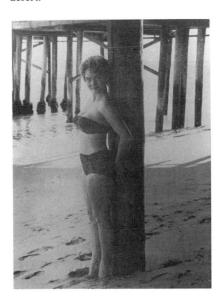

"I smiled a little. They had met at the beach."

Medical Association dismissed the *Pageant* article as "basically self-promotion," noting that an investigation sparked by the article had concluded that the unnamed product was probably the Ivalon (or polyvinyl) sponge with which other surgeons were already experimenting. According to *JAMA*, Franklyn's history and credentials were as suspect as his "new" invention. He had graduated from the New York University College of Medicine sometime in the 1940s and had been licensed in New York in 1942 and in California and New Jersey the following year. There were "indications"—but no proof—that he had served residencies in anesthesiology and dermatology. He was neither a member of a specialist society nor a diplomate of a specialist board, and he had not joined the local or national medical societies. But it was Franklyn's self-aggrandizing behavior that most troubled his colleagues. It was "strange indeed," the article concluded, "that a physician would permit publication of the details of a surgical procedure in a popular magazine when such procedure does not appear to have the benefit of exhaustive tests on animals to establish its safety and efficacy," but perhaps no stranger than the fact that Franklyn's Hollywood phone number was listed in the Miami, Florida, classified pages under "Physicians and Surgeons—Plastic Surgery."[17]

Dr. Walter C. Alvarez, in 1954 an emeritus consultant to the Mayo Clinic, tackled Franklyn on his own turf with a January 11, 1954, article in the *Los Angeles Times* headlined "Operations on Bosoms Dangerous," in which he warned women of the dangers such surgery might pose. William Kiskadden, another Los Angeles plastic surgeon, carried the message to medical professionals. In a January 1955 article by the same name, Kiskadden summarized for plastic surgeons the debate over the Ivalon sponge and advised that they refrain from performing the operation. Other surgeons, too, advocated a cautious approach, in part because sponge augmentation continued to generate problems. In 1958, two surgeons reported that they had begun to use the Ivalon sponge after finding that augmentation with fat grafts failed when the grafts liquefied. For a time, Ivalon had seemed a satisfactory alternative, and the surgeons were pleased to report "good results" in twelve women (a total of twenty-four breasts). They noted, however, that one patient complained of hardening, and all were disappointed that a 25 percent reduction occurred in the initial breast volume they had achieved when the sponges shrank. This, combined with the possible cancer risk, led these surgeons to recommend against mammary augmentation using sponges.

Much of the outcry, however, appeared to center on the messenger rather than the product. Franklyn himself commented on this, attributing other surgeons' less-than-favorable reaction in part to professional jealousy and in part to the age-old prejudice against cosmetic surgery. Gradually, sponges of varying synthetic sorts entered the arsenal of cosmetic surgery; in addition to Ivalon, several others (including Polistan, discovered in 1959, Etheron, introduced in 1960, and Hydron, a latecomer in 1961) were used throughout the 1950s and early 1960s.[18]

When he tried to explain why he had devoted so much time and energy to developing a technique for breast augmentation, Franklyn, like other surgeons, pointed directly to American consumer culture, which (in the years after World War II) raised the "sweater girl" to a cultural icon. Movie posters and *Playboy* magazine glorified breasts that defied gravity; brassiere and bathing suit manufacturers employed innovative structural engineering techniques that made this defiance possible; Sears, in its 1951 catalog, offered twenty-two different kinds of "falsies" for those who were unable to fill out these new garments unaided. The vogue of the "hourglass figure," Franklyn explained, meant that thousands of "girls and women whose neuroses had been traced definitely to the fact they were flat-chested" were desperate for new techniques that would release them from the bondage of inferiority.[19]

Popular magazine articles suggest that many Americans viewed breast augmentation surgery in this light. Under the heading "Monroes on the Increase," *Cosmopolitan,* in 1956, noted, "Emphasis in our society on the beautiful bust has become so extreme that there was little surprise in psychological circles when a teen-aged girl just recently committed suicide because she was flat-chested. How much misery this condition causes is not known." A similar article in *Lady's Circle* carried the following information under the heading "Flat-Chested Females": "Women who feel socially inferior because of small breasts and flat chests have resorted to plastic operations in which resilient pads of inert plastic-foam sponge are placed beneath the wall of the chest and the glandular tissues. This builds up the breasts to satisfactory proportions." Both of these articles noted that breast augmentation techniques were still experimental: *Cosmopolitan* specifically advised women that the new technique of augmentation with plastic sponges, which was generating "a great deal of excitement among lay people," was unpredictable, while *Lady's Circle* cautioned that plastic surgeons were increasingly dubious about operations involving sponges, concluding, "a woman who feels her marriage is in jeopardy because of small breasts is best treated, together with her husband, by a competent psychiatrist." At the same time, however, the articles expressed sympathy for women so afflicted and hope that new solutions would be forthcoming.[20]

The combination of increasing demand and more publicity called surgeons' attention to the psychological implications of breast surgery. In 1958, plastic surgeon Milton T. Edgerton and psychiatrist A. R. McClary, both of the Johns Hopkins University, published a pioneering article on the psychiatry of breast augmentation. "Literally thousands of women, in this country alone," they wrote, "are seriously disturbed by feelings of inadequacy in regard to concepts of the body image. Partly as a result of exposure to advertising propaganda and questionable publicity, many physically normal women develop an almost paralyzing self-consciousness focused on the feeling that they do not have the correct size bosom. Whether one views them as the victims of the attitudes of a crass society, or as uniquely distorted character problems in a psychiatric sense, none-the-less, their lives and often the lives of their husbands and families are made miserable by the development of such conflicts." The questions this raised for surgeons were several. What procedure would be "safe, simple and satisfactory"? If such a procedure were found, would it solve patients' emotional problems? And how were surgeons to predict which cases might be solved surgically?[21]

In an attempt to shed light on these questions, the authors had studied thirteen women who had received Ivalon sponge implants since 1950; the study was supplemented with random observations drawn from nineteen additional cases. All of the thirty-two women shared a conviction that "wearing padded bras or falsies was 'phony,' 'cheating,' and made the feeling of inadequacy even worse." Recalling the justification for clean underwear parroted by generations of American mothers, one patient explained, "One might be in an accident and be found out and feel so ashamed that one couldn't face people again." More than half of the women had first learned of the operation through popular magazines. Despite these patients' diversity—there was "no uniformity of psychiatric diagnosis, social position, economic or education level, occupation or religion"—the investigators found that results in all cases were "unusually satisfactory," suggesting that breast augmentation could cure a variety of ills. All but two of the patients were "extremely pleased," and comments like "changed my entire life" were common. The authors noted that while they had initially suspected that such changes in self-image would not hold up over time, in all patients they had. Despite their positive findings, Edgerton and McClary ended on a cautious (and as later experience would prove, eerily prophetic) note that acknowledged the still-experimental status of this technique: "Every patient must be clearly apprised of the newness of the method and the possibility of being recalled to the hospital at some future time for removal of the implants, if any late unfavorable tissue reaction should develop. Any surgeon not willing to shoulder this responsibility should probably not use the material on patients with a long life-expectancy."[22]

Three years later, citing the "startling amount of interest" generated by the first article, Edgerton again addressed breast augmentation's psychological effects. Although he remained cautious about the physical ramifications, the mental ones were clear. In many cases, he wrote, women "have actively used the operation to catalyze a series of effective changes in their living situations. It is important that plastic surgeons continue to learn more about this latter group in hopes that we may understand how anatomic changes that produce 'happiness' may be reflected in the lives of the patients and those close to them."[23]

Silicone Produces the Perfect 36

Most patients who had had their breasts augmented with sponge implants were happier postoperatively, Edgerton and his colleagues found, but porous materials like Ivalon continued to cause problems. The most significant problem was hardening: over time, recipients and surgeons found, breast tissue would not only contract around the sponges but would infiltrate them, filling in the pores. Removal became difficult, if not impossible, and often resulted in significant scars and deformities. Surgeons thus kept searching for a better solution.

The injection of liquid silicone as a means of augmenting the female breast has been, since its very beginning, largely an underground practice, and its roots are difficult to trace. Board-certified plastic surgeons seem not to have adopted this practice in large numbers, and they were among the most vocal and committed critics once problems began to surface. But while plastic surgeons, in general, did not inject silicone, patients and other doctors perceived this practice as within the realm of cosmetic surgery. In many ways the story of liquid silicone recalls the earlier story of paraffin. Like that story, it is concerned with the widespread popularization of an experimental technique with disastrous results. Then, too, it shows clearly the limits of authority wielded by the members of organized medicine: plastic surgeons could neither control the practice nor prevent it from being connected with their specialty. More significantly, however, it suggests the ways in which American attitudes toward vanity have shaped American responses to medical practices. Unlike other augmentation techniques, reconstruction seems never to have been an issue in silicone injection. The practice was, from the beginning, acknowledged as purely cosmetic, and its early association with topless dancers and Las Vegas showgirls generated jokes, laughs, and shoulder shrugs rather than serious medical consideration.

If penicillin was the wonder drug of American medicine at mid-century, silicones were a wonder product of American industry. Chemists had been exploring the world of silicones for years, but not until 1943, when the Corning Glass Works and Dow Chemical Company joined to form Dow Corning Corporation to make silicone materials needed for the war effort (such as an engine lubricant that would not break down at high temperatures) did the product come of age. By the war's end, researchers had begun to identify other applications. In 1946, several researchers reported that storage in siliconized bottles prolonged the clotting time of blood. In 1950, silicone rubber tubing was used to replace a damaged urethra, and in 1955 Dow Corning again used silicone rubber to manufacture the first successful shunt for draining excess cerebrospinal fluid in hydrocephalic children. Requests for samples and for specific products and information were so numerous that in January 1959 Dow Corning's board of directors established the Dow Corning Center for Aid to Medical Research to coordinate the diverse requests and the company's efforts.[24]

Accounts differ as to when, and by whom, liquid silicone was first used to enlarge small breasts, but all locate it around World War II and most locate it in Japan (according to one report, Japanese surgeons first used silicone to plump out legs withered by polio). The widespread publicity later accorded the Japanese sakurai formula, invented in 1954, supports the attribution of this technique to Japanese physicians, although several other accounts place the invention earlier. According to the *New York Times,* Japanese cosmetologists pioneered the use of silicone to enlarge the breasts of Japanese prostitutes during the war, after such solutions as goats' milk and paraffin were found wanting.[25]

American physician Harvey D. Kagan claimed to have used Dow Corning 200 Fluid, an industrial silicone, as a means of breast augmentation as early as 1946, but not until the mid-1960s did the practice of injecting liquid silicone first receive widespread attention in the United States. Some of this attention was generated by doctors themselves. At the 1964 annual scientific meeting of the American Oto-rhinologic Society for Plastic Surgery, for example, a *Chicago Daily News* reporter found that doctors talked freely among themselves about liquid silicone, the "amazing liquid chemical that turns old faces into new." Doctors also discussed the technique's drawbacks—primarily that long-range effects were unknown—and, fearful of publicity, clammed up when they found a reporter in their ranks. According to this reporter, surgeons were more enthusiastic than they were willing to let on; even one of the most conservative surgeons present admitted, "It would appear to signal a definite revolution in the area of cosmetic surgery."[26]

Some surgeons and physicians continued to voice their optimism about liquid silicone, but widespread revelations about negative sequelae had begun, by the mid-1960s, to cool the ardor of others. In 1964, concerned about such reports, Dow Corning had voluntarily listed liquid silicone with the Food and Drug Administration as a drug rather than an implant material; the FDA reclassified liquid silicone as a new drug in early 1965, in an attempt to restrict its use. Only the seven plastic surgeons and one dermatologist who had agreed to participate in the experimental studies sponsored by Dow Corning's Center for Aid to Medical Research were allowed access to medical-grade silicone manufactured by Dow Corning; others were required to file an affidavit with the company certifying that the material would not be used for injection into humans.[27]

The actions of Dow Corning and the FDA generated a wave of publicity about the silicone injection industry. Because silicone injections had been particularly popular with dancers and showgirls, the practice of silicone injection had been most popular on the west coast, and much of the publicity surfaced there. In November 1965, for example, the *San Francisco Chronicle* reported on the new industry that silicone had spawned. Two dancers at Big Al's, a popular North Beach topless club, had set the city on fire with their silicone-enhanced bosoms. Carol Doda and another unnamed woman had each received weekly injections of one-half ounce of liquid silicone over a period of about twenty weeks. In all, each woman had received nearly a pint of liquid silicone

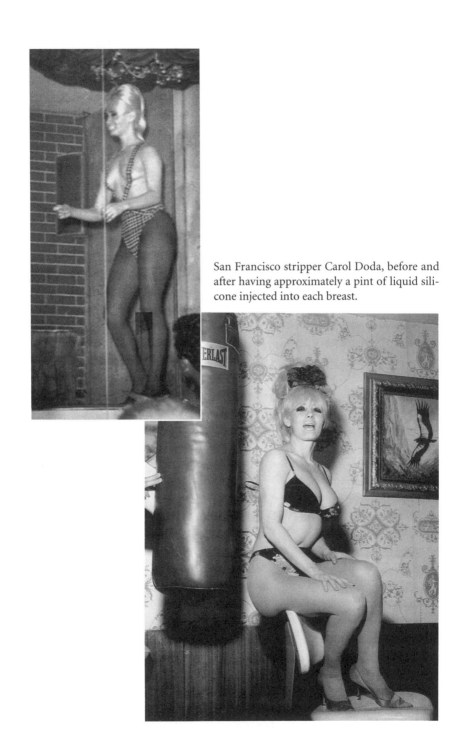

San Francisco stripper Carol Doda, before and after having approximately a pint of liquid silicone injected into each breast.

in each breast. To accommodate and protect their new accoutrements, the women wore special support garments twenty-four hours a day when not on stage. Both women were proud of their achievement. As Doda explained, "I believe in self improvement. If you don't make yourself better, you might just as well be dormant." And they were happy to share their experiences with others: "Why lots of times a man will come in here with his wife or date; she'll be kind of flat and I can see her looking at me all through my act," the other dancer explained. "Then she'll write me a letter—she's ashamed of her looks and wants to know who my doctor was. I always tell them."[28]

By the time this article appeared, however, the injections were hard to find in San Francisco. Only Big Al's house doctor would admit to having given them at all, and even he insisted that he had dropped the practice six months before. Surgeons Mark Gorney of San Francisco and Paul Schneider of Oakland, with Dow Corning's Silas Braley, cautioned the paper's readers that, with the exception of the registered members of the Dow Corning study group, anyone who was injecting liquid silicone was either using up medical-grade fluid that had been legally available until 1964 or using toxic or illegal substances. New side effects were still being discovered, but this at least was known: silicone, after injection, tended to migrate, turning up in lymph nodes and other areas of the body; it also formed lumps (which surgeons, recalling paraffin's similar tendency, termed granulomas) that could mask (and prevent early detection of) breast cancer. At worst, then, silicone injections could result in amputation, and at the very least all recipients were expected to have "pendulous breasts" by the time they were forty. Despite this knowledge, the *Chronicle* asserted, women continued to demand and to receive injections, often resorting to the flourishing black market that had grown up in cities like Los Angeles and Las Vegas.[29]

As a lighthearted editorial entitled "Abreast of the Times" (published in *JAMA* in 1966) suggests, some medical practitioners had trouble taking the silicone injection industry seriously. "We live in a 'mammoriented' world," *JAMA* noted. "Breast size, within certain expanding limits, has become an aesthetic criterion." The editorial reminded doctors that due to "some evidence of problems" silicone was considered a drug and the practice of mammary injection was illegal, but concluded humorously, "the ladies must await either the clearance of the drug by the FDA . . . or a return to fashion of the less voluptuous figure characteristic of the 1920's and 1930's." As problems continued to surface, however, medical practitioners took notice. Franklin Ashley, a Los Angeles plastic surgeon and participant in the Dow Corning study, warned his colleagues in 1967 that "the high incidence of carcinoma of the breast and the large number of women who had silicone injections into the breasts present a combination of circumstances that unquestionably will pose future problems." Two years later, Khoo Boo-Chai cited Japan's long experience with silicone-injected breasts as a reason for caution. Horror stories continued to surface as surgeons attempted to treat women who had received injections. In November 1969, a North Carolina plastic surgeon reported the case of a thirty-one-year-old Caucasian female who had received injections from an osteopath in Las Vegas in 1965. When he saw the woman approximately a year and a half later, both breasts were infected and had to be amputated. Such stories multiplied throughout the late 1960s and early 1970s. By 1971 the FDA had determined that at least four women had died from silicone embolisms that had formed after injection.[30]

Despite negative publicity, however, women continued to seek out, and seemed to have little trouble finding, practitioners willing to inject their breasts with silicone. The affidavit program instituted by Dow Corning did restrict access to Dow Corning–manufactured medical-grade silicone, but even in this limited arena it was not foolproof. In at least one case, the company stuck to its guns, refusing to supply medical-grade silicone to a California plastic surgeon who requested it to continue his breast augmentation business and threatened to use industrial-grade silicone if the company would not comply. In 1967, however, Dow Corning pled no contest and paid a $5,000 fine for having shipped liquid silicone illegally three years earlier. And, as Dow Corning frequently pointed out in response to criticism, industrial grades of liquid silicone were readily available from at least three—and perhaps as many as fourteen—manufacturers in the United States alone.[31]

Legislation to limit the practice seemed only to drive it underground or over the border. In 1974, for example, the new disease of "Tijuana Silicone Rot" surfaced in the press. Since 1967, the *San Francisco Chronicle* reported, surgeons in San Diego and Tijuana had seen almost four hundred women who had received injections with industrial-grade silicone in several Mexican border cities. In one case, a forty-year-old divorcée had answered a personal advertisement in a suburban San Diego newspaper that promised "silicone for a beautiful bust." A woman visited her at home and sang the praises of a "perfectly wonderful safe treatment" that did not involve surgery. For $800, the divorcée went from flat to a 38B. Her initial joy gave way to despair when, just eighteen months later, both breasts—now infected and gangrenous—had to be amputated. In 1975, the *Chronicle* reported, surgeons suspected that more than twelve thousand women had received silicone injections in Las Vegas alone; more than a hundred women a year were seeking help for conditions ranging from discoloration to gangrene that developed anywhere from one to fourteen years later. That same year, *Esquire* profiled an itinerant orthopedist who had begun injecting breasts after dabbling in psychotherapy, hypnosis, cybernetics, and acupuncture (he had then lost his license and served time for performing an illegal abortion). "Dr. Jack" claimed to have injected five thousand breasts in ten states since 1963.[32]

Despite attempts at regulation, the industry continued to flourish for several reasons. Silicone injection was relatively easy for both patients and practitioners. It seemed the ultimate solution for cosmetic purposes because it appeared to provide all the benefits of surgery, without the dangers and inconveniences, in an outpatient setting. Then, too, reports about the dangers of the practice varied widely. Although they were not sure about medical-grade silicone's effects on the body, medical and lay commentators often attributed problems to the use of impure, industrial silicone, to the use of additives such as peanut or olive oil, or to the use of other substances altogether. The connection with breast cancer followed this path. Surgeons almost unanimously advised against using silicone in the breast not because it might cause cancer but because it might mask cancer. Physicians did not see much difference, but women did, and this explanation did not deter them; they weighed the options and chose the short-term advantage of breast enlargement over the longer-term disadvantage that cancer might go undetected. In the euphoric, confident world of postwar America, surgeons and patients alike seemed to share a conviction that every discovery meant progress and a concurrent belief that nothing could go seriously wrong. As surgeon John Conley put it in 1968, the "unfortunate use of paraffin" in the early twentieth century and its terrible sequelae were "a tragedy of injectional augmentation," but "there is little chance of this happening today, with the excellent protection provided by public health controls and the higher standards of the practitioner." Finally, and perhaps most important, for some women, this faith in progress was accompanied by

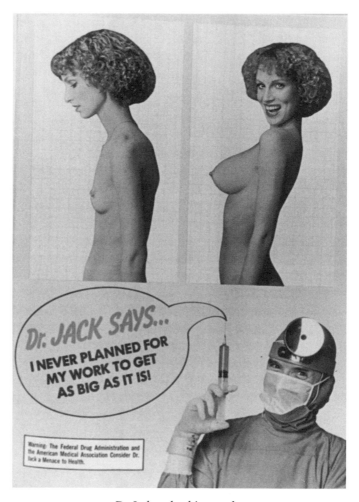

Dr. Jack makes his rounds.

a distrust of organized medicine. These women, desperate for larger breasts, believed that a perfect method for breast enlargement existed and that the only reason hospitals did not offer it was that physicians did not take women's concerns seriously. By going "outside" regular channels, these women believed, they were criticizing organized medicine for not responding to their needs at the same time they were getting those needs met—a heady and unfortunate combination that, among other things, suggests how wide was the gulf that had developed between women and their doctors.[33]

While surgeons concurred that injection into breast tissue was ill-advised, the information prospective patients received varied widely: many doctors and surgeons continued to rely on liquid silicone as a solution to other cosmetic problems, and magazines continued to tout it as a potential miracle cure. In 1967, for example, *Harper's Bazaar* reminded its readers that in 1964 it had run a "carefully considered, ultimately cautionary piece" about silicone injections, but that it was now, with the publication of an extremely laudatory article, revising its advice: "Less than two and a half years later, we can state on excellent authority that silicone injection therapy is here—and now. No longer in the throes of original experiment, it has become accepted procedure among some highly respected doctors as cosmetic rehabilitation." *Vogue*, in 1971, described silicone as a marvelous product on the forefront of medical history, limited only by the puritanical stance of the FDA. In 1972, *W,* the fashion industry bible, credited "a relatively inexpensive and quickly produced network of silicone"—not leisure and money—with "keep[ing] Beautiful People beautiful." Michael Kalman, a dermatologist with New York's Orentreich Group who had been using silicone since 1967, assured *W* readers that the use of pure medical-grade silicone guaranteed success. The article specified that faces only were under discussion and quoted Kalman as saying "we prefer not to inject it into the breast," but the headline—"Silicone isn't a youth pill and it can't work miracles. But injections, doctors say, can do everything from filling up facial lines to perking up sagging breasts"—encouraged speculation. An article in *Newsweek* that same year painted silicone as popular among the glamourous, adventurous set: "The cosmetic wonders of liquid silicone have been discovered by jet-set sophisticates. And while the use of silicone remains highly controversial, such injections have become increasingly popular for shaping up other parts of the would-be body beautiful." *Newsweek* noted that access to medical-grade liquid silicone was restricted, but asserted that "more than a dozen U.S. and overseas firms make the product and hundreds of American doctors use it for cosmetic purposes." Phyllis Diller, one of the few injectees willing to talk, put a humorous spin on her experience that typified many commentators' attitude toward this practice. "It gave my psyche a big lift and helped my career," she told *Newsweek*. "I just hope to hell it isn't the type of silicone that travels. I don't want swollen ankles."[34]

The question of why the story of silicone injections developed in the way it did is difficult to answer. Whether one psychoanalyzes this desire or not, it seems clear that postwar fashions played a role in shaping women's wish for, and commitment to getting, larger breasts. The relative ease and low cost of silicone injections made them more appealing than surgery, particularly for insecure young women. Ginny, who was profiled in *Ms.* magazine's exposé of the injection industry, fit this bill. In 1970, Ginny was seventeen and frantic. She could not afford surgery and instead found a local pediatrician with a sideline in silicone who told her that the "chances [of something bad happening] are so minimal that you shouldn't even think about it"; she received three injections at $50 each.

The medical profession's response, which was initially lighthearted and never consistent, probably played a role in the way the story developed, as did the nation's journalists, who joked about the practice even as they reported its drawbacks and dangers. By the 1970s, the baby boom generation's tendency to distrust authority figures—sparked by Sputnik and fanned by Lyndon Johnson and Richard Nixon—may have come into play; the generation that was injecting itself was the most likely to discount the federal government's advice not to. *Esquire,* in its 1975 profile of Dr. Jack, seemed to exemplify this attitude. Silicone gel implants, the author conceded, had an advantage in that they did not appear to mask cancer, as injections often did. "Beyond that," the author asserted, "it's pretty questionable whether implants are, necessarily, inherently, safer than injections (as the A.M.A. likes to contend), except insofar as implantations are performed under uniform circumstances by answerable physicians, which is clearly not the case with injections." And aesthetically, *Esquire* noted, injections were much more pleasing.[35]

The injection debacle, however, was shaped as much by American cultural attitudes toward beauty and vanity as by the specific episode itself. To some degree, the medical profession's initial response, the FDA's seeming inability to put forth a coherent story, and the nation's journalists' refusal to take the issue seriously merely testified to the delicacy of the tightrope on which American women have historically balanced in their pursuit of beauty. Being beautiful, American women learn, is important, but caring too much and trying too hard (and letting that desperate effort show) destroys the effect: true beauty must be (or at least look) effortless; a too-obvious effort reveals vanity. Insisting that the personal is in no way political—a stance that would be challenged, albeit briefly, by feminism's second wave—this framework requires that women fight these embarrassing battles alone and preferably in the dark. The women who revealed their infected and traumatized breasts in the glare of media attention also exposed the impossible dilemma American women have faced. The response—that women who were silly enough to get silicone injections deserved what they got—rebuked them for this trespass. Significantly, this view resurfaced in the recent controversy over implants, when several commentators, including the *Wall Street Journal*, proposed that America's emphasis on free will and self-determination mandated that women be able to determine for themselves the risks they will take. Although this is clearly an important strand in American culture, it is one that has been applied selectively. Its application in this case seems to suggest that some Americans believe that those who would risk health for beauty forfeit the right to protections routinely afforded other Americans.

Ginny's case suggests something of how this has played out. In 1978, after experiencing significant health problems, Ginny filed suit against Dow Corning and against the doctor who had injected the silicone eight years earlier. At that time, Dow Corning had been named as co-defendant in fifteen to twenty civil cases but had lost only once; in Ginny's case the judge dismissed the company from the case, and, despite the fact that half a dozen similar cases were pending against him, the jury decided in favor of the doctor. According to Patricia Kayajanian, Ginny's attorney, some jurors thought the doctor was at fault, but most simply had no sympathy with a woman who subjected herself to silicone breast injections. "Usually, way down deep inside," Kayajanian observed, "people feel that anybody who has cosmetic surgery deserves what she gets—especially when the juror can't afford it." When the trial ended, Ginny's physician was still in practice.[36]

The Invention of the Sac

Twenty-some years of less-than-satisfactory results might have persuaded patients and surgeons that women's breasts should be left alone, but patients continued to clamor for a solution and surgeons continued to search for one. In February 1961, disappointed with the results they had achieved and observed with sponge implants, plastic surgeon

Thomas D. Cronin, then chief of plastic surgery at St. Joseph Hospital in Houston, Texas, and his resident, Frank Gerow, visited Dow Corning to discuss alternatives. The eventual result—the first Silastic® mammary prosthesis, a silicone rubber envelope filled with liquid silicone—was implanted in March 1962. The implant was introduced the following year at the Third International Congress for Plastic and Reconstructive Surgery.[37]

New models were introduced almost yearly between 1964 and 1994, but the operation remained substantially the same. As in augmentation with open-pore sponges, the surgeon makes an incision of approximately two inches in the crease beneath the breast and inserts the implant. (Some surgeons prefer to make the incision around the areola or in the armpit, believing this creates a smaller scar, although others contend these incisions are not long enough to allow the surgeon to see and control bleeding adequately.) Because silicone implants are generally smooth-shelled, flesh does not permeate the implant, as occurred with open-pore sponges. In most cases, implants are placed between the pectoral muscle and the breast tissue, although some surgeons prefer to place the implant beneath the pectoral muscle.[38]

Early implants were not perfect. In the first designs, the rubber envelope was thick and had a wide edge that was palpable after implantation, and a sponge in the center (an attempt to reduce the weight of the implant) tended to harden. Varying amounts of dacron cloth attached to the sac in an attempt to ensure that it remained in place caused excessive scarring. Dow Corning, however, continued to refine the design. The amount of dacron fabric was reduced several times (eventually to nothing), and the edge was made still finer; in 1969 a seamless design was perfected, and in subsequent years scientists developed a thinner silicone for the envelope and a more fluid gel for the filling, in an attempt to achieve a more natural feel. In 1965, Dr. H. G. Arion introduced an alternative, the Simaplast inflatable prosthesis, which the surgeon would fill with saline after implantation, but the saline implant displayed a troubling tendency toward spontaneous deflation, and silicone had already conquered the market. That year, in a widely publicized study, surgeon Ralph Blocksma and Silas Braley of Dow Corning concluded that silicone fulfilled most if not all of the criteria defining the ideal soft tissue substitute for which surgeons had long been searching: it was, they asserted, not physically modified by soft tissue, chemically inert and noncarcinogenic; it produced no inflammation, no foreign body reaction, no stage of allergy or hypersensitivity. Unlike sponges, which surgeons had to carve and sterilize individually for each patient, silicone implants could be fabricated in the form desired and sterilized by the manufacturer before shipping.[39]

Although later significantly modified, the first implant offered to the profession after Cronin and Gerow's presentation—a sac with a narrow seam and a single patch of dacron on the back—was well received. In December 1964, two Salt Lake City surgeons reviewed seventy-four cases and concluded that (while not without complications) the Cronin-type silicone gel prosthesis was superior to all of the open-pore sponges then in use, including Ivalon, polyurethane, Etheron, Teflon, and silicone. Montreal surgeon Colette Perras came to a similar conclusion the following year. "The past two decades have centered such attention on this feminine loveliness [the breast]," Perras wrote in 1965, "that the small breasted woman is sometimes disturbed by a feeling of inadequacy, even though she may be happily married and have children." Perras had taken seriously women's "desire to be normal" and had experimented with a variety of alloplastic materials including "glass balls, terylene wool, ox cartilage, polyvinyl sponge, polyester sponge, and silastic sponge," but the new Cronin prosthesis, she found, was preferable to all.[40]

Surgeons' enthusiasm quickly found its way into the popular press. As *Time* reported in early 1964, "Whether a woman's motive is mere vanity or the need to restore the appearance after injury or surgery, there is an increasing variety of materials for building up the bosom. Doctors have tried everything from paraffin and glass balls to synthetic sponges and the patient's own body fat," but at the recent meeting of the American College of Surgeons, Dr. John R. Lewis Jr. of Atlanta had reported better results with Cronin's dacron-backed prosthesis. In 1970, in typical breathless style, *Cosmopolitan* summarized the new knowledge: "Silicone breast augmentation is the operation that everybody whispers about . . . yet it is actually among the leading 'cosmetic' operations today. . . . COSMO has received several hundred letters asking just these questions, usually from girls with fairly minuscule breasts. (Wouldn't *you* be concerned?)" According to "a leading plastic surgeon," Cosmo girls learned, women from all walks of life, from strippers to housewives, were having their breasts enlarged. Half were married and half were trying; 98 percent were very happy with the results. The implant,

Cosmo assured its readers, was inert and did not react to the body; post-operative sensation would be normal. Reflecting America's postwar fascination with all things plastic, the article concluded, "The fact of the matter is that surgically augmented breasts have a *better* contour than the real thing. They stand up . . . will not sag or droop or get flaccid. They're firm and solid."[41]

Though some accounts of breast implants were less positive than this one, throughout the 1970s and 1980s the information that women received about silicone implants was largely reassuring. Writer Simona Morini, in 1972, asserted that the silicone implant was the "modern solution" to the problem of small breasts: "a soft, resilient material, resembling real breasts in consistency and weight, that is non-allergenic, can safely be sterilized, cannot be absorbed by the body, and, above all, is not carcinogenic." Drs. Arthur and Stuart Frank, who wrote *Mademoiselle*'s "Health" column in the 1970s, also exuded confidence: "Although the Women's Movement has effectively de-emphasized the shape and size of women's breasts as objects of sexual attraction or derision, there has nevertheless been an unprecedented interest in methods and devices which alter the appearance of the breast, and an increasing frequency of requests for elective plastic surgery. . . . The surgery now is safe, relatively simple, effective and has few side effects." A slightly more cautious *Cosmo* noted in 1978 that "some ultraconservative doctors feel the evidence isn't all in yet [and advise against it]," but continued, "Like so many *other* medical matters today, there is no absolute unanimity of opinion, and so you must really assess the possible (faint) risks and decide for *yourself!*" In 1981, Dr. Charles E. Horton, professor of plastic surgery at the Eastern Virginia Medical School and former chairman of the American Board of Plastic Surgery, assured Cosmo girls that "Silicone implants . . . are still a good option." Four years later, New York surgeon Steven Herman described for *Glamour* readers the "psychological and vocational [modeling, for example]" benefits of breast augmentation; the article noted that capsular contraction occurred in 40 percent of cases but did not explain what this meant.[42]

Breast Reconstruction

Although authorities estimate that 80 percent of breast augmentations are undertaken for cosmetic reasons, the 20 percent sought for reconstruction after breast cancer has historically constituted a sizable and increasingly vocal minority. Medical factors, in part, account for the increased interest in breast reconstruction in the 1970s. The Cronin implant, which was then widely regarded as the first safe, simple, and successful technique, was significant: it caused doctors who had previously regarded reconstruction as too complicated to think again. The trend away from radical mastectomies (in which surgeons remove not only the breast and lymph nodes but the pectoral muscle as well) toward modified radical mastectomies (in which the breast and lymph nodes are removed but muscle and flesh are left in place) and more recently lumpectomies (in which only the tissue known to be cancerous is removed) played a role, as the more moderate operations left surgeons more to work with.

Cultural developments, however, played at least as significant a role. The women's movement of the 1970s called attention to issues of women's health in general and to the problems of breast cancer and breast reconstruction after cancer in particular. More significantly, women began to demand that medical caregivers take women's needs into account when treating breast cancer. Some women demanded that surgeons operate only to the extent necessary (in other words, perform a radical mastectomy only if the cancer had spread so far that a modified radical would endanger a woman's health). Others wanted surgeons to alter the practice, peculiar to the United States, of performing an immediate mastectomy if a biopsy indicated cancer. Women found this practice particularly callous because it gave them no time to adjust their expectations. A woman scheduled for a biopsy would go under the anesthetic not knowing whether she would be missing a breast when she woke up. Above all, however, women demanded that the medical profession revise its definition of vanity. Women wanted physicians to take seriously their need to put the experience of cancer behind them and begin life again with a reconstructed breast, rather than simply tell them how lucky they were to be alive.[43]

In 1975, both *Time* magazine and *Good Housekeeping* took up the issue of breast reconstruction; both articles tackled the issue of vanity and framed reconstruction as a feminist issue. According to *Good Housekeeping*, the number of women who had pursued reconstruction was still small, "probably fewer than 500." The fact that the technique was new and time-consuming, as well as the fact that so many surgeons "persisted" in performing radical mastectomies rather than the newer modified radicals, accounted for the low number, the magazine asserted, but more important was that "virtually all plastic and reconstructive surgery has been stigmatized as 'cosmetic,' associated with nose-bobbing and face lifting so that many successful surgeons dismiss it as 'vanity of vanities.'" *Time* emphasized the fact that more women were pursuing the option of reconstruction, rather than the fact that numbers were still low, but also mentioned the vanity problem: "In the past, many doctors dismissed such surgery as frivolous (some major insurance companies still refuse to pay for such 'vanity' operations)."[44]

Jean Zalon, whose book *I Am Whole Again* was excerpted in several magazines, and Betty Rollin, an NBC correspondent whose account of her battle with breast cancer, entitled *First You Cry,* became a bestseller as well as a made-for-TV movie starring Mary Tyler Moore, were among the many women who went public in the 1970s both to help women deal with the illness and to effect changes in the way the health care system dealt with breast cancer. Both had undergone breast reconstruction themselves and were ardent advocates of the procedure. In 1976, Rollin told *Family Circle* readers how the removal of a breast had affected her. After she had recovered from the mastectomy, she recalled, "I was not having the kind of sexual problems that I . . . had heard and read about. I did not worry that my husband would no longer find me attractive. He found me attractive; he wanted me. The crazy thing was I didn't want *him.* He still found me attractive . . . but . . . I no longer found *me* attractive. I was damaged goods now and I knew it. For me, feeling sexy had a lot to do with feeling beautiful. Those narcissistic feelings were short-circuited now. The fuse had blown." Given the physical and emotional trauma that breast cancer patients experienced, it is not surprising that many quickly came to see the silicone implant as a savior and attempted to ensure that all patients would have access to this option. Breast reconstruction was so important to Massachusetts women that in 1977 they formed the Betsy Coalition (named for the mannequin used to demonstrate breast self-examination) and undertook a letter-writing campaign to convince Blue Cross/Blue Shield to reinstitute coverage for breast reconstruction after cancer. Although the insurance company did not acknowledge the group's contribution, it did reinstitute coverage for reconstruction on June 1, less than three months after discontinuing it.[45]

Just as they waxed enthusiastic over breast implants for cosmetic purposes, popular magazines assured women that breast reconstruction using silicone implants was safe and effective. *Harper's Bazaar,* in 1976, told women that the implants "have already been used for cosmetic purposes in over 100,000 women, including cancer patients, with no reports of harmful effects." Two years later, *People* similarly noted that nearly five thousand women had had reconstruction with silicone implants and that complications were rare: "Sometimes the body extrudes the implant or scar tissue forms inside the breast and makes the implant very rigid. But if something like that happens it is correctable." *McCalls,* in 1980, told mastectomy patients that "The operation itself can be a simple procedure, consisting of a single incision and the implantation of a silicone gel-filled sac." *Ms.,* in 1983, offered one of the only alternatives to the rosy picture painted by other magazines. In a well-researched, lengthy article, writer Abby Avin Belson painted an unusually complete, balanced picture of the psychological benefits and physical risks of all implants. This article, however, was an exception, and most magazines continued to downplay the drawbacks. In 1987, *Life* magazine reported on the case of Peggy McCann, who had received silicone breast implants from Frank Gerow, their co-developer, in 1985. Before the surgery, McCann had asked Gerow whether the implant might break. "It's possible," Gerow had replied, "but rare, not dangerous, and fixable." McCann ended up undergoing more than four separate surgeries to deal with problems like unanticipated fluid buildup, but still concluded that the process was worth it, and many women agreed with her. Between 1981 and 1987, the annual number of reconstructions quintupled.[46]

During the 1970s, fear of breast cancer and enthusiasm for the silicone gel implant hit such high levels that for a time surgeons advocated a preventive measure called subcutaneous mastectomy. As reporter Jack Star explained in *Look* magazine in 1971, subcutaneous mastectomy developed in part because of the American practice of immediate mastectomy following a biopsy. The woman whose case he described had both a family history of breast cancer (her mother and aunt had both died of it and her sister had recently had a mastectomy) and a tendency to develop cysts. By her mid-thirties she had undergone five excisional biopsies, never knowing if she would wake up without a breast. Eventually, she elected to have a subcutaneous mastectomy, in which 95 percent of "possibly cancerous" tissue was removed and replaced with a silastic implant. According to Star, the procedure was useful not only for patients with a tendency toward cysts but also for those whose only problem was "cancer phobia."[47]

There are no statistics on how many American women underwent subcutaneous mastectomies in the 1960s and 1970s, but the procedure

was widespread enough by 1972 to generate heated debate among surgeons. In an editorial published in *Plastic and Reconstructive Surgery,*
Houston surgeon Bromley S. Freeman cautioned his colleagues that subcutaneous mastectomy was "not a panacea for all ills of the female breast."
The progressive increase in this procedure, he wrote, "may be evidence
of a situation similar to the epidemic of caecal resections of the early
1900's, the wholesale use of tonsillectomies in the 1930's, and (possibly)
the present-day pattern of hysterectomies." Many surgeons continued
to advocate the procedure—surgeon Donald T. Moynihan, in 1979,
wrote, "There can be complications but I personally feel it is worth the
risk for women who are constantly developing new lumps that can't be
distinguished from cancer"—but by the mid-1980s the procedure was
losing favor. In 1984, Washington, D.C., surgeon C. Lawrence Slade
published a report on long-term results, covering eighty-eight women
who had received subcutaneous mastectomies (sixty-nine for fibro-
cystic disease, thirteen for silicone granulomas resulting from injections
received in Asia) between 1965 and 1979. Most of the women (seventy-
six) received silicone implants (four received a local flap and eight were
not reconstructed); all had had complications, and one had developed
cancer. And, as San Diego surgeon Jack C. Fischer commented, patient
dissatisfaction might well have been higher than the 50 to 100 percent
rate of capsular contracture Slade had reported. "Plastic surgeons know
women whose results would display well at a national meeting, yet the
patient would tell us (if we asked) that her breasts no longer serve the
function of sexuality they were destined for throughout adulthood."[48]

Sequelae and Side Effects

As the number of women carrying silicone gel-filled implants in their
breasts continued to increase, surgeons kept an eye on potential problems. Given the fact that implants were often requested as reconstructive measures after cancer—and, in the case of subcutaneous mastectomy,
as a preventative measure—it is not surprising that much of their interest focused on the cancer connection. This focus, however, limited surgeons' vision, as most surgeons agreed that cancer was not a risk
associated with silicone implants. As three Baltimore surgeons pointed
out in 1967, as it was "generally accepted that 5½% of all women develop
breast cancer," it was inevitable that "at least 2,000" of the 40,000 women
with augmented breasts would develop cancer. In 1970 another surgeon

similarly reported that a survey of 10,941 patients augmented by 265 surgeons revealed that silicone injections led to the highest rate of complications, followed by open-pore sponges; only seven cases of cancer had turned up. Both articles mentioned that information on other side effects was insufficient.[49]

Although anecdotal reports of complications surfaced consistently in medical journals, the first large-scale report appeared not in a medical journal but in *Ms.* in 1978. Inspired in part by plastic surgeon John Goin's comment in *Medical Economics* that surgeons knew little about side effects because "like the victims of rape, most of these patients refuse to come forward," reporters Marjorie Nashner and Mimi White placed a notice in *Daily Variety*, which promised anonymity in exchange for information. From the thirty interviews they conducted, Nashner and White concluded that breast augmentation offered a 60 percent complication rate in exchange for "an operation you don't need."[50]

Nashner and White's groundbreaking article generated a significant amount of discussion. Dr. Dale B. Dubin of Tampa, Florida, wrote to congratulate them on an accurate, up-to-date, well-researched, and well-documented article, the "first article of its kind I have ever seen in a lay magazine." An anonymous woman, who had scheduled implant surgery for August, was also thankful. "Although the doctor I had chosen was probably ethical and competent," she wrote, "I realize now that he de-emphasized the negative aspects of the operation. Thank you for saving me from a possible disaster." Some surgeons agreed with the conclusions Nashner and White drew. Dr. Dennis Thompson, for example, told them, "According to the latest statistics, more than 60 percent will develop a problem, the most frequent one being breasts that harden." Recalling Milton Edgerton's advice about life expectancy, David White, a surgeon who went on record as opposing the use of existing implants, asserted that the studies on which surgeons and patients based their belief in the safety of implants were completely inadequate: "You cannot compare a test of any implant on a rabbit for eighteen months with a breast implant a young woman may have in her body for thirty or forty years. It would seem that the patients are serving as rabbits for testing these implants."[51]

Others, however, were not as appreciative of the reporters' work. M. E. Nelson, who responded for Dow Corning, took issue with the article's negative tone. Gerald Imber, a New York plastic surgeon, was also displeased. Imber admitted that the article was accurate and the horror stories true, but criticized the authors for extrapolating too much from a small number of cases: "Qualified plastic surgeons and self-styled plastic surgeons alike are performing this procedure at a rate that exceeds 150,000 procedures per year in the United States alone," he wrote. "For every 'awful' result depicted, there are likely 250,000 graceful and pleasant post-surgical results." Imber acknowledged that capsular contracture was a common side effect, but he insisted that in only 12 percent of cases was it really bad; the others were either minor or could be treated. Neither "inflammatory statements and sensational reports" nor an insistence on perfection should define accounts of the operation; rather, journalists should provide "adequate, intelligent, and honest information" so that women "may be able to make a qualified and intelligent judgment in [their] own best interests."[52]

The tension Imber identified—between how surgeons, journalists, and women defined concepts such as success, complication, and women's own best interests—was the focal point of an article the following year by Las Vegas surgeon Gregory Hetter. Hetter surveyed women with breast implants and found numerous complications. Firmness occurred in 74 percent of the women who had received silicone gel implants and 40 percent of those who had received saline. A surprisingly high percentage (41%) had some loss of nipple sensation; 15 percent had some numbness; another 15 percent were dissatisfied with the shape of their breasts; 10 percent were disappointed that the scars showed. Despite these problems, however, most women were pleased. Ninety-one percent said they felt better about themselves; 60 percent had changed their clothing styles; 47 percent were more outgoing. Only 9 percent of those who had lost sensation were bothered by the loss, and only three women (2%) were "very bothered." An overwhelming 96 percent said they would do it again; a few were undecided, and only 1 percent said no. Other surgeons confirmed Hetter's findings. In 1983, two surgeons reported that breast augmentation had slowed a patient's free-style swim time by almost one-fourth. The patient—a forty-six-year-old physical education teacher and competitive swimmer—was satisfied with the trade-off.[53]

Some protested that complications were not a reasonable trade-off for larger breasts. In 1980 Madalyn Eisenberg told *Good Housekeeping* that augmentation was "the biggest mistake a woman could make." She had returned to college at thirty-seven, and the sight of thousands of tanktopped students made her insecure. She persuaded her husband, and at her surgeon's suggestion chose the largest implants available, despite her diminutive size. After a miserable few months, in which she had to wear a size 14 top to accommodate her new shape, couldn't jog, find clothes that fit, or sleep on her stomach, and had no sensation at all in her breasts, she decided to have the implants removed. "Now I can jog, shop, sleep on my stomach and wear sweaters without embarrassment. And I love my new freedom—the freedom of being *me*," she concluded.[54]

Positive accounts, however, were much more common. *Glamour*, in 1981, assured readers that fears of cancer were completely groundless: "Breast augmentation surgery is a simple, safe procedure. It is not without some risk and discomfort, of course, but the results are usually rewarding." *Vogue*, in 1984, told readers that all risks of breast augmentation had been reduced and side effects were controllable, and in 1986 went further: "The American Society of Plastic and Reconstructive Surgeons has monitored breast-implant procedures for more than twenty years," readers were told. "In more than a million implants . . . no relationship has been found between the implants and cancer, spontaneous abortion, or birth defects. No illnesses or deaths have been associated with the presence of silicone implants in the body," and contracture could be treated. As late as 1989, *Good Housekeeping* said simply, "Occasionally minor complications may occur."[55]

The most common side effect—the one that resulted in the 60 percent complication rate reported in the 1978 *Ms.* article, as well as in the development of various types of implants designed to prevent or minimize it—was capsular contracture. The body reacted to an implant by forming a capsule of dense, fibrous scar tissue around it. In some women, this simply resulted in slightly firmer breasts. Many others, however, experienced a range of effects including severe discomfort, pain, and bizarre appearance (what one surgeon called the "baseball in a sock" effect).

Although this complication was documented and discussed early on, surgeons tended to minimize it and patients tended to believe it was a small price to pay for larger breasts. Two books published in the early 1970s designed to explain cosmetic surgery to lay readers made this point. Harriet LaBarre, for years the beauty editor of *Ladies Home Journal*, wrote, "Occasionally a woman will notice that as healing progresses, the breasts become a little firmer than she would like." LaBarre assured her readers, however, that they would relax, and besides, "Breasts aren't a fad . . . to have breasts, *real* breasts, is vitally important to women." Plastic surgeon Kurt Wagner simply noted that "this is part of the surgical aesthetics of mammaplasty to fashion it so that this does not happen."[56]

Surgeons were unable to ensure that capsular contraction did not occur, but through a fluke of social intercourse they discovered what for a time became the preferred method of dealing with it. In 1976, several Orlando, Florida, surgeons introduced the "Closed Compression Technique for Rupturing a Contracted Capsule around a Breast Implant." On February 22, 1975, a patient who had been scheduled for surgical release of the capsule attended a party. (In this technique, often called an open capsulotomy, a surgeon, depending on what he found when he opened the breast up, would either remove or simply loosen scar tissue in an attempt to soften the breast.) "We were having a grand time," she recounted, "when a large professional football player suddenly hugged me and squeezed me very tightly. We heard a loud pop and he said 'what was that?' I said, 'I think my beads broke,' and I ran to the bathroom. When I examined myself, my breasts had become soft." The closed capsulotomy technique was not without its own complications. First, it was extremely painful for women, and the effects were often of limited duration, meaning it had to be repeated, often more than once. Second, as a surgeon reported in 1981, it often resulted in rupture of the implant, although how often was unclear as surgeons and women alike did not find out if an implant had ruptured unless the breast was surgically reopened. (Saline implants that ruptured were easily detectable because the body absorbed the saline, resulting in an obviously deflated breast; silicone gel, in contrast, simply remained inside the fibrous capsule the body had formed.) Still, as the only available solution, closed capsulotomy was quickly adopted by surgeons all over the United States. As Richard Boies Stark, professor of clinical surgery at Columbia University's College of Physicians and Surgeons and former chairman of the American Board of Plastic Surgery, told *Cosmopolitan* in 1981, "In augmentation, scar tissue occasionally causes undesirable hardness. This can often be softened or broken up by vigorous massage."[57]

In the early 1980s, Los Angeles surgeon Franklin L. Ashley was instrumental in the development of a different solution, based on the work of celebrity surgeon William J. Pangman in the 1950s and 1960s. The new invention—a silicone gel-filled implant covered with polyurethane foam—was introduced in medical journals and popular magazines under the slogan "the contracture stops here" (a lighter implant based on the same principles, called the Même, was developed in the early 1980s and manufactured in turn by Aesthetech, Cooper Surgical, and Surgitek, a division of Bristol-Myers Squibb). Tucson, Arizona, surgeon B. R. Burckhardt was one of the skeptics: he wrote to *Plastic and Reconstructive Surgery* protesting the advertising practices of Natural Y Surgical Specialties, Inc., and cautioned, "We are all looking for the magic bullet, but there is no present reason to believe that it will, when found, be coated with polyurethane." Burckhardt's warning would later prove prophetic, but at the time it fell on deaf ears. In just ten years, polyurethane-covered implants captured 25 percent of the market. By 1991, when the FDA released a report suggesting that polyurethane might break down in the body and in the process release the chemical 2,4-toluenediamine (TDA), a known animal carcinogen, more than two hundred thousand women carried the Même.[58]

Capsular contracture is the most common and most publicized, but not the only, "side effect" of breast augmentation. Perhaps the most ironic, given that breast augmentation seems tied so tightly to women's sense of femininity and sexuality, is the possible loss of nipple sensation. No one seems to know just how often this occurs, and surgeons agree that it is impossible to predict whether or not it will occur. The documentation problem is exacerbated by the fact that many women lose sensation temporarily (sensation returns in many, but not all, of these patients in the first years or so after surgery) as well as by the fact that many claim not to care. In 1976, surgeons Eugene Courtiss and Robert M. Goldwyn noted that they were aware that loss of nipple sensation was common after breast reduction but were surprised to find it had occurred in 15 percent of the augmentation patients they studied; three years later, surgeon Gregory Hetter put the incidence at 41 percent, but noted that only 9 percent of these complained about it.[59]

Silicone bleed may also be a problem. Although surgeons and Dow Corning were aware of this much earlier, it garnered little attention until the late 1980s, when Ralph Nader's Public Citizens' Health Research Group and several dissatisfied patients brought it to the attention of the press. Although exactly what the surgeons and the manufacturer knew and when they knew it remain in dispute, it seems clear that everyone involved in breast implants, with the exception of the patients, knew enough to know that they did not have any definitive answers. Several Dow Corning memos, the earliest of which bore a date of 1967, were released during the 1991 battle with the FDA. These memos suggest that Dow Corning was informed several times that animal studies raised the question of whether silicone was as chemically inert and stable in the body as everyone had assumed. By the 1970s the medical literature treated this finding as common knowledge. In 1977, for example, surgeon Garry S. Brody noted, "The transport of materials across any silicone rubber membrane is inevitable. The quantities and the fate of the material that passes through the membrane of the implanted breast prosthesis is difficult to quantify by current analytical technology, and this has not been done. Inferential evidence suggests that the quantities are minute, and their physiological significance remains unclear."[60]

Like many surgeons, Brody emphasized surgeons' lack of concrete negative knowledge and extrapolated from that to conclude that implants were probably safe. By the time his summary of surgeons' colossal lack of knowledge was published, however, surgeons knew more than they thought they did. They knew that implants often ruptured (and that ruptured implants could remain undetected, sometimes for years), thus putting significant quantities of silicone in direct contact with tissue. Surgeons also knew that even intact implants "bled" minute quantities which, over a period of years, would add up, although to an unknown amount. Years of experience with silicone injections had also taught them that liquid silicone, introduced into women's breasts, often had horrifying results. It formed lumps, and it traveled, showing up in distant places like lymph nodes. Animal studies had suggested that silicone was not necessarily inert. Reflecting medical schools' emphasis on technical expertise rather than broad analytic thinking, as well as their own optimistic faith in the progress of modern medicine, however, surgeons failed to put these pieces of information together. Rather than take seriously the pieces of negative information that were available, or pursue more concrete findings, most surgeons took the absence of conclusive, negative information at face value and continued to implant silicone gel-filled sacs in women's breasts.

Not until the late 1980s, in fact, did surgeons, medical caregivers, and the FDA begin to take seriously the questions some researchers had raised about silicone. In 1986, several surgeons published a cautious, pioneering article in *Plastic and Reconstructive Surgery* suggesting that their colleagues take note of the growing number of questions about silicone. Although silicone was "relatively inert chemically," they wrote, "it is becoming clear that [it] is not biologically or chemically inactive." Echoing other reports that had appeared in the medical press, the surgeons called for more studies and more evidence, but their time-frame was more immediate. "We must remember," they cautioned, "that these reports will not go away if we ignore or deny them." At the same time, however, these surgeons believed that at least one conclusion could be drawn from the information presently available: "It seems reasonable to suggest that silicone implants could precipitate autoimmune phenomena in the susceptible host."[61]

Gradually, as the FDA focused its spotlight, this information began to find its way into the popular press. *Science News* mentioned it as a concern in 1988; *Newsweek* reported that leaking silicone seemed, in some women, to cause "an arthritis-like inflammation" in 1989. Many medical practitioners, however, continued to defend silicone breast implants. An article in the March 1990 issue of *Indiana Medicine*, for example, argued that concern about silicone was unwarranted: "Although minute quantities of silicone-gel are known to 'bleed' over time, it is estimated that use of silicone-lubricated syringes by insulin-dependent diabetics results in a similar amount of silicone in their tissues over a lifetime, as would be found in a woman with breast implants. No studies to date have demonstrated a higher incidence of sarcomas in diabetics or in patients with pacemakers or artificial joints made with silicone."[62]

A similar tone dominated discussions of the more common side effects. Capsular contracture was recognized as a problem significant enough to mandate the development of new implants, but it was also widely regarded as something women simply lived with in exchange for cleavage. Surgeons who accepted this definition claimed to do so in deference to women's evaluation of risk versus benefit. As Garry S. Brody wrote in 1984 after the FDA's initial move to reclassify implants as medical devices, because breast augmentation receives such "prolonged, intense, and continuous public interest," surgeons should be careful about the effect their words might have on "special interest groups such as feminists and Naderites." In the case of capsular contracture, he asserted, the FDA was using surgeons' words against them in quoting complication rates of 40 to 70 percent. But, as Brody pointed out, "Very few patients are deterred by the prospect of firmness as a trade for size and appearance, just as few patients are deterred from appendectomies because of the resultant abdominal scar. They do not like it, but they accept it as a small price to pay for the desired results." Therefore, he suggested, surgeons should think of a new name for the condition.

An expected result should not be termed a complication; instead, he suggested phenomena, sequela, consequence, expected result, or side effect.[63]

Reports of reduced or lost sensation generated little concern for the same reasons. As Goldwyn and Courtiss put it, because sensuality has "a considerable psychic component," the possibility of sensation loss deterred neither them nor their patients, who "after surgery felt more secure in their sexual roles and said that they were able to respond with less inhibition and more sensuality." The surgeons concluded, "Fortunately, patients undergoing plastic surgery of the breast are concerned more with getting rid of a deformity and achieving a desired body image than with maintaining or improving mammary sensation." Reflecting the tendency of surgeons and patients to downplay this drawback, popular magazine articles seldom mention it; when they do, it receives little attention. *Good Housekeeping,* in 1989, said simply, "Some patients may lose nipple sensitivity after the operation."[64]

Such attitudes suggest that the tendency to commodify the body that has attracted so much discussion in recent years surfaced in the specialty of plastic surgery as well. Surgeons defined breasts as both valuable commodities and independent entities, attached to but seemingly separate from the women who carried them. Side effects were thus always weighed against the known, if not precisely quantifiable, benefits of larger breasts. When they did look more closely at side effects, surgeons tended to look only at the breasts rather than at the body as a whole. The tendency to see breasts as depersonalized entities, rather than as body parts sharing blood and oxygen, as well as impurities, with the rest of women's bodies, may have encouraged them to discount the possibility that augmentation might affect the rest of the body.

Personal Politics (or, the Psychology of Breasts)

While surgeons were assuring each other and their patients that silicone gel-filled breast implants were, in columnist Anna Quindlen's words, "not unsafe," what were women thinking? One of the most publicized statements during the recent controversy was from an American Society of Plastic and Reconstructive Surgeons document originally filed with the FDA on July 1, 1982; ten years later it was reprinted, and almost universally derided, in publications including *Mother Jones* and the *New York Times.* Responding to the FDA's renewed interest in breast implants, the society had argued that implants functioned to augment "a female breast that has not developed sufficiently to give the patient a normal concept of breast image. . . . There is a substantial and enlarging body of medical opinion to the effect that these deformities are really a disease which in most patients results in feelings of inadequacy." With this statement, the ASPRS did no more than summarize almost a century's worth of thought on this issue. Similar pronouncements permeate both medical and lay writings about cosmetic surgery, but until the early 1990s the suggestion that this statement was, if not ludicrous, at least questionable, was never made.[65]

Popular sources have for years described the psychological torture small-breasted women endure. In her 1970 guide to cosmetic surgery, Harriet LaBarre asserted that in western culture "the flat-chested woman or girl is made to feel inadequate, unwomanly." As a result, LaBarre wrote, such women have low self-esteem, are wracked by anxiety at the beach, in clothing stores, or "when wearing low-cut dresses"; they are particularly anxious about getting married and suffer a "subconscious feeling of deformity." Although "flat-chested women and girls are generally . . . alive, attractive, with lots of verve and dash," a psychiatrist LaBarre consulted explained that this is accompanied by "repressed hysteria and emotional problems, all tied up with misery over their inferior condition." Writer Simona Morini had a similar message for *Vogue* readers. "When frustration, discomfort, acute self-consciousness become more unbearable than the fear of major surgery or stronger than the discouraging words of an old-fashioned physician," Morini wrote, the modern woman knew it was time for a breast job. Women who chose to have their breasts augmented confirmed this view.[66]

Surgeons, too, have long been cognizant of the psychological problems associated with small breasts. The inferiority complex, which surgeons found so persuasive in the 1920s and 1930s, was not originally understood to stem from small breasts, but as surgeons' armamentarium expanded, so did their frame of reference: just as surgeons in the 1940s and early 1950s began to see that an inferiority complex could be caused by wrinkles and cured by a face-lift, surgeons in the late 1950s and 1960s found that an inferiority complex that stemmed from small breasts could be cured by the new technique of breast augmentation. As surgeon John R. Lewis Jr. asserted in 1965, "underdevelopment" was a clear indication for surgery. Surgeon Hugh A. Johnson observed four years later that the new techniques were particularly welcome because the fashions of the day meant that breasts were the only thing that differentiated women from men. "Nothing says quite so well, 'I am feminine,'" Johnson wrote, "as a nicely formed breast."[67]

By 1972, in an evaluation of the new saline prosthesis, a group of surgeons from Canada, Georgia, and California could simply refer to "the inferiority complex characteristic of the flat-chested woman." Several Orlando, Florida, plastic surgeons confirmed this finding. They had taken the increased demand for augmentation, the surgeons wrote, as an indication that thousands of women have "feelings of inadequacy about the size of their breasts." A survey of 132 breast augmentation patients demonstrated that the effect of small breasts on self-esteem was "obvious." Before augmentation, 43 percent of the women suffered from depression; 47 percent reported feelings of inferiority and low self-worth; 65 percent reported moderate to strong feelings of inadequacy; and a striking 89 percent were self-conscious. Dr. Jack, the itinerant injector profiled in *Esquire* in 1975, reported similar findings: "My patients aren't a bunch of preening neurotics; they just feel a need for better looks. A real need. What about all those people who're living in a corner because they don't look the way they want to look? That can be a very confining thing for some people. It prevents them from living more fully, from really living at all."[68]

And, surgeons reported, augmentation cured these problems. As Dr. Jack put it: "I get a beautiful feeling when I see them coming out of the corners they've been hiding in. It's kinda like freeing them from something they never thought they could escape. It's better than watching people get up from a sickbed." Surgeon A. Richard Grossman put it this way: "The results of augmentation mammaplasty are beautiful and fascinating." The combination of a "more desirable physical contour" and a "tremendous improvement in self-image" led to better sexual adjustment and a happier life. Both men and women, he reported, noted that husbands became more sexually aggressive after their wives' surgery. "Why? Because the mother of their children, housewife, and confidante is now a new 'chick.' She is sexually desirable again, she has all the qualities that were present when he married her, and now she has fulfilled his idea of sexuality again." Perhaps basking in this reflected glory, Grossman hazarded, women felt more sexual too.[69]

Although surgeons continue to stress, in both medical and popular journals, that the only acceptable reason for a woman to augment her breasts is personal satisfaction—to feel better about herself—this insistence has always coexisted with an eye to changing fashions. In the years after World War II, medical and lay commentators alike attributed the new interest in breasts to cultural currents. Syndicated newspaper columnist Josephine Lowman, in 1953, attributed increased interest in breast surgery "to the impact of the 'sweater girl' and to strapless, low-cut evening gowns and swim suits." In 1954, newspapers reported, fashion designers and manufacturers of falsies united to protest Christian Dior's new line, which reintroduced the "flat look." At the 1957 annual meeting of the ASPRS, New York surgeon Gustave Aufricht cautioned his colleagues not to jump too quickly on the augmentation bandwagon, because while Americans were currently fixated on breasts, fashions were changeable. "My waiting room used to be full of women wanting smaller breasts," he commented. "Now, doubtless because of people in the public eye, without mentioning any names, it's the opposite."[70]

Surgeons have also recognized that fashions differ according to season and geographic location. In the 1970s, surgeons often commented that west coast women not only had more interest in breast augmentation than women in the rest of the country, but routinely selected implants ranging from 25 percent to 300 percent larger than those chosen in the East and Midwest. In 1976, Dr. V. Michael Hogan of New York University commented that west coast surgeons used implants almost three times larger than those commonly used in the East. Los Angeles surgeon and breast enlargement pioneer Robert Alan Franklyn put it differently: "We're 10 to 15 years ahead of the East Coast." *Newsweek* noted in 1985 that nearly one hundred thousand breast augmentations had been performed over the past year "for a total addition to the nation's mammary capacity of some 13,000 gallons (of silicone gel)"; women in the West and South, the article added, routinely get implants 25 percent larger than those in northern areas. Surgeons have also noted that the approach of the Christmas season—when women decide they need more cleavage for their formal gowns—and the approach of summer, when bathing suits become a concern—lead to higher numbers of surgeries.[71]

But if fashions, seasons, and geography are recognized as factors, the most significant change surgeons have noted is an overall trend toward larger breasts. In 1973, several New York surgeons pointed to Miss

America's changed and changing measurements—from 30–25–32 in 1921, when the contest began, to 34–21–34 for 1970's proud winner—as evidence of the national fixation on breasts. Model agent Eileen Ford publicly criticized the trend toward increased breast size in the 1980s even as she admitted augmentation was epidemic at her agency. Fashion designer Norma Kamali commented too: "When I'm thinking about fashion, I think of perky little firm breasts that can go braless and not bounce or hang, and then I talk to men and realize that they like big tits." Los Angeles surgeon Garry Brody explained in 1986 that augmentation was becoming more extreme simply because surgeons had discovered that breasts would tolerate larger implants than was once thought possible. In a comment on the advantages of the inflatable (saline) implants he had developed, West Palm Beach surgeon Hilton Becker explained, "when women have the chance to adjust their breast size after surgery, it's been my experience that almost all of them will change it, usually to a larger size."[72]

Throughout the 1960s, 1970s, and 1980s, the paradigm of the inferiority complex found new life as a justification for breast augmentation as surgeons and patients alike reported that patients' preoperative feelings of inferiority gave way to postoperative confidence. The remarkable consistency of this rhetoric is its most striking aspect. One wonders if feminism had any effect at all.

Feminism and fashion have a long history. In 1851, just three years after the Seneca Falls Convention, Elizabeth Cady Stanton and Amelia Bloomer launched a crusade that reflected their and other reformers' conviction that women would never be fully emancipated until they no longer displayed their oppression in the clothes they wore. The first feminist mass meeting, held in New York in 1914, proclaimed—along with the right to work, the right to one's own name, and the right to organize—the "right to ignore fashion." Feminist critiques of cosmetic surgery have generally agreed that the silicone sacs invented by Thomas Cronin and Frank Gerow in 1961 belonged in the same Freedom Trash Can into which young women threw other "objects of female oppression" at the infamous 1968 demonstration. From this perspective, feminism and cosmetic surgery are unalterably opposed: cosmetic surgery represents capitulation to the cultural ideologies and beauty myths that have historically victimized women, while feminism, by framing beauty as a social rather than an individual issue, empowers women to resist such pressures.[73]

Yet in 1988, in an article entitled "Cheers for Cher," the editors of *Ms.* magazine heralded the dawn of "an era that's not afraid to applaud real women" and designated Cher an authentic feminist hero. The article continued: "Women who dare to be themselves, who dare to take control of their lives and reinvent themselves according to their own dreams, needs, and specifications are still all too rare. And those who are among the brave must be willing to risk all. Cher's done that. . . . This is a woman who defies the conventions and expands her personal horizons." That in Cher's case the reinvention was surgical was explicitly acknowledged and applauded.[74]

In the 1970s, women insisted that the personal is political; they defined appearance and beauty as social issues rather than individual problems. A decade later, however, popular conceptions of feminism began to reflect the same emphasis on individual achievement and fulfillment that swept through the larger culture. The fact that cosmetic surgery was framed as individual self-realization long before feminism's second wave helps to explain how it could so easily be reframed that way after that wave crested. In this sense the embrace of cosmetic surgery appears to be consistent with the liberal, individualist strand of feminism that emerged after the suffrage battle and surfaced again in the wake of the battle for the ERA. As media critic Susan Douglas notes, with this reemergence, "political concepts and goals like liberation and equality were collapsed into distinctly personal, private desires," and feminism itself was reframed as individual self-realization. In this self-actualizing context, Cher is indeed an authentic hero and columnist Barbara Kerbel's more recent assertion that surgical enhancement is "a totally feminist thing to do" makes perfect sense.[75]

All of the available evidence suggests that cosmetic surgery can indeed empower individual women. But while they are neither antithetical nor mutually exclusive (and have, at key historical moments, overlapped), feminism and individualism remain separate and distinct from each other. Our commitment to honoring women's voices—to listening to their own interpretations of their actions and their lives—should not obscure our ability to place these voices in context. Many women have chosen to buy into the celebration of the breast (and up a cup size or two), and to some degree popularized feminism has incorporated this practice. Cosmetic surgery may empower individual women by curing their inferiority complexes or, in less technical terms, making them feel

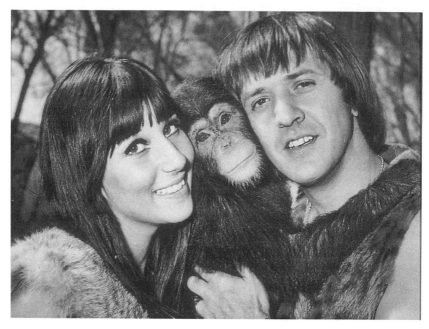

Cher (with Sonny and Toto), from *Bang Bang*, their first movie.

better about themselves. Overall, however, its history offers a compelling reminder of just how limited has been the range of options that women have perceived to be available to them—and of how provocative that angry and incisive feminist critique of the tangled relationship between consumer culture and sexism and beauty was.[76]

In 1977 a group of researchers undertook a comparative study that, while it confirmed other studies that had found implants an effective solution for women who believe bigger breasts will cure them, suggested that there was more to this interpretation than met the eye. This group devised a study of 370 women in the Midwest that enabled them to compare women seeking breast implants with women who were satisfied with themselves the way they were. The women were divided into three groups: small-breasted women seeking breast augmentation (denoted by the letters AUG); average-sized women not seeking augmentation (ABC); and small-breasted women not seeking augmentation (SBC). "Taken as a whole," the study concluded, "the results show the SBC subjects to be the most statistically deviant. They scored in more

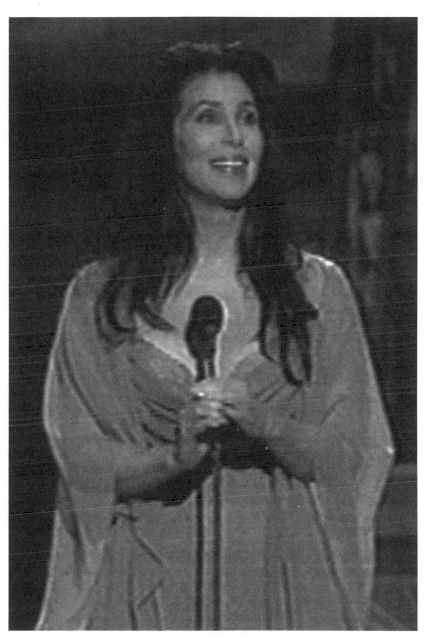

Cher, 1997 (video frame still).

liberated, feminist, assertive, independent, and adventuresome directions on the CPI (California Psychological Inventory) and Attitudes Toward Women Scale" than either of the other two groups. While altering one's body may be an act of self-assertion, this study seems to suggest, the qualities we might expect to see in an "authentic feminist hero" are more commonly shared by those who see no need for surgery.[77]

The Controversy

The controversy over breast implants that resulted in the almost total ban on silicone prostheses thus has a long history. Throughout the twentieth century, surgeons and women have been searching for solutions, and since the Second World War both groups have become more daring about experimenting. The controversy of the early 1990s, too, has a longer history than might initially appear to be the case, and a review of this history helps to place it in context. Breast implants are classified as "medical devices," which before the passage of the 1976 Food, Drug, and Cosmetics Act did not require FDA approval. They stayed on the market because the law applied only to new products, not to established ones. (Each of the various permutations through which the gel-sac moved was regarded as "substantially similar" to existing implants and was thus not classified as a new product subject to regulation; this process is referred to as "grandfathering.") Over the years, the FDA made several half-hearted attempts to assert control over the breast implant situation. In January 1982, the FDA proposed that implants be reclassified because they "present a potential unreasonable risk of injury" and because "insufficient information is available to provide reasonable assurance of [their] safety and effectiveness," but the move went no further. Three years later, in December 1985, the FDA instituted a program called Medical Device Reporting, which required surgeons to notify a central registry if devices failed. Because "failure" was not clearly defined, however, and because physicians did not maintain careful, long-term records, data did not materialize. As of 1987, surgeons had registered a mere 719 reports, most of which dealt with broken implants. Some regulatory bodies went further than the FDA. At the urging of the Maryland Women's Health Coalition, the Maryland House of Representatives passed a bill requiring surgeons to supply patients with standardized information about benefits, risks, and potential side effects. Most states, however, did not follow suit.[78]

The recent phase of the controversy began in two stages. In the June 1988 issue of *Ms.*, Sybil Niden Goldrich published a short article entitled "Restoration Drama," in which she reported her own experience with breast implants. In 1983, after two mastectomies and a lot of research, Goldrich chose silicone implants, which all the surgeons she interviewed recommended as the "simplest and least traumatic procedure." She experienced complications ranging from hardened, misshapen breasts to decay of skin grafts designed to create the nipple/areola complex. After five operations in ten months requiring more than fifteen hours under anesthesia, she opted for a transverse abdominal island flap reconstruction but remained committed to finding out why her implants had failed. "The crux of the problem," she found, "was defining the word 'failure.' To most doctors, a failed implant is a 'broken' implant—one literally damaged in the manufacturing; to a patient, a failed implant is one that causes her pain or discomfort or requires its removal or change." Manufacturers' package inserts, Goldrich found, contain warnings that "plastic surgeons do not routinely share with their patients," including the possibility of infection, blood clots, and decay. The two most common were encapsulation and "rupture of the implants from stress or trauma, causing them to leak, which then results in pain, toxicity, or possibly an autoimmune disease, like scleroderma, lupus, or rheumatoid arthritis"—the problems she herself had had.[79]

Goldrich's article generated a flood of mail from women in similar situations, but not until six months later did a related incident—which John E. Sherman, assistant clinical professor of plastic surgery at New York's Mount Sinai School of Medicine later dubbed the "Tempest in a Petri Dish"—spark national interest. In November 1988, the FDA released a study showing that silicone gel caused cancer in rats. Alarmed, the Public Citizens' Health Research Group associated with consumer advocate Ralph Nader called on the FDA to ban the sale of silicone implants, but scientists concluded that the study had "little, if any, relevance to humans." Critics made much of the fact that plastic surgeons, who had a vested interest in implants, were among the study's most assiduous debunkers; comments like that of John H. Davis, chair of plastic surgery at the University of Vermont Medical School, who called implants "a great boon to women," generated sniggers. The FDA, however, agreed with Dr. Sherman's explanation. "Granted," Sherman wrote, "plastic surgeons might be expected to refute the study," but "general consensus asserts the study is inaccurate because the breed of rats it used is known to develop cancers in response to almost *any* kind of implant, and the types of cancers developed by these rats have never been found in humans who've had implants. Also, the study contradicts all previous research in the field, some of which has involved humans." In December 1988, an FDA advisory panel voted against the ban.[80]

As it turned out, the FDA's December decision signaled a hiatus in, rather than a cessation of, its interest in breast implants. Although most scientists concurred with the finding that the rat study should not be applied to humans, the very fact that experts had disagreed called attention to how little concrete knowledge was available. And although the FDA attempted to reassure anxious consumers, it did not rule out the possibility of further investigation. "At this point, FDA does not believe there is cause for alarm about breast implants, nor is there sufficient justification to take them off the market," the agency noted in March 1989: "But answers are needed to questions about the frequency of short-term adverse effects related directly to the breast, and also about the possibility of long-term risks from silicone in the body." In a move that set the stage for the later controversy, the FDA also notified manufacturers that they had thirty months in which to submit data demonstrating the implants' safety.[81]

Popular periodicals, which had in years past heralded implants as one of medicine's great success stories, began to raise more questions. As *Mademoiselle* noted in February 1989, "As consumers, we would like to think that doctors—and the federal agencies that monitor them—are all-knowing. The rat-study controversy is proof that this is not so. It is up to you to weigh all the information you can gather to determine which procedure, if any at all, is the right one for you." Later that summer, *Vogue,* too, picked up the story, warning readers that the "price tag for breast implants may be much higher than their stated cost of $4,000 a pair." Government officials and plastic surgeons seemed untroubled, writer Robin Henig noted, but others were less sanguine. Douglas R. Shanklin, a pathologist at the University of Tennessee in Memphis, had said grimly, "We have performed a natural experiment on millions of American women. . . . We're just going to have to sweat it out." Richard Chiacchierini, a statistician with the FDA, had similar qualms. The studies that indicated no cancer risk were based on examinations of patients at six or sometimes eleven years, he pointed out, but the FDA believed that "the question of whether implants cause cancer can't be answered for at least ten to fifteen years." *Vogue* readers were left with a much more sobering conclusion than they were accustomed to. The clearest risk, they were told (in addition to those of surgery), was hardening. The uncertain risks, "including, for example, autoimmune disease, are more difficult to gauge."[82]

Surgeons viewed the increasingly critical stance of the lay press with alarm, and many continued to insist that the implants were perfectly safe; some went so far as to voice publicly their frustration with the microscope under which they found themselves. Several surgeons, in 1990, reasserted their belief in the safety of implants and reviewed the studies they found persuasive. "Why then," they asked, "in light of sound laboratory and clinical evidence, has there been such controversy in the lay press?" Largely, they asserted, because of "a combination of misinterpretation of the Dow Corning study by a consumer activist group, the Public Citizen Health Research Group, and media sensationalism." To the question, "Is there cause for concern?" the surgeons answered, "The information from responsible analysis of the laboratory data, as well as the long-standing record of clinical safety, would indicate there is not." The FDA might have agreed with them, but by then the topic had generated too much attention. At congressional hearings, on prime-time news shows, and in the pages of the nation's press, Americans asked questions and demanded answers. Finally, the FDA put manufacturers on a ninety-day notice, and in late 1991—a quarter of a century after the first silicone gel-filled breast implants hit the market and nearly ten years after the FDA first turned its spotlight on breasts —the hearings began.[83]

The Aftermath

Over the course of the twentieth century, surgeons and women came to see breast augmentation—like other cosmetic surgical operations—as simply another form of self-improvement. No objective difference seemed to exist between surgery to compensate for a missing breast and surgery to compensate for a small breast. The only determining factor was the patient's subjective diagnosis of how her condition made her feel. Some women who lost a breast to cancer viewed their scars as symbols of survival, and some women with small breasts were happy with them. Many others, however, felt deformed, self-conscious, and inferior and chose a surgical solution. The ASPRS definition of small breasts as deformities, which received so much attention during the controversy, was thus not a new definition or even a clarification; it merely recapped the agreement women and surgeons had negotiated over the course of the twentieth century.

The tendency in American culture to view the body as a commodity that can either help or hinder its inhabitant's success contributed to this development. Increasingly, surgeons and patients defined breasts as independent entities that could be altered by the purchase and installation of implants. This helps to explain why, once concern about breast cancer was resolved, broader questions went unaddressed, and why women's inquiries about a possible connection between implants and autoimmune diseases were initially greeted with such skepticism. It was ridiculous, most surgeons seemed to agree, to think that something in women's breasts could have any effect on the rest of their bodies— and in any case, as this was elective surgery undertaken out of vanity, the question was not worth studying. The initial recommendation of the FDA advisory panel similarly reflected fifty years of accumulated experience in abdicating control. Like surgeons, who for years had thrown up their hands in frustration, insisting that such decisions were not theirs to make, the advisory panel did not want the responsibility of deciding who deserved continued access to breast implants and for what reasons.

The FDA's final decision signaled several things—first, a more activist stance on the part of the FDA, which had seemed, during the Reagan years, to be dying the same slow death deregulation brought to other federal agencies. Granted, the FDA decision raised more questions than it answered. Although critics of breast implants welcomed the FDA's intervention, some took umbrage at what they interpreted as the implication that women had in the past flippantly sacrificed health for vanity and could be expected to continue this behavior without legal intervention. The problem, these critics asserted, was not that women valued breasts above all else but that information on "all else" had been systematically withheld. The solution they proposed was not protective legislation but rather full disclosure, which would enable women to make truly informed decisions. Surgeons, too, held to this view, insisting, in the words of ASPRS president Jim Hoehn, that "the manufacturers did hoodwink the doctors" and that full disclosure and informed consent, not regulation, would solve all problems.[84]

The fact that few were happy with the ultimate decision testifies to the complexity of the problem. But despite the chorus of criticisms, the FDA decision meant that, for the first time in almost a century, the issue had been addressed in a broader forum than medical journals and women's magazines and brought to public attention. Most important, the FDA's decision signaled a willingness to tackle significant, troubling issues, inspired by a conviction that abdication was not the answer. The thirty-year window provided by the initial multibillion dollar settlement negotiated by implant manufacturers and the continuing negotiations about responsibility suggest that discussion will continue. What questions this discussion will entertain, however, remains to be seen.

For the fundamental question here is not whether cosmetic surgery is feminist or antifeminist. Neither is it whether or not implants cause illness, though this question surely deserves further study. Nor is it why so many Americans, despite what some scientists consider compelling scientific evidence, continue to believe that implants cause illness (or why so many scientists, despite what many women see as convincing, if unquantifiable, evidence, insist that there is sufficient proof to conclude that they do not). The real question is how it happened that so many women became convinced that their lack of mammary endowment constituted a disease in the first place and why implants were so universally heralded—by the companies that manufactured them, by the surgeons who implanted them, by the women who wanted them, and by the men who wanted their women to have them—as a cure.

As the likelihood that the FDA would limit or ban silicone breast implants increased, surgeons began to explore (or reexamine) alternatives. In the late 1980s, the technique of autologous fat transfer sparked renewed interest, with liposuction providing a new twist: Why couldn't fat that had been liposuctioned from other areas simply be reinjected into the breast? This was found to be ill-advised, but the idea of relying on a woman's own body for material with which to rebuild or augment her breasts has received new attention, and techniques using flesh from the buttocks, back, and abdomen are currently in use. Many surgeons have simply decided that saline implants hold more promise than they originally thought. Others are turning their sights toward new horizons. An implant containing a biocompatible substance such as peanut oil was first suggested in the mid-1980s; work on this possibility continues, as do efforts to develop an implant filled with soybean oil. The latest suggestion, at this writing, is an implant of "engineered tissue" described, only partly in jest, as a "grow-your-own" alternative. Some women are hedging their bets. Like Atlanta housewife

P. J. Brent, who told the *New York Times*, "I love my small, 'deformed' breasts," at least thirty thousand women in 1992 chose "explantation" (implant removal) over the other alternatives available. Many of those who have not yet had implants are waiting: while the total number of cosmetic surgical procedures increased by 37 percent between 1990 and 1993, breast augmentations decreased by 48 percent. But should a promising new technique come on the market, these trends may prove temporary. When *Glamour* magazine, in 1995, asked men, "If it were painless, safe, and free, would you encourage your wife or girlfriend to get breast implants?" 55 percent said yes.[85]

The Eye of the Beholder

On November 11, 1960, Rod Serling once again invited CBS viewers to enter *The Twilight Zone*. The episode that aired that night was called "The Eye of the Beholder"; devotees remember it as one of the series' most memorable. The story begins as a woman, her head shrouded, mummylike, in gauze, chats with her nurse in what is obviously a hospital room. Patient 307, whom we learn is Miss Janet Tyler, has undergone a procedure to make her look normal, and she is anxiously wondering what she will see when the bandages come off. Evoking the subjective camerawork that distinguished noir films such as Robert Montgomery's adaption of Raymond Chandler's *The Lady in the Lake* (1946) and Delmer Daves's *Dark Passage* (1947), the doctors and nurses are filmed from behind or below, or in silhouette. Their faces are not shown.

As we wait with Janet Tyler, we learn something of the tragedy that has haunted her life. "I never really wanted to be beautiful," she tells the doctor. "I just wanted people not to scream when they looked at me." Later she says longingly, "I want to belong; I want to be like everybody else." The doctor is sympathetic and hopeful that the outcome will be positive. He cautions her gently, however, that because this is her eleventh procedure, it will not be possible to try again. Should the effort prove unsuccessful, she will be "allowed" to move into a "special area" where people of her kind have been "congregated." Tyler protests: "The state hasn't the right to penalize someone for an accident of birth . . . hasn't the right to make ugliness a crime!" Later, to a sympathetic nurse, the

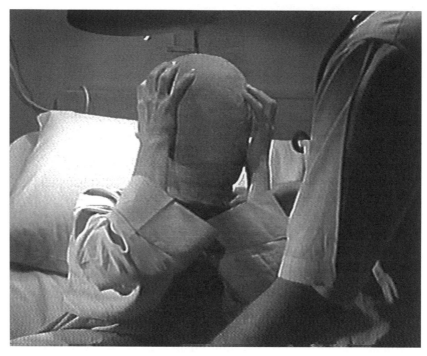

Patient 307 waits for the bandages to come off.

doctor muses over Tyler's predicament—"What is the dimensional difference between beauty and something repellent? . . . Why shouldn't people be allowed to be different?"—but it is clear that there is nothing he can do. When Rod Serling interrupts the story to ask, "What kind of world where ugliness is the norm and beauty the deviation from that norm?" we begin to see where we are headed.

The twist—in typical *Twilight Zone* fashion—comes toward the end, and, although we know what to expect, it is startling. The doctor slowly unwraps the bandages to reveal the beautiful face of Donna Douglas (like Sandra Dee or Barbara Eden, an icon of desire to the boys of the baby boom). But the doctors and nurses gasp, and their horror and disappointment are immediately mirrored in the face of Patient 307; the camera finally pulls back—to reveal that the faces of the doctors and nurses are bulbous, piglike, and hideous (and, reflecting the "glorious conformity" so prized in this culture, virtually identical). Tyler screams and tries to run, but to no avail; she is exiled to live out her days with others of her kind.

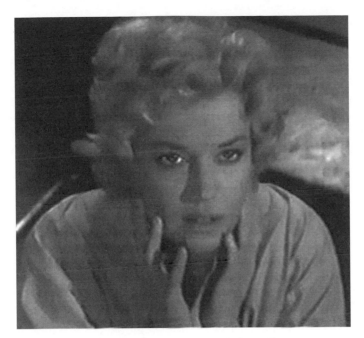

Miss Janet Tyler is unveiled . . .

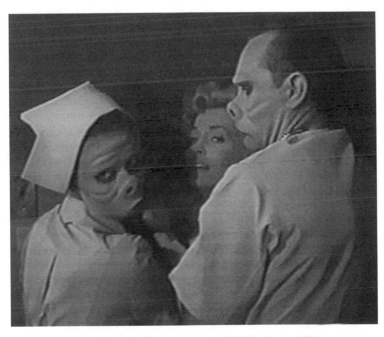

. . . and the beholders are revealed (video frame stills).

The singular appeal of this episode became apparent to me almost as soon as I began working on this book. On a plane or at a party, people would ask eagerly: "Do you remember that *Twilight Zone* episode? The one where the woman has cosmetic surgery and is all bandaged up, and the surgeons are filmed from the back so you can't see their faces, and then they take off the patient's bandages and she's beautiful and the camera pulls back and they're all ugly?" I hadn't seen it, until recently—and when I did, my first thought was, "But it's not even about cosmetic surgery!" (It's not: the procedure Patient 307 has undergone is identified only as a series of injections; at one point the doctor even expresses regret that, because of her bone structure and flesh type, plastic surgery is not appropriate in her case.) But by 1960, when this episode first aired, cosmetic surgery had become the lens through which Americans examined and thought about issues of beauty and ugliness. In some sense, then, "The Eye of the Beholder" is very much about cosmetic surgery, if only because everyone who watched it assumed it was and remembers it that way.

In 1960, when this episode ran, Americans might have "read" it as a comment on the McCarthy years: the pig faces of the doctors and nurses and of their "fearless leader" recall nothing so much as George Orwell's *1984*, while the homogenized society they so fiercely defend evokes a vision of conformity as chilling as the one Kurt Vonnegut described in "Harrison Bergeron," in which piercing noises prevent writers from concentrating and weights tie dancers to the ground. Then, too, with its clear message about the kind of society that practices such as segregation perpetuate, it might have played as a statement about the burgeoning civil rights movement. But the collective memory of those who watched it in 1960 is that it was about beauty and about the particularly unforgiving culture of modern America, which seemed to require that those who would be truly part of it meet certain standards of appearance—and had invented cosmetic surgery to help them do so.

Cosmetic surgery is no longer the peculiarly American phenomenon it seemed in 1960. American surgeons now import as well as export techniques: liposuction, perhaps the most significant phenomenon in recent years, originated in France. Surgeons in other countries—unhampered by the regulatory framework provided by institutions such as the FDA and by the litigious nature of modern America, which has, among other things, driven malpractice insurance costs sky-high—claim to be freer to experiment and to indulge in more dramatic procedures. Brazilian celebrity surgeon Ivo Pitanguey, in the 1970s, prided himself on pioneering surgical body-sculpting techniques that American surgeons were afraid to try. Russian surgeon Igor A. Volf told the *New York Times* in 1995, "Surgeons in the West work in a very rigid frame. They are afraid of being sued by their patients—they fear complications, they fear leaving bruises. I do the big, bold operations Western doctors are afraid to do." American citizens who go overseas seeking more adventurous surgeons (and less expensive surgeries) account for some part of the international surgical boom. But as the recent increase in interest and procedures in Argentina suggests, the fact that Americans are now not the only citizens of the world who see cosmetic surgery as a means of self-improvement is a more significant factor.[1]

Never an exclusively American phenomenon, cosmetic surgery has, in recent years, come to seem more universal than particular. This development, however, should not obscure the fact that for many decades it was widely perceived to be—if not exclusively, then especially—American. American surgeons were the first to spot its potential; American citizens as quickly (and as enthusiastically) grasped its promise. A poignant letter that a young midwestern woman wrote to the American Board of Plastic Surgery in 1961 offers an illustrative case:

> Dear Sirs,
>
> I read the article on plastic surgery and what it can do for your face in a syndicated column on Sunday, August 13.
>
> What I am about to ask you is very important to me, more important than anyone really knows, so please don't laugh and cast my letter aside, or tell me to write someplace else. . . .
>
> My face suits me fine. I want to know if anything can be done about the lower part of my legs. From the knees on down, to be specific. Surely there is something somebody can do, isn't there? I've become terribly self-conscious and have developed a severe complex. And it keeps getting worse. Exercise doesn't work. I inherited my legs from my father, and he, from his mother. And I've tried every exercise in the book for a long time. . . .
>
> I am seventeen and life is passing me by. The only time I'm happy is when I'm driving a car and people can't see my legs. If my calves were bigger, everything would be fine. This is the only light of hope I know. Please don't put it out.[2]

By the end of the decade, "Plastics" would come to symbolize everything that Benjamin Braddock's generation found wrong with American culture. In 1961, however, this young woman's expressed faith in plastic surgery as the embodiment of the plasticity of American culture marked her as typically American even more surely than did the fact that she was happiest in her car. And in many ways, this writer is still representative of the millions of Americans who have sought cosmetic surgery to correct perceived flaws. She learned about cosmetic surgery from a newspaper article, she believed so fervently that physical appearance equated to social value that she developed a psychological complex, she believed that if her calves could be altered, her entire life would be changed, and she dared to hope that modern medicine would provide a solution.

This case is exemplary, too, in that in 1961 plastic surgeons could offer no solution to the letter writer's problem. Much had changed since the turn of the century. New educational and occupational opportunities had attracted growing numbers of surgeons, and publicity about cosmetic surgery's wide-ranging benefits had generated ever larger numbers of patients. First with nose jobs, then with face-lifts and eye lifts, then with chin reshaping, and finally with breast augmentation and tummy tucks, surgeons and patients had sought, and often found, new remedies for what were perceived to be problems of human inferiority and inadequacy. In 1961, however, there was no solution for an unattractive lower leg. The pathetic case of Sadye Holland, who in the 1920s had sought help from a plastic surgeon for the same problem and had ended up having to have both legs amputated at the knee, discouraged patients from pursuing this path (and the significant judgment against her surgeon served as a warning to medical practitioners). Some began to rethink these techniques in the late 1950s, but body sculpture left large, visible scars, and only the most obese—or the most obsessed—found the trade-off worth it.[3]

Today, if she could convince her parents to sign the consent form and pay the price, that young woman would be able to get out of her car. Liposuction of the knees and ankles would be a start. Introduced to the United States in 1981, liposuction quickly became, and has remained, one of the most-requested procedures. Despite problems ranging from pulmonary embolisms (which killed about a dozen patients during the early 1980s) to uneven skin tone and texture, it has been judged hugely successful by doctors and patients alike: as one suctionee put it, "WASP-y knees" are now available to all. Liposuction was the top cosmetic procedure chosen by American women in 1993. Although men still prefer hair transplants, liposuction has lured many to the surgeon's office (the notorious terrorist Carlos the Jackal was finally caught when the surgeon he had contracted to reduce his love handles recognized him and turned him in). For the letter writer, a calf implant, using a carved piece of solid silicone or a cigar-shaped implant filled with silicone gel, would complete the job.[4]

Liposuction is an obvious example, but it is only one of many. Today, medical or surgical intervention can solve myriad other problems for which there was once no solution. Some of these are only minimally invasive: permanent eyeliner enables women "to liberate themselves from the daily task of applying eye makeup"; injections of saline solution can erase varicose veins; injections of collagen fill out lines and plump lips.[5] More recently, an enterprising surgeon in Los Angeles began offering injections of botulinum toxin, which prevent wrinkles by effecting localized paralysis.[6] Many interventions, however, are "real" surgical procedures. Cheekbone implants promise that Faye Dunaway look without the pain and danger of having molars extracted.[7] A craniofacial structure judged less than ideal can be taken apart and put back together according to plan.[8] Surgeons have pioneered new techniques to minimize the distinctive facial characteristics of Down's Syndrome.[9] Men, too, are being offered a wider range of surgical options. Pectoral implants, like calf implants, offer the perfect body without the pesky problem of daily workouts.[10] Surgical penile enlargement and lengthening are now widely available, although horror stories and lawsuits are becoming numerous enough to inspire

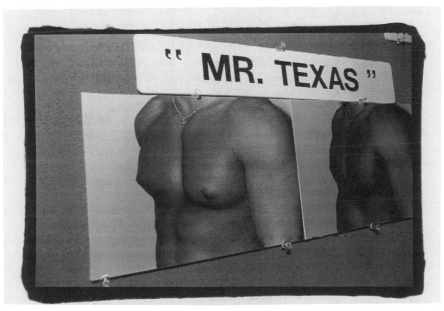

Mr. Texas, after and before.

caution about this particular procedure.[11] And of course, the breast implant scandal has created an entirely new specialization in cosmetic surgery: explantation.[12]

In a sense, cosmetic surgery has come full circle. Cosmetic surgery was pioneered in the early twentieth century by adventurous practitioners urged on by eager patients who believed fervently that beauty could be created through surgery. To patients, cosmetic surgery promised a more attractive appearance and a changed life; to surgeons, it offered a lucrative and rewarding practice and a limitless supply of patients. This combination created a free-for-all atmosphere that encouraged experimentation, and practitioners did not hesitate to promote themselves and their practices through articles, advice books, advertisements, and public performances.

The specialty coalesced, in the century's middle decades, around an ideal of professional control, organization, and regulation. Plastic surgeons who held to an ideal of professional medicine and specialization joined together to claim the field. Their most important achievement occurred in 1939 with the formation of the American Board of Plastic Surgery. For the first time, board certification offered practitioners and consumers alike a means to distinguish between who was, and who was not, a plastic surgeon.

For several reasons, this control was never complete. In practical terms, although the American Board of Plastic Surgery was able to govern certification, it never ruled practice: anyone, it seemed, could call himself a plastic surgeon and anyone who could find patients could be one. More important was that surgeons discovered very early on that it was cosmetic, not reconstructive, surgery that made them popular and prosperous—and cosmetic surgery found its authority in the wider world, not in the plastic surgeon's office. Self-described reputable surgeons' commitment to driving "quacks" from the field is understandable. Yet, perhaps inevitably, by moving to take over this territory, these surgeons tacitly acknowledged the authority that was already located in the adventurous practitioners on the fringes of organized medicine and in the press. These reputable surgeons liked to claim medicine as their cultural framework. But the fact that they so quickly came to share their patients' conviction that the beholder's eye became more discerning with the advent of consumer culture locates them very much in the mainstream of American culture. As they increasingly emphasized the social and economic importance of appearance, surgeons strengthened normative standards, thus locating authority in this larger world. Even the inferiority complex—which, by making cosmetic surgery medical, seemed, at least initially, to offer a middle ground between medicine and culture—ultimately undermined surgeons' authority. When psychological health was at stake, diagnosis was shaped as much by the patient's subjective feelings as by the surgeon's judgment.

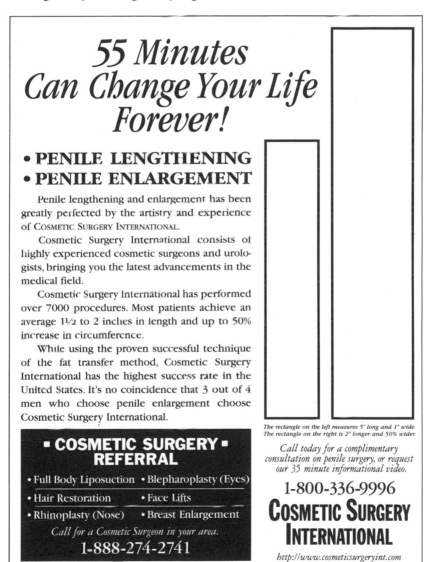

An advertisement for Cosmetic Surgery International, one of the leading providers of penile enhancement.

But if it was incomplete even at its peak, the degree of control held by the American Board of Plastic Surgery has decreased even more since the late 1970s. In part, this is simply a function of numbers: in 1948, fewer than three hundred board-certified plastic surgeons were in practice; today there are more than four thousand. It is also, however, a function of the decentralization of American medicine. In 1977, inspired by physicians who alleged that being excluded from the American Society of Plastic and Reconstructive Surgeons and denied the opportunity to publish in the journal *Plastic and Reconstructive Surgery* unfairly interfered with their right to earn a living (as well as by a distrust of organized medicine informed by the broader cultural urge to Question Authority), the Federal Trade Commission (FTC) began investigating the society. Reliance on certification by the American Board of Plastic Surgery in awarding membership or otherwise judging quality, the FTC asserted, amounted to unfair restraint of trade.[13]

Plastic surgeons rallied energetically, and the FTC dropped the case in 1980, but by then the point was moot. In 1978, the year after it had first focused its sights on plastic surgeons, the FTC took on the American Medical Association, alleging that the association's ban on advertising was illegal because it denied consumers "the opportunity to obtain the information they need to select a physician." The U.S. Supreme Court upheld the ruling in 1982, and although the ASPRS did not sign the consent decree, the AMA did, with predictable results. Despite pointed reminders from surgeons like New York's Arthur G. Ship that the law now "*permits,* but does not *require,* physicians to advertise," since 1982 advertising by physicians has increased markedly.[14]

Just as predictably, plastic surgery has generated not only a greater number of advertisements than other specialties but a disproportionate share of misleading and fraudulent ones. The American Society of Plastic and Reconstructive Surgeons remains the specialty's largest and most important organization, but it now competes with several others for public recognition. None of these has had an easy time formulating policies on advertising; all have had less success at enforcing such standards. Moreover, despite several well-publicized exposés, Americans remain fairly unsophisticated when it comes to making sense of medical terminology and evaluating physicians' credentials. Practitioners who offer cosmetic surgery continue to derive benefits from calling themselves "board-certified" without specifying which board and by giving their practices official-sounding names like the "Academy of Facial

Surgery." In 1971 a study found that of 3,200 medical practitioners offering plastic surgical services, only 1,441 were certified by the American Board of Plastic Surgery; more than half, in other words, were self-designated. Twenty years later, an image audit conducted for the ASPRS found that, to the public, the terms *plastic surgery* and *cosmetic surgery* were practically synonymous. Consumers were also confused about the difference between and significance of terms such as *board certification* and *state licensing*.[15]

The strange case of New York plastic surgeon Richard L. Dombroff exemplifies the situation that developed as a result of all this. As journalist Mark Holoweiko noted in his 1989 exposé, Dombroff's start was promising (Columbia University and the Johns Hopkins University School of Medicine), but he never achieved board certification. In 1982, the year the Supreme Court ruled that physicians could advertise, Dombroff began advertising to the tune of $1,000 a week. He presented himself as a populist committed to democratizing the nation (or at least the New York metropolitan area) by bringing the benefits of plastic surgery—and with these, the possibilities of self-improvement and transformation—to the masses (at discount prices). This he in fact did: by the mid-1980s, a variety of employees at his chain of "Personal Best" clinics were performing five thousand operations a year, and his annual advertising budget reached $1.5 million, most of which went for TV spots that featured his wife, Pamela, with whom he lived in extravagant style.[16]

At the same time, malpractice suits were mounting: more than half a dozen as early as 1983; nine by 1984, when Dombroff's insurance carrier dropped his malpractice coverage; eighty by mid-1986; two hundred and twelve—a possible world record—by mid-1989, when Holoweiko's article ran in *Medical Economics*. Because Dombroff was not board certified, neither the American Board of Plastic Surgery nor the American Society of Plastic and Reconstructive Surgeons had any authority over him; state licensing boards' commitment to due process makes them by nature slow to act; while the Medical Society of the State of New York was able to persuade one malpractice carrier not to renew coverage, it could not prevent Dombroff from obtaining a new policy (from New York's joint underwriting association, which, Holoweiko explained, by law could not refuse). Retribution thus came not from organized medicine but from the same source as Dombroff's success: the media and, eventually, the public. After declaring bankruptcy, Dombroff plea-bargained a three-month jail term (for "the felony of scheming to defraud in the first degree and aiding and abetting the unlicensed practice of medicine") and surrendered his New York license.[17]

Granted, Dombroff's case, like that of Henry Junius Schireson, is an extreme example. But as this example suggests, the environment in which cosmetic surgery now exists—which surgeon Mark Gorney once likened to "the midway of a cheap carnival, complete with flashing colored lights, gaudy trappings, and loud barkers"—comes close to replicating the atmosphere into which cosmetic surgery, in this country at least, was born. Now, as then, surgeons seemingly will do anything to promote themselves and their practices, and experimentation thrives, often along lines pioneered decades earlier by the most adventurous, and adventuring, practitioners. J. Howard Crum scandalized his colleagues in the 1920s by performing public face-lifting operations at beauty conventions. Today surgeons do not operate in public, but they are happy to appear in public to promote their specialty and their practices. Since 1972, when Gimbels sponsored its first public lecture on cosmetic surgery, such presentations have become routine features at department stores, hospitals, and women's clubs around the country. Charles C. Miller, perhaps the most visionary among early-twentieth-century practitioners, advocated dissecting women's facial muscles to prevent movement and the wrinkling that would result. Today, there is Botox, which, when injected, produces the same results.[18]

In the second decade of this century, surgeons adopted the practice of injecting paraffin and then abandoned it in horror when they discovered its long-term results. Liquid silicone and collagen have gone in and out of favor, but now we are offered a new solution. The injection of autologous fat (sometimes called microlipoinjection) is currently being touted as a solution for everything from wrinkles to small penises. The results previously reported for similar fat-transfer techniques would seem to be less than promising: when introduced into new parts of the body, surgeons found in previous experimental episodes, fat can atrophy, liquefy, reabsorb unevenly and lump, even rot. Whether these new techniques will produce better results remains to be seen, but current indications are that, while they may produce some satisfactory results, they will also generate a significant amount of reparative work.[19]

Surgeons' traditional emphasis on artistry has come back in a particularly haunting manner. The infamous Henry Schireson, in 1938, asserted that a plastic surgeon could reproduce, in thirty minutes, the eyes of the Mona Lisa, on which Da Vinci had labored for four years. Today, Parisian body artist Orlan lives out Schireson's claim. In separate operations, all done as performance pieces and videotaped, Orlan has had surgeons use her face as a sculptural medium to recreate Diana's eyes, Europa's lips, Psyche's nose, the chin of the Venus de Milo, and the forehead of the Mona Lisa. European surgeons, according to Orlan, had trouble with this project, but American surgeons understood it immediately.[20]

Americans have responded to these developments in a variety of ways. Recalling a character in a 1923 novel about youth serum treatments, who despite her disapproval was insatiably curious and "read everything that appeared in the newspapers and magazines about it, not neglecting the advertisements," some are content just to imagine. A growing number, however, are moved to pursue one or several of these procedures, often with the most laconic of explanations. Mary Roach's recent article on Botox embodies this attitude. "You mess around with neurotoxin, you want to have a pretty good reason. You bet I do. It goes like this: I'm noticing ugly little lines between my eyebrows, and they bug me." Roach's summary of the injections' effect is equally disquieting: "I'm planning a murder, and it looks as if I'm thinking about my grocery list."[21]

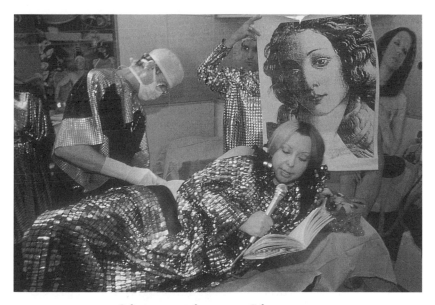

Orlan prepares for surgery, February 1991.

That many Americans have become more comfortable with cosmetic surgery suggests that surgeons' and patients' attempts to demystify it have been largely successful. As one surgeon termed it, cosmetic surgery is sanity, not vanity; it is simply the fast lane on the American highway to self-improvement. America, these days, admittedly seems an unpleasant place: competitive, critical, demanding, dangerous. As Americans have come to view their faces and bodies as entities that may be altered for social advantage or economic benefit, cosmetic surgery has become simply a realistic response to life in this most Darwinian of worlds. Most Americans probably would not go so far as to deem the decision not to have cosmetic surgery antisocial, but they are more ready than ever to concede that it may be impractical. And as Americans and their surgeons have come to see cosmetic surgery as the most practical solution for an ever-larger number of problems, not having surgery, like tilting at windmills, can seem hopelessly naive, at the very least outdated.

For this development, critics have been quick to point the finger at surgeons, and they may be held accountable to some extent. Clearly,

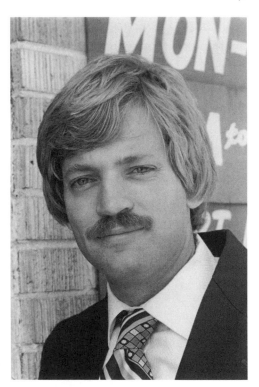

The future of politics? David Duke as Klansman, 1980 . . .

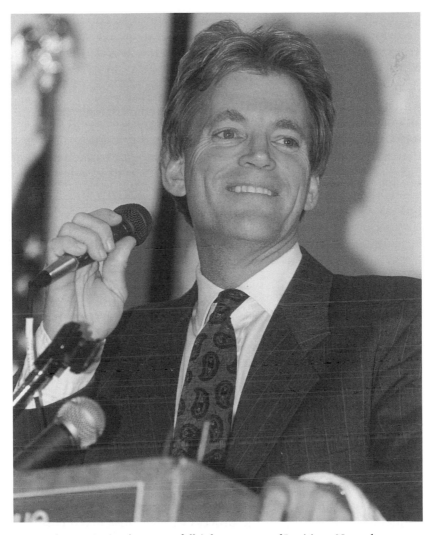

... and campaigning (unsuccessfully) for governor of Louisiana, November 1991.

plastic surgeons have led the trend toward marketing medical services to particular groups of consumers. They have not created the process called medicalization, but they have contributed to it by inventing new names for a growing number of deformities. An entirely new category, "hereditary lipodystrophies," derived from liposuction alone: "bat wing deformity" is characterized by "redundant skin and tissue hanging from the upper arms"; "spare tire deformity" is defined by excess adipose tissue around the waist and abdomen; most commonly, "violin deformity" (also called "saddlebags" or "riding breeches") is characterized by deposits of adipose tissue on the lateral (outer) thigh where it meets the hip. And, surely, surgeons are guilty of encouraging their patients' dreams. True, all but the most self-promoting admonish patients to be realistic (calf implants, they might have told the author of that desperate letter, will give you bigger calves, but they cannot guarantee that "everything will be fine"). But the readiness with which they acknowledge that in many cases a seemingly cosmetic change does result in a new outlook and a new life means that even the most conservative surgeons have fostered visions of total transformation. That it is these tales that shape patients' hopes and expectations should not surprise us.

Still, in moving toward an endorsement of cosmetic surgery, not just to improve appearance but to remedy deformities that adversely affect patients' health (in the new, larger sense of the word), surgeons have been driven by their patients' self-diagnoses. The patients who wrote plaintive letters to Jerome Webster and to the American Board of Plastic Surgery in the 1930s and 1940s—the patients who today tell their surgeons that their small breasts, or their big noses, or their riding breeches, make them feel ugly, self-conscious, ill at ease in the world (in a word, deformed) and insist that cosmetic surgery will cure their inferiority complexes or, in current terminology, improve their self-esteem—must also be considered responsible. Without the thousands of Americans who begged their surgeons to devise solutions to the problems that distressed them, cosmetic surgery would not be the phenomenon it is today.

Surgeons and patients, in short, together constructed a pragmatic, sensible, affordable image of cosmetic surgery—an American image of cosmetic surgery—and in the process they reconstructed cosmetic surgery as a peculiarly American solution to the inequalities of the modern world. From the beginning, cosmetic surgery has been shaped by pressures and priorities within American culture as well as within the profession of medicine, and its history illuminates the complex interplay between medical and cultural imperatives. With time it may lose its national flavor, but there is still something quintessentially American about cosmetic surgery; in it we see reflected the promise of individual transformation, the American dream of re-creation and reinvention writ large. Yet if we look carefully, we also see that, in cosmetic surgery, medical and cultural values have intertwined to produce a practice that subverts our most cherished hopes even as it seems to fulfill them, that is both cause and consequence of a loss of faith in the possibility of transformation on a broader scale. Because the pressures on them weighed more heavily, women were the pioneers in this individualizing process, but men are no longer immune; their recent rush to the scalpel suggests just how strong these cultural currents are. For Americans and for their cosmetic surgeons, the individual, external self offers a last, and apparently everlasting, frontier. As to whether this particular frontier is worthy of exploration, there may be, after all, a "lesson to be learned" in the Twilight Zone.

$\mathcal{N}otes$

Abbreviations

AAPS   American Association of Plastic Surgeons
ABPS   American Board of Plastic Surgery
ASPRS   American Society of Plastic and Reconstructive Surgeons, Inc.
JAMA   *Journal of the American Medical Association*
JPW   Jerome Pierce Webster Library of Plastic Surgery
NAPS   National Archives of Plastic Surgery
PRS   *Plastic and Reconstructive Surgery*

Archival Sources

National Archives of Plastic Surgery
Special Collections
Francis A. Countway Library of Medicine
Harvard Medical School
Boston, Massachusetts

Citations reflect the folder designations in use at the NAPS in 1991. Names of surgeons are their own. Patients or prospective patients are herein identified by initials only; the key is held by the archivist.

Jerome Pierce Webster Library of Plastic Surgery
Columbia University Libraries
Health Sciences Library
Special Collections Section
New York, New York

When I conducted my research in 1994, the Jerome Webster Collection was unprocessed; citations reflect the folder designations in use at that time. I reviewed correspondence and clipping files, in addition to 1,806 records, chosen at random, out of a total whose number was then unknown. Because I could not be certain that

I had a representative sample, I elected not to do a statistical study of these records, although the large number of rhinoplasty cases encouraged me to undertake some preliminary statistical evaluation (see Chapter 5).

Anecdotal evidence is taken from case files and from correspondence. All names of patients or prospective patients used herein are pseudonyms; the key is held by the archivist.

INTRODUCTION   *Present at the Re-Creation*

1. Josleen Wilson, *The American Society of Plastic and Reconstructive Surgeons' Guide to Cosmetic Surgery* (New York: Simon and Schuster, 1992), 13, 26, 191, 192.

2. Both quotations from Richard B. Stark, "The History of Plastic Surgery in Wartime," *Clinics in Plastic Surgery* 2:4 (October 1975), 509–510.

3. Ibid., 511; Anthony F. Wallace, "The Early Development of Pedicle Flaps," *Journal of the Royal Society of Medicine* 71 (November 1978), 834–835; Arthur J. Barsky, "A Personal Memoir: Plastic Surgery in the Twentieth Century," *Surgical Clinics of North America* 58:5 (October 1978), 1019.

4. The WHO definition is quoted by David C. Thomasma, "The Goals of Medicine and Society," in *The Culture of Biomedicine*, ed. D. Heyward Brock (Newark: University of Delaware Press, 1984), 51.

5. Joan Jacobs Brumberg, *Fasting Girls: The History of Anorexia Nervosa* (New York: New American Library, 1988), 3–6.

6. *New York Times*, December 12, 1978, C 10:1. This phenomenon is unique to the United States. British, French, and American surgeons participated equally in World War I, but at the onset of World War II Britain claimed only four plastic surgeons and France, two. The United States, in contrast, had almost fifty. This pattern has continued in the intervening decades.

7. JPW/Cecily Clemons.

8. *San Francisco Chronicle*, November 1, 1993, 11.

9. Sharon Romm, *The Changing Face of Beauty* (St. Louis: Mosby Year Book, 1992), 6; *San Francisco Chronicle*, November 1, 1993, 11; Calvin Colton, *Junius Tracts*, 1844, quoted in John G. Cawelti, *Apostles of the Self-Made Man* (Chicago: University of Chicago Press, 1965), 39.

10. Mary Lou Weisman, "The Feminist and the Face-Lift," *San Francisco Chronicle*, January 5, 1984, People section, 2; Dr. Gabe Mirkin's study, published in the *San Diego Union*, July 13, 1982, C1 is quoted in Terry Todd, "Anabolic Steroids: The Gremlins of Sport," *Journal of Sport History* 14:1 (Spring 1987), 89; "33,000 Women Tell How They Really Feel about Their Bodies," *Glamour*, February 1984, is quoted in Naomi Wolf, *The Beauty Myth: How Images of Beauty are Used against Women* (New York: William Morrow and Co., 1991), 10; Brumberg, *Fasting Girls*, 231.

11. JPW/Hilda Novak; Jacques W. Maliniak, *Sculpture in the Living: Rebuilding the Face and Form by Plastic Surgery* (New York: Romaine Pierson, 1934), 57; Henry Junius Schireson, *As Others See You: The Story of Plastic Surgery* (New York: Macaulay Co., 1938), 70–71; Frances Cooke Macgregor, *Transformation and Identity: The Face and Plastic Surgery* (New York: Quadrangle Press/New York Times Book Co., 1974), 60.

12. *HouseCalls,* Winter 1992. *HouseCalls* is a "community newsletter" published by St. Luke's Hospital, 3555 Army Street [now Cesar Chavez], San Francisco, CA 94110.

13. The American Society for Plastic and Reconstructive Surgery admitted its first female member in 1943. In 1980, Alma Dei Morani found approximately one hundred female plastic surgeons worldwide, of whom forty-one were in the United States; most were in private practice. See Alma Dei Morani, "Women Plastic Surgeons: An International Survey," *PRS* 66:5 (November 1980), 774–778. Maxwell Maltz, *Dr. Pygmalion: The Autobiography of a Plastic Surgeon* (New York: Thomas Y. Crowell Co., 1953).

14. Gustave Aufricht, "Philosophy of Cosmetic Surgery," *PRS* 20:5 (November 1957), 397.

15. The "homeliest girl" contest ran for the entire month of December 1924; the winner was announced in April 1925. The contest is noted in John D. Stevens, *Sensationalism and the New York Press* (New York: Columbia University Press, 1990), 135. I am indebted to Jesse Berrett for this reference. For information on films, I am grateful to Kristine Krueger, National Film Information Service, Academy of Motion Picture Arts and Sciences, and to Madeleine Mullin, National Archives of Plastic Surgery; for Oprah, see Journal Graphics Transcript #1468.

16. "Cheers for Cher," *Ms.,* July 1988, 53; on the therapeutic ethos, see Elaine Tyler May, *Homeward Bound: American Families in the Cold War Era* (New York: Basic Books, 1988), 14, 27; see also Robert N. Bellah et al., *Habits of the Heart: Individualism and Commitment in American Life* (Berkeley: University of California Press, 1985).

ONE   *Plastic Surgery Before and After*

1. Max Thorek, *A Surgeon's World: An Autobiography* (Philadelphia: J. B. Lippincott, 1943), 164.

2. This first society was founded in 1921 as the American Association of Oral Surgeons, renamed the American Association of Oral and Plastic Surgeons in 1931, and continues to exist as the American Association of Plastic Surgeons (AAPS), the name it took in 1942. The Society of Plastic and Reconstructive Surgery was organized by Jacques Maliniak in 1931 and in 1941 changed its name to the American Society of Plastic and Reconstructive Surgeons, Inc. (ASPRS), although it was sometimes referred to as the American Society of Plastic and Reconstructive Surgery. For the sake of clarity, throughout this book I use the names American Association of Plastic Surgeons and American Society of Plastic and Reconstructive Surgeons to refer to these organizations.

3. Historians have written extensively on the transformation in American culture that occurred between 1880 and 1920. Two concise treatments are Richard Wrightman Fox and T. J. Jackson Lears, eds., *The Culture of Consumption: Critical Essays in American History, 1880–1980* (New York: Pantheon, 1983), ix–xiv; and Joan Shelley Rubin, "Salvation as Self-Realization," *Reviews in American History* 20 (1992), 505–511.

4. Robert H. Ivy, "Personal Recollections of the Organization and Founders of the American Association of Plastic Surgeons," *PRS* 47:5 (May 1971), 438–439.

5. Maurice H. Cottle, "John Orlando Roe, Pioneer in Modern Rhinoplasty," *Archives of Otolaryngology* 80 (July 1964), 22–23; John B. Roberts, "The Cosmetic Surgery of the Nose," *JAMA* 19:8 (August 20, 1892), 231–233; "Society Proceedings, San Francisco County Medical Society, July 1903," *Occidental Medical Times* 17:10 (October 1903), 393. Jacques Joseph of Berlin, often credited with devising the intranasal operation, acknowledged Roe as the originator and as late as 1904 continued to voice preference for the extranasal incision.

6. Allan M. Brandt, *No Magic Bullet: A Social History of Venereal Disease in the United States since 1880* (New York: Oxford University Press, 1987), 10, 40, 161.

7. Joseph Safian, "Ethical Plastic Surgery vs. the Quack Beauty Doctor," Radio Lecture, Station WEAF, New York City, June 30, 1926, given under the auspices of the Gorgas Memorial Institute (NAPS, Safian Correspondence); James T. Campbell, "The Subcutaneous Injection of Paraffin More Particularly for the Correction of Nasal Deformities," *Illinois Medical Journal* 6:4 (September 1904), 381.

8. Perhaps because paraffin reached its zenith as a solution to cosmetic problems, Gersuny, who pioneered its use in this arena, is generally remembered as having popularized its use; see Robert M. Goldwyn, "The Paraffin Story," *PRS* 65:4 (April 1980), 517–524; F. Gregory Connell, "The Subcutaneous Injection of Paraffin for the Correction of Deformities of the Nose," *JAMA* 41:12 (September 19, 1903), 697–699 and *JAMA* 41:13 (September 26, 1903), 781; "Society Proceedings, San Francisco County Medical Society," *Occidental Medical Times* 17:10 (October 1903), 393; see also Harmon Smith, "Paraffin Injected Subcutaneously for the Correction of Nasal and Other Deformities," *JAMA* 41:13 (September 26, 1903), 773–776.

9. Goldwyn, "The Paraffin Story"; J. Carlyle DeVries, "The Surgical Correction of Featural Deformities," *American Journal of Dermatology and Genito-Urinary Diseases* 13:9 (September 1909), 427–428; Joseph C. Beck, "Chicago Laryngological and Otological Society Meeting of October 13, 1908," *Illinois Medical Journal* 15:1 (January 1909), 104; Blair O. Rogers, "A Chronologic History of Cosmetic Surgery," *Bulletin of the New York Academy of Medicine* 47:3 (March 1971), 269.

10. Seymour Oppenheimer, "A Condemnatory Note on the Use of Paraffin in Cosmetic Rhinoplasty," *Laryngoscope* 30:9 (September 1920), 595. For examples of reports of negative results, see Benjamin Franklin Davis, "Coal and Petroleum Products as Causes of Chronic Irritation and Cancer," *JAMA* 62:22 (May 30, 1914), 1716–1720 and "Paraffinoma and Wax Cancer," *JAMA* 75:25 (December 18, 1920), 1709–1711.

11. Goldwyn, "The Paraffin Story," 517.

12. Lois W. Banner, *American Beauty* (Chicago: University of Chicago Press, 1983), 205. According to Banner, the demise of the female moral superiority argument in the 1920s "seriously undermined" the identification of beauty with natural and democratic ideals. Character dropped out of the equation, but, once raised, the possibility that every woman might be beautiful did not disappear, "leaving the commercial beauty culture the major claimant to the means of beauty for all women." While today early feminists' moral superiority argument appears outdated, and, "with its overtones of asexuality, counterproductive to the movement for full sexual

expression," it "had raised an important barrier to the commercial exploitation of women in the area of physical appearance. With its demise, the modern commercial beauty culture scored a significant triumph" (207–208).

13. Ibid., 213–215, 217–219.

14. Ibid., 219–225.

15. First developed in 1886, face peeling involved applying acid (and in some cases electric current) to remove the upper layers of skin. As Banner notes, biographies of Helena Rubenstein and Elizabeth Arden "make clear that they did not use toxic substances in their cosmetics nor did they offer services for which their staffs were not trained" (214), but other sources suggest that many beauty parlors and doctors' offices offered similar types of services.

16. Rogers, "Chronologic History," 267; Kathryn Lyle Stephenson, "The 'Mini-Lift': An Old Wrinkle in Face Lifting," *PRS* 46:3 (September 1970), 226.

17. John B. Mulliken, "Biographical Sketch of Charles Conrad Miller, 'Featural Surgeon,'" *PRS* 59:2 (February 1977), 175–184; Rogers, "Chronologic History." Terms like *quack* and *irregular physician* are difficult to define in the years before medical education and certification were standardized. In general, they were used to denote physicians or practices that fell outside the boundaries of standard practice, such as they were at that time. Miller may have been regarded as a quack because the school he attended was not highly regarded, but his reputation is probably due more to the fact that he was extremely self-aggrandizing in a time when physicians were supposed to eschew publicity and to his interest in cosmetic surgery, which most doctors regarded as a subject unworthy of serious medical interest. The label *quack drugstore* appears to have derived from allegations that his employees, who were not doctors, wrote prescriptions for drugs they then dispensed.

18. Mulliken, "Biographical Sketch"; Rogers, "Chronologic History"; also see Miller articles cited below.

19. Charles C. Miller, *Cosmetic Surgery: The Correction of Featural Imperfections* (Chicago: Oak Printing Co., 1907), xxiv.

20. Charles C. Miller, "Outstanding Nasal Alae," *American Journal of Dermatology and Genito-Urinary Diseases* 11:6 (June 1907), 286–287; "Cosmetic Surgery of the Face," *International Journal of Surgery* 20:10 (October 1907), 312; "Semilunar Excision of the Skin at the Outer Canthus for the Eradication of 'Crow's Feet,'" *American Journal of Dermatology and Genito-Urinary Diseases* 11:11 (November 1907), 483–484.

21. See previous and Miller, "The Proper Treatment of the Nose with the Bulbous Tip," *Medical Council, Philadelphia* 12:8 (August 1907), 273; Miller, *Cosmetic Surgery*, 3.

22. Miller, "Outstanding Nasal Alae," 287.

23. Mulliken, "Biographical Sketch," 182.

24. Miller, "Subcutaneous Section of the Facial Muscles to Eradicate Expression Lines," *American Journal of Surgery* 21:8 (August 1907), 235; "Triangular Excisions of the Mucosa for Overcoming Operation for Downturning of the Angles of the Mouth," *Medical Council, Philadelphia* 13:4 (April 1908), 123.

25. *New York Times*, August 4, 1916, 4:4; B. K. Rank, "The Story of Plastic Surgery, 1868–1968," *Practitioner* 201(July 1968), 115; Anthony F. Wallace, "The

Development of Plastic Surgery for War," *Journal of the Royal Army Medical Corps* 131 (1985), 29; John Marquis Converse, "The Extraordinary Career of Doctor Varaztad Hovhannes Kazanjian," *PRS* 71:1 (January 1983), 140; Varaztad Kazanjian, "Remembrance of Things Past," *PRS* 35:1 (January 1965), 5–13; Hal B. Jennings, "Plastic Surgery in the Army: A Short Historical Account," *PRS* 48:5 (November 1971), 413–418.

    26. Converse, "Extraordinary Career"; and Kazanjian, "Remembrance."

    27. Converse, "Extraordinary Career," 140; Kazanjian, "Remembrance," 10; Jennings, "Plastic Surgery in the Army," 413–414; *New York Times,* August 4, 1916, 4:4.

    28. On Sidcup, see previous citations and Frank McDowell, "Plastic Surgery in the Twentieth Century," *Annals of Plastic Surgery* 1:2 (March 1978), 217–220; Arthur J. Barsky, "A Personal Memoir: Plastic Surgery in the Twentieth Century," *Surgical Clinics of North America* 58:5 (October 1978), 1019–1029; Richard Battle, "Plastic Surgery in the Two World Wars and in the Years Between," *Journal of the Royal Society of Medicine* 71 (November 1978), 844–845; Ivy, "Personal Recollections"; Richard B. Stark, "The History of Plastic Surgery in Wartime," *Clinics in Plastic Surgery* 2:4 (October 1975), 512. Among the Americans working at Sidcup were Vilray P. Blair, who in 1917 was offered the post of chief of head and neck (maxillofacial) surgery with the U.S. Army. He later persuaded the army's surgeon general to change his title to chief of plastic surgery, the first time the specialty was recognized by the army. Blair combed the country, recruiting physicians from hospitals and medical schools, and established four hospitals in the United States for the treatment of plastic surgical cases: Jefferson Barracks, Missouri, Walter Reed Hospital in Washington, D.C., Fort McHenry, Baltimore, and Camp May, New Jersey; three training programs were also established.

    29. Peter Bodley, "Development of Anaesthesia for Plastic Surgery," *Journal of the Royal Society of Medicine* 71 (November 1978), 841–842; Anthony F. Wallace, "The Early Development of Pedicle Flaps," *Journal of the Royal Society of Medicine* 71 (November 1978), 837–838; Rank, "Story of Plastic Surgery," 115–116; Wallace, "Development of Plastic Surgery for War," 30.

    30. *New York Times,* June 14, 1918, 6:2; Lawrence Ryan, "Plastic Surgery," *Illinois Medical Journal* 34:2 (August 1918), 69.

    31. Mrs. William K. Vanderbilt, "Miracles of Surgery on Men Mutilated in War," *New York Times Magazine,* January 16, 1916, 6:1; *New York Times,* July 27, 1919, 12:1.

    32. Dr. William Seaman Bainbridge, "Restoration of the Warrior's Lost Face," *Current Opinion* 67:3 (September 1919), 169; *New York Times,* December 29, 1918, III 4:1; *New York Times,* June 1, 1918, 6:5.

    33. Vanderbilt, "Miracles of Surgery"; *New York Times,* July 27, 1919, 12:1; Ernest Hemingway, *A Moveable Feast* (New York: Charles Scribner's Sons, 1964), 82.

    34. McDowell, "Plastic Surgery in the Twentieth Century," 220–221; Battle, "Plastic Surgery in the Two World Wars," 845.

    35. Converse, "Extraordinary Career"; Kazanjian, "Remembrance"; Barsky, "Personal Memoir," 1019–1020.

    36. Gustav J. E. Tieck, "New Intranasal Procedures for Correction of Deformities of the Nose Successfully Applied in Over 1,000 Cases during the Past Twelve Years," *American Journal of Surgery* 34:5 (May 1920), 117; M. F. Arbuckle, "Plastic Surgery of the Face: Its Recent Development and Its Relation to Civilian Practice," *JAMA*

75:2 (July 10, 1920), 102; Seymour Oppenheimer, "The Surgical Correction of the Aquiline or Hump Nose," *American Journal of Surgery* 34:5 (May 1920), 121.

37. Tieck, "New Intranasal Procedures," 117; Oppenheimer, "Surgical Correction," 121.

38. Oppenheimer, "Surgical Correction," 121; Ferris Smith, "Plastic Surgery: Its Interest to Otolaryngologists," *JAMA* 75:23 (December 4, 1920), 1556.

39. John Staige Davis, "Plastic and Reconstructive Surgery," *JAMA* 67:5 (July 29, 1916), 338.

40. Ibid., 338–339; Ralph St. J. Perry, "The Principles of Cosmetic Surgery," *American Journal of Clinical Medicine* 22:2 (February 1915), 152. On necessary training and qualifications, see also Vilray P. Blair, "The Aims of the SubSection of Plastic and Oral Surgery," *Surgery, Gynecology, and Obstetrics* 25:6 (December 1917), 730–731; Rea P. McGee, "The Maxillofacial Surgeon in a Mobile Hospital," *JAMA* 73:15 (October 11, 1919), 1118; Smith, "Plastic Surgery," 1555.

41. Ralph St. J. Perry, "Cosmetic Surgery," *American Journal of Clinical Medicine* 22:1 (January 1915), 49; Tieck, "New Intranasal Procedures," 117; Oppenheimer, "Surgical Correction," 122.

42. Mary Sharon Webb, "Beyond Beauty: Philosophy, Ethics and Plastic Surgery" (Ph.D. diss., Yale University, 1985) offers a cogent discussion of how the developing specialty dealt with these values.

43. Davis, "Plastic and Reconstructive Surgery," 339.

44. Tieck, "New Intranasal Procedures," 117; on women see Kathy Peiss, *Cheap Amusements: Working Women and Leisure in Turn-of-the-Century New York* (Philadelphia: Temple University Press, 1986), 139, for the Veiled Beauty story; Christina Simmons, "Modern Sexuality and the Myth of Victorian Repression," in *Passion and Power: Sexuality in History,* ed. Kathy Peiss and Christina Simmons (Philadelphia: Temple University Press, 1989), 157–177; Elaine Tyler May, *Great Expectations: Marriage and Divorce in Post-Victorian America* (Chicago: University of Chicago Press, 1980); Lillian Faderman, *Odd Girls and Twilight Lovers: A History of Lesbian Life in Twentieth-Century America* (New York: Penguin, 1991), esp. 37–61.

45. Tieck, "New Intranasal Procedures," 117; Joseph C. Beck, "Present Status of Plastic Surgery about the Ear, Face and Neck," *Laryngoscope* 30:5 (May 1920), 264; Oppenheimer, "Surgical Correction," 122. Beck conceded that "only in a small minority [of such cases] will one succeed" in dissuading the potential patient.

46. Adalbert G. Bettman, "Plastic and Cosmetic Surgery of the Face," *Northwest Medicine* 19:205–209 (1920), reprinted in *Aesthetic Plastic Surgery* 12:5–7 (February 1988).

47. Bettman, "Plastic and Cosmetic Surgery of the Face"; Rogers, "Chronologic History," 280–281.

48. Miller, *Cosmetic Surgery,* 3.

49. McDowell, "Plastic Surgery in the Twentieth Century," 220.

50. *New York Times,* August 4, 1920, 17:4; and "The Vanity That Becometh," August 6, 1920, 8:4.

51. *New York Times,* December 12, 1920, VI 6:2. In an undated list of foreign plastic surgeons, surgeon H. O. Bames of Los Angeles noted of Bourguet, "Good esthetic results; very questionable ethics" (NAPS, ABPS #277).

52. Banner, *American Beauty,* 269–271.

TWO   *The Specialty Takes Shape*

1. See "Archival Sources" preceding the start of the notes.

2. Paul Starr, *The Social Transformation of American Medicine* (New York: Basic Books, 1982), 98–123, 357.

3. One of the AMA's goals in this campaign was to curb Americans' tendency to choose practitioners and treatment methods from advertisements. The financial support provided by its growing membership, combined with its increasing authority, enabled the AMA to launch a campaign aimed at convincing magazines and newspapers to refuse advertisements having to do with medicine. By 1919, some nineteen thousand of the twenty thousand periodicals surveyed by the U.S. Public Health Service refused to carry advertisements from doctors. On quacks and quackery, see James Harvey Young's classic *The Medical Messiahs: A Social History of Health Quackery in Twentieth-Century America* (Princeton: Princeton University Press, 1967) and Starr, *Social Transformation,* 129–132. Gerald Carson's *The Roguish World of Doctor Brinkley* (New York: Rinehart & Co., 1960) recounts the brilliant career of a goat-gland transplanter and radio doctor brought down only by the combined efforts of the American Medical Association, the U.S. Post Office, the State Department, and the Federal Communications Commission.

4. See Advisory Board for Medical Specialties, *Directory of Medical Specialists Certified by American Boards* (New York: Columbia University Press, 1942), 1450–1473; editor's foreword to Samuel Iglauer, "Correction of Outstanding and Cauliflower Ears," *Hygeia,* April 1926, 196. The AMA-recognized school requirement did not apply to founding members. On the hospital, see Charles Rosenberg, "Inward Vision and Outward Glance: The Shaping of the American Hospital, 1880–1914," *Bulletin of the History of Medicine* 53 (1979), 346–391 and *The Care of Strangers: The Rise of America's Hospital System* (New York: Basic Books, 1987). The literature on professionalization and organization continues to expand; see W. Bruce Fye, *American Cardiology: The History of a Specialty and Its College* (Baltimore: Johns Hopkins University Press, 1996).

5. On the general state of medicine, surgery, and plastic surgery during these years, see, for example, Gustave Aufricht, "Story of the Foundation of the Plastic and Reconstructive Surgery Journal and Reminiscences of the Early Formative Years of Plastic Surgery as a Specialty," *PRS* 68:3 (September 1981), 370–375; Arthur J. Barsky, "A Personal Memoir: Plastic Surgery in the Twentieth Century," *Surgical Clinics of North America* 58:5 (October 1978), 1019–1029; Bradford Cannon, "The Flowering of Plastic Surgery," *JAMA* 263:6 (February 9, 1990), 862–864; Claire G. Fox and William P. Graham III, "The American Board of Plastic Surgery, 1937–1987," *PRS* 82:1 (July 1988), 166–185; William G. Hamm, "The Development of Plastic Surgery during the Past Sixty Years," *Annals of Plastic Surgery* 12:2 (February 1984), 102–104; Frank McDowell, "Plastic Surgery in the Twentieth Century," *Annals of Plastic Surgery* 1:2 (March 1978), 217–224; Joseph C. Beck, "Some Conclusive Remarks regarding Plastic Surgery from Personal Experience," *Annals of Otolaryngology, Rhinology, and Laryngology* 44:1 (March 1935), 93; and Pam Hait, "History of the American Society of Plastic and Reconstructive Surgeons," *PRS* 94:4 (September 1994), 1A–100A. Accounts of which schools, hospitals, and physicians were recognized as providing acceptable training differ, but most count those run by Blair and Davis.

Opthalmology, otolaryngology, and obstetrics and gynecology, in 1916, 1924, and 1930, respectively, were the first specialties to create examining boards that credentialed their members.

6. In midlife, Maliniac changed the spelling of his name to Maliniak. I have respected this change but have cited articles and statements as they were published at the time.

7. Richard J. Walsh, "The Divine Right to Look Human," *Woman's Home Companion,* October 1927, 29–30, 70.

8. Joseph Colt Bloodgood, "The Possibilities and Dangers of Beauty Operations," *Delineator,* October 1927, 20, 60; Maxine Davis, "Does Plastic Surgery Work?" *Pictorial Review,* December 1937, 18–19, 76–78.

9. Thyra Samter Winslow, "Beauty for Sale," *New Republic,* November 25, 1931, 40–42; Boyden Sparkes, "New Faces for Old," *Popular Mechanics,* July 1932, 66–71.

10. Dorothy Cocks, "What about Plastic Surgery?" *Good Housekeeping,* June 1930, 109, 150, 152, 155–156.

11. Jerome P. Webster, "In Memoriam: Vilray Papin Blair, 1871–1955," *PRS* 18:2 (August 1956), 83–103. The obituary carried in the *St. Louis Post Dispatch,* November 21, 1955, states that Blair received his M.D. degree from Washington University in 1893 (NAPS, ABPS #180).

12. Webster, "In Memoriam"; Fox and Graham, "The American Board," 166–168; Frank McDowell, "History of the American Association of Plastic Surgeons, to 1963," *PRS* 32:2 (August 1963), 243.

13. Webster, "In Memoriam," 88.

14. See Webster, "In Memoriam"; Fox and Graham, "The American Board"; and Robert H. Ivy, "Some Circumstances Leading to Organization of the American Board of Plastic Surgery," *PRS* 16:2 (August 1955), 77–85; also see Francis X. Paletta, "The American Board of Plastic Surgery Examinations," *PRS* 44:6 (December 1969), 558–563.

15. Webster, "In Memoriam"; Fox and Graham, "The American Board"; Ivy, "Some Circumstances"; Paletta, "The American Board."

16. Jerome P. Webster to Vilray P. Blair, March 8, 1937 (NAPS, ABPS #465).

17. Vilray P. Blair to John Staige Davis, November 1, 1937 (NAPS, ABPS #465); December 23, 1937 (NAPS, ABPS #237).

18. Vilray P. Blair to John Staige Davis, October 11, 1938 (NAPS, ABPS #232); Vilray P. Blair, notes, sixth meeting, American Board of Plastic Surgery Executive Committee, November 11, 1938 (NAPS, ABPS #15).

19. Albert D. Davis, "The Value and Limitations of Plastic Operative Procedures," *Medical Times* 67:4 (April 1939), 162–163; Vilray P. Blair, "Plastic Surgery of the Head, Face and Neck: The Psychic Reactions," *Journal of the American Dental Association* 23 (February 1936), 236–240; Kathryn Lyle Stephenson, "The 'Mini-Lift': An Old Wrinkle in Face Lifting," *PRS* 46:3 (September 1970), 226–235.

20. Francis X. Paletta, "History of the American Society of Plastic and Reconstructive Surgeons, Inc., 1931–1981: Its Growth, Change, Unity," *PRS* 68:3 (September 1981), 292–296; obituary, *PRS* 58:2 (August 1976), 261–265.

21. Jacques Maliniac, "American Society of Plastic and Reconstructive Surgery: Its Beginning, Objectives and Progress, 1932–1947," *PRS* 2:6 (November 1947),

517–521; obituary. The name City Hospital, Welfare Island comes from Maliniak himself, who remembered being assigned there in the late 1920s.

22. Maliniac, "American Society," 517–521; obituary; and Aufricht, "Story of the Foundation," 371.

23. *New York Times,* October 29, 1932, 10:6; May 27, 1933, 15:8.

24. *New York Times,* January 27, 1930, 23:4; January 29, 1930, 17:3.

25. *New York Times,* February 3, 1930, 21:6; June 12, 1930, 27:3.

26. JPW/Rose Brumberg; "Repairing Accident-Damaged Faces," *Literary Digest,* February 13, 1937, 17–18.

27. Minutes, American Board of Plastic Surgery Executive Committee, October 16, 1939 (NAPS, ABPS #16); Minutes, American Board of Plastic Surgery Annual Meeting, June 5, 1941 (NAPS, ABPS #18); John Staige Davis to Vilray P. Blair, June 26, 1941 (NAPS, ABPS #239); Vilray P. Blair to Jerome P. Webster, August 1, 1941; Vilray P. Blair to Jerome P. Webster, August 8, 1941; Vilray P. Blair to Jacques Maliniac, August 8, 1941; Jerome P. Webster to Vilray P. Blair, August 15 and 20, 1941 (all in NAPS, ABPS #465); John Staige Davis to Vilray P. Blair, August 2, 1941 (NAPS, ABPS #239); Minutes, American Board of Plastic Surgery, September 21, 1941 (NAPS, ABPS #19).

28. Andrew R. Boone, "Human Faces Remodeled," *Popular Science,* June 1934, 24–26 (Drs. Howard L. Updegraff of Hollywood and Ferris Smith of Grand Rapids, Mich., were also mentioned); Gretta Palmer, "When Plastic Surgery Is Justified," *Ladies Home Journal,* December 1939, 20–21.

29. A. F. (Mrs.) to American Board of Plastic Surgery, April 2, 1949 (NAPS, ABPS #313). On the Webster-Maliniak link, see Jerome P. Webster to James Barrett Brown, December 12, 1932 (JPW/Brown, Dr. James Barrett); Jerome P. Webster to Howard Patterson, February 6, 1939 (JPW/ P-General); Jerome P. Webster to John Staige Davis, August 20, 1941 (JPW/Joan Stott).

30. Harmon T. Rhoads, Jr., "As I Remember: Clarence R. Straatsma," *Annals of Plastic Surgery* 7:4 (October 1981), 329; Harry H. Orenstein, "How Excellent a Showman: Joseph Eastman Sheehan, 1885–1951," *Bulletin of the New York Academy of Medicine* 59:3 (April 1983), 327–330.

31. *New York Times,* March 30, 1927, 21:1; and Orenstein, "Showman."

32. On Dillinger, see John Edgar Hoover, "Plastic Surgery and Criminals: The Surgeon's Responsibility," *American Journal of Surgery* 28:1 (January 1935), 156, 159 and "The Practitioner's Responsibility When Fugitives Attempt to Conceal Identity by Means of Surgery," *JAMA* 104:18 (May 4, 1935), 1663–1664; *New York Times,* April 12, 1935, 18:4. See also *New York Times,* August 23, 1925, VII 5:1; May 9, 1928, 27:4; May 10, 1928, 26:6; August 14, 1932, II 4:2; and Harry Hayes, Jr., "Cops, Robbers, and Plastic Surgery," *PRS* 76:4 (October 1983), 645–648.

33. "Plastic Surgeon," *Time,* May 13, 1935, 44–45; Minutes, American Association of Oral and Plastic Surgeons, 1935 Annual Meeting (NAPS, HMS c86, #2). Also see McDowell, "History of the American Association of Plastic Surgeons," 255. Jerome Gelb, in "As I Remember: Clarence R. Straatsma," *Annals of Plastic Surgery* 7:4 (October 1981), 331 calls him "the Brooklyn-born British-accented plastic surgeon"; Hector Marino, in "Reminiscences of the American Society of Plastic and Reconstructive Surgeons, Inc., and Some of Its Members," *PRS* 68:3 (September 1981), 377, calls him "flamboyant." Also see Orenstein, "Showman."

34. Surgeons J. Eastman Sheehan, H. Lyons Hunt, and Arthur T. McCormack, as well as dermatologist Howard Fox, were quoted by name in Walsh, "The Divine Right to Look Human."

35. Minutes, American Board of Plastic Surgery Executive Committee, October 16, 1939 (NAPS, ABPS #16); John Staige Davis to Vilray P. Blair, January 24, 1940 (NAPS, ABPS #238).

36. The correspondence concerning these cases is incomplete but nonetheless revealing. See Jerome P. Webster to Vilray P. Blair, April 1, 1941; Clarence R. Straatsma to Vilray P. Blair, April 3, 1941; Gustave Aufricht to Vilray P. Blair, April 4, 1941; Thomas G. Orr to Joseph Eastman Sheehan, May 9, 1941; Joseph Eastman Sheehan to Thomas G. Orr, May 24, 1941 (NAPS, ABPS #329); Minutes, American Board of Plastic Surgery, September 21, 1941 (NAPS, ABPS #19). A story in *True Detective* magazine was the source of the abortionist connection; see Vilray P. Blair to Claire L. Straith, July 9, 1941 (NAPS, ABPS #329). Like Sheehan, Coakley and Safian became members of the founders' group; Pomerantz did not (see *Directory of Medical Specialists,* 1464, 1467).

37. Joseph Eastman Sheehan, obituary, *PRS* 8:1 (July 1951), 77–78. A woman complained to the American Board of Plastic Surgery in March 1945 that Sheehan had botched her nose job and yelled at her when she complained; the photographs she sent in support her claim that the surgical result was not aesthetically pleasing. The Board's response has not been preserved. See M.M.C. to American Board of Plastic Surgery, March 18 and June 3, 1945 (NAPS, ABPS #313). Louis Hall (attorney) to Jerome P. Webster, August 24, 1948 (JPW/Patients through 1949).

38. Jane A. Bowden, ed., *Contemporary Authors* 67 (Detroit: Gale Research Company, 1972), 383–384; Maxwell Maltz, *Dr. Pygmalion: The Autobiography of a Plastic Surgeon* (New York: Thomas Y. Crowell Co., 1953), 1, 5, 50–51, 53–54, 145.

39. *New York Times,* January 27, 1930, 23:4; January 29, 1930, 17:3; February 3, 1930, 21:6; June 12, 1930, 27:3; October 6, 1930, 25:4. On the prison project, see Elmer J. Leterman and Thomas W. Carlin, *They Dare to Be Different* (New York: Meredith Press, 1968), 85–87; and Maxwell Maltz, *New Faces, New Futures: Rebuilding Character with Plastic Surgery* (New York: Richard R. Smith, 1936), 254–255. Maltz must have met some of the other surgeons involved in the New York project, including Gustave Aufricht at Lincoln and Clarence Straatsma at City, but this association does not appear to have been maintained. Few surgeons refer to Maltz's work. Alma D. Morani, in "Reflections," *Clinics in Plastic Surgery* 10:4 (October 1983), recalls "observing the techniques of . . . Maxwell Maltz . . . and many others" (670). Reviews: see *Booklist* 32 (June 1936), 283; *New York Times,* April 26, 1936, 20; *Scientific Book Club Review* 7 (May 1936), 4. Jerome P. Webster saw a number of patients whose visits were inspired by Maltz's writings; he also saw some who were dissatisfied with Maltz's work (JPW/Marvin Bernhardt; Marie Boyer; Josie Farber; Anna Martin; Robert Patrick; Mary Rogers).

40. See, for example, *Vogue,* May 1, 1931, 26; June 1, 1931, 16; February 15, 1932, 36; March 15, 1935, 38; March 1, 1936, 40; also see clippings in JPW/Morgue 3.

41. *Vogue,* February 1, 1935, 22.

42. Jerome P. Webster to Vilray P. Blair, April 6, 1939 (NAPS, ABPS #465). For a recap of the case, see also Jerome P. Webster to John Staige Davis, February 29, 1944 (NAPS, ABPS #343).

43. Joseph Tamerin to Bob [Robert] Goldwyn, no date (NAPS, HMSc 84, #8); see also Vilray P. Blair to John Staige Davis, August 17, 1942 and John Staige Davis to Vilray P. Blair, August 26, 1942 (NAPS, ABPS #239). The following fall, New York surgeon Lyndon Peer wrote to Jerome P. Webster, "Dr. Ivy suggested that I destroy all correspondence relating to the ethics of an individual recently considered by the [ABPS]. This request has been complied with." Peer to JPW, October 26, 1943 (JPW/ASPRS 1938–1944).

44. See *Contemporary Authors.* Also *New York Times,* February 12, 1939, II 10:2 and March 12, 1944, 7:7. Maltz published several articles from 1939 to 1944: "New Method of Tube Pedicle Skin Grafting," *American Journal of Surgery* 43:2 (February 1939), 216–222; "New Method of Tube Pedicle Skin Grafting," *Journal of the International College of Surgeons* 3 (December 1940), 526–531; "Surgical Treatment of Recent Facial Wounds," *Journal of the International College of Surgeons* 5 (July/August 1942), 334–342; "Reconstruction of Thumb: New Technic," *American Journal of Surgery* 58 (December 1942), 429–433; "Reconstruction of Nasal Tip: New Technic," *American Journal of Surgery* 63 (February 1944), 203–205; "Surgical Treatment of Recent Wounds of the Face," *Eye, Ear, Nose and Throat Monthly* 23 (February 1944), 60–68. These articles are listed in the Ivy Index, vol. 3 of the *McDowell Series of Plastic Surgery Indexes* (Baltimore: Williams & Wilkins), 643. All the journals in which Maltz's articles appeared are recognized professional journals, but they are not the specialty journals, probably because he was not a member of the specialty organizations.

45. "John Crosby on TV," *New York Herald Tribune,* May 29, 1958 (JPW/ Maltz, Maxwell); "The Theatre," *New Yorker,* January 19, 1963, 60; *Newsweek,* January 21, 1963, 57; Maltz, *The Time Is Now* (New York: Simon and Schuster, 1975). I am indebted to Jesse Berrett for background on Frank Slaughter and for tracking down a copy of *The Magic Scalpel.*

46. Leterman and Carlin, *They Dare to Be Different,* 89–91; Robert Coles, "Dr. Maltz's Lifemanship," *New York Times Book Review,* February 26, 1967, 8, 10. Maltz's 1946 *Evolution of Plastic Surgery* received a less-than-favorable review in the *Bulletin of the History of Medicine* from Josiah Charles Trent, then an instructor in thoracic surgery at the University of Michigan at Ann Arbor.

47. On Bames, see Vilray P. Blair to Earl C. Padgett, December 27, 1938; Vilray P. Blair to Curt O. Von Wedel, December 27, 1938; Earl C. Padgett to Vilray P. Blair, December 29, 1938; Curt O. Von Wedel to Vilray P. Blair, January 3, 1939 (NAPS, ABPS #180). On Bettman, see Vilray P. Blair to John Staige Davis, May 5, 1941 and John Staige Davis to Vilray P. Blair, May 8, 1941 (NAPS, ABPS #239).

48. J. Howard Crum, *The Making of a Beautiful Face, or, Face Lifting Unveiled* (New York: Walton Book Co., 1928); *New York Times,* March 13, 1931, 48:3; Winslow, "Beauty for Sale." Apparently, little is known about Crum. Judith B. Zacher, M.D., included a short discussion of his book in "Plastic Surgery in the Late 1920s: Three Points of View," *Clinics in Plastic Surgery* 10:4 (October 1983), 667.

49. Winslow, "Beauty for Sale."

50. Crum, *Making of a Beautiful Face,* 5, 20.

51. Jacques W. Maliniak, "Facts and Fallacies of Cosmetic Surgery," *Hygeia,* March 1934, 200–202.

52. The school is now fully accredited as the Loyola University School of Medicine in Chicago. On Brinkley, see Carson, *The Roguish World*, 18. On Crum, see JPW/Eleanor Carroll; Claire Conway; Mildred Flanner; Sylvia Thatcher.

53. *New York Times*, March 18, 1932, 13:2; March 11, 1937, 25:4.

54. Davis, "The Value and Limitations," 158; also see Medical Society of the State of New York, *Medical Directory of New York, New Jersey, and Connecticut* (New York: Federal Printing Co., 1929), 75, and American Medical Association, *American Medical Directory* (1931), 80, 1114; (1961), 757; (1973), 2921. The episode is reminiscent of Crum's previous performances, and the doctor's quoted comment about artistry recalls much of Crum's book. Many if not most plastic surgeons, however, claimed and still claim to be artists, and the 1938–39 incident may have involved someone else entirely.

55. Alice Virginia Rogers to Jerome P. Webster, March 1937; Jerome P. Webster to Iago Galdston, March 1937; Iago Galdston (wire) to Alice Virginia Rogers, March 29, 1937 in JPW/Morgue 1. *Saturday Review of Literature*, January 31, 1942, 19. For examples of the letters received by the ABPS, see Mrs. I.D.S. to American Board of Plastic Surgery, May 18, 1944 and D.D. to American Board of Plastic Surgery, May 1, 1951 (NAPS, ABPS #313).

56. Henry Junius Schireson, *As Others See You: The Story of Plastic Surgery* (New York: Macaulay Co., 1938), xi.

57. Neither of these was approved by the American Medical Association. See *JAMA* 140:6 (June 11, 1949), 552; *New York Times*, March 27, 1927; 3:1; Carson, *Roguish World*, 3. Brice's nose job generated a great deal of publicity; see *New York Times*, August 2, 1923, 10:2; August 15, 1923, 10:3; August 16, 1923, 2:3 and 14:4. Also see Norman Katkov, *The Fabulous Fanny* (New York: Alfred A. Knopf, 1953), 141–142; Herbert G. Goldman, *Fanny Brice: The Original Funny Girl* (New York: Oxford University Press, 1992), 112, 127–128, 185–186; and Barbara W. Grossman, *Funny Woman: The Life and Times of Fanny Brice* (Bloomington: Indiana University Press, 1991), 147–151. Although both the *Philadelphia Record* and *Hygeia* assert that Schireson's first successful practice was in New York, the *New York Times* in 1923 identified him as a "Chicago plastic surgeon."

58. *New York Times*, March 26, 1927, 1:2; March 27, 1927, 3:1; Jacques W. Maliniak, *Sculpture in the Living: Rebuilding the Face and Form by Plastic Surgery* (New York: Romaine Pierson, 1934), 197–198. The Rubin episode is covered in the *JAMA* reports; the outcome is not stated.

59. *JAMA* 90:5 (February 4, 1928), 387–388. A similar case against a French surgeon, Dr. Dujarrier, received a great deal of publicity in the United States. In 1929 the Tribunal de Paris awarded Mme. LeGuen 200,000 francs (then $8,000). LeGuen had allegedly threatened to commit suicide if Dujarrier did not operate to reduce her legs. He agreed, but contracture and gangrene set in, and amputation resulted. The judge explained that Dujarrier "had made the serious mistake of offering to perform an operation which was not necessary to save the patient's life." The threat of suicide was no explanation, the judge continued; Dujarrier should have referred her to a psychiatrist. In 1931 the verdict was upheld by the Paris court of appeals, not because the court condemned non–life-saving operations but because the court found a lack of informed consent. See *New York Times*,

February 26, 1929, 29:3; *JAMA* 92:14 (April 6, 1929), 1198–1199; 96:21 (May 23, 1931)1809.

60. *JAMA* 90:5 (February 4, 1928), 387–388.

61. *JAMA* 93:4 (July 27, 1929), 303; *JAMA* 94:12 (March 22, 1930), 873; *New York Times,* June 24, 1930, 25:5; *JAMA* 96:22 (May 30, 1931), 1883.

62. Kevin Sweeney, "A Brief History of Plastic Surgery Movies," *Plastic Surgery News* (July 1990); *Science News Letter,* September 17, 1938, 185 and November 11, 1939, 312.

63. *JAMA* 112:5 (February 4, 1939), 435; 112:24 (June 17, 1939), 2543; 114:22 (June 1, 1940), 2228–2229; 117:16 (October 18, 1941), 1369; Robert Maris, "King of the Quacks," *Hygeia,* June 1944, 414–415, 454. *Hygeia* gave 1939 as the date Schireson declared bankruptcy.

64. Maris, "King of the Quacks"; *JAMA* 123:12 (November 20, 1943), 772.

65. "King of Quacks," *Time,* May 1, 1944, 43–44; Maris, "King of the Quacks"; *JAMA* 125:2 (May 13, 1944), 161; 125:10 (July 8, 1944), 730; 126:2 (September 9, 1944), 116; 126:15 (December 9, 1944), 972; 129:13 (November 24, 1945), 895; 131:9 (June 29, 1946), 769; 131:14 (August 1946), 1163; 135:6 (October 11, 1947), 365; 140:6 (June 11, 1949), 552. After the *Record's* accusation, the state board of Medical Education and Licensure stated that the investigation was continuing under a new director.

66. *JAMA* 125:10 (July 8, 1944), 730; 126:2 (September 9, 1944), 116; 126:15 (December 9, 1944), 972; 129:13 (November 24, 1945), 895; 131:9 (June 29, 1946), 769; 131:14 (August 1946), 1163; 135:6 (October 11, 1947), 365; 140:6 (June 11, 1949), 552.

67. Jerome P. Webster's papers contain numerous references to Schireson: see JPW/Schireson, Henry J.; Jerome P. Webster to Dr. Warren B. Davis, May 18, 1944 (JPW/D-general, 1931–1960); Jerome P. Webster to Miss Mary Reid, superintendant, Presbyterian Hospital, January 10, 1947 (JPW/Patients to 1947); also see JPW/Lois Brandt; Paula Freedman.

68. Katkov, *The Fabulous Fanny,* 141; Maris, "King of the Quacks." Davis, in "The Value and Limitations," 158, noted that publicity about plastic surgery reached a high point with the Sadye Holland case, dropped, revived with Frederick Collins's 1928 *Delineator* piece, "The Truth about Face Surgery," dropped, and did not revive until Dillinger's capture in 1935.

THREE   *Consumer Culture and the Inferiority Complex*

1. Hazel Rawson Cades, *Any Girl Can Be Good-Looking* (New York: D. Appleton-Century Co., 1927), 3, 7, 10. Cades (Mrs. John Simpson Pearson) was beauty editor of *Woman's Home Companion* from 1922 to 1956 and contributed to other national magazines. She was a member of the National Girl Scouts' public relations committee; her other books for young women were *Good Looks for Girls* (1932) and *Handsome Is as Handsome Does* (1938).

2. *New York Times,* March 8, 1925, 18:2 (also see December 5, 1926, 27:4; January 25, 1928, 20:5; and December 21, 1934, 15:2); George C. Schaeffer, "Plastic Surgery, Its Relation to General Surgery," *Ohio State Medical Journal* (January 1925), 14.

3. Cades, *Any Girl*, 9–10, 34, 156–157; Celia Caroline Cole, "Lost and Found," *Delineator*, June 1926, 22, 66; Letters, *Photoplay*, June 1923, 10 and December 1923, 24. See also Joseph Colt Bloodgood, "The Possibilities and Dangers of Beauty Operations," *Delineator*, October 1927, 20, 60.

4. *New York Times*, March 4, 1925, 21:6; "Hi-Jacking the Face," *Collier's*, November 16, 1929, 26.

5. Joseph C. Beck, "Review of Twenty-five Years Observations in Plastic Surgery, with Special Reference to Rhino-Plasty," *Laryngoscope* 31:7 (July 1921), 489; John Staige Davis, "Art and Science of Plastic Surgery," *Annals of Surgery* 84:2 (August 1926), 203–210; Vilray P. Blair, "Plastic Surgery of the Head, Face and Neck: The Psychic Reactions," *Journal of the American Dental Association* 23 (February 1936), 236–240.

6. Advertisement, *Photoplay*, February 1923, 113.

7. Cecil Barton, "Hollywood," *Vogue*, February 15, 1930, 59; Frederick Lewis Allen, *Only Yesterday: An Informal History of the Nineteen-Twenties* (1931; New York: Harper and Row, 1957), 101–102; Lary May, *Screening Out the Past: The Birth of Mass Culture and the Motion Picture Industry* (Chicago: University of Chicago Press, 1980), 164–165; *New York Times*, April 28, 1929, 24:8.

8. Mrs. Nesta E. Harris to *Photoplay*, *Photoplay*, June 1923, 10.

9. Norman Katkov, *The Fabulous Funny* (New York: Alfred A. Knopf, 1953), 141; *New York Times*, August 15, 1923, 10:3 and August 16, 1923, 14:4; on Brice's nose job, also see Herbert G. Goldman, *Fanny Brice: The Original Funny Girl* (New York: Oxford University Press, 1992), 112, 127–128, 185–186; and Barbara W. Grossman, *Funny Woman: The Life and Times of Fanny Brice* (Bloomington: Indiana University Press, 1991), 147–151; "The Tragedy of Valentino's Brother's Nose," *Literary Digest*, September 21, 1929, 43, 46. After being disfigured in an automobile accident, vaudeville star Josephine Rochlitz was regarded with sympathy when she underwent plastic surgery with John Staige Davis (*New York Times*, April 28, 1929; 24:8).

10. Sylvia Ullback [Sylvia of Hollywood], *No More Alibis* (Chicago: Photoplay Publishing Co., 1935), 138 (I am indebted to Megan Heath and Kristine Krueger of the National Film Information Service, Academy of Motion Picture Arts and Sciences, for this reference).

On face peeling, see Harold J. Brody, *Chemical Peeling* (St. Louis: Mosby Year Book, 1992); Robert Kotler et al., *Chemical Rejuvenation of the Face* (St. Louis: Mosby Year Book, 1992); H. O. Bames, "Truth and Fallacies of Face Peeling and Face Lifting," *Medical Journal and Record* 126:2 (July 20, 1927), 87; *New York Times*, February 20, 1928, 25:7 and November 14, 1933, 4:2; Jacques W. Maliniak, *Sculpture in the Living: Rebuilding the Face and Form by Plastic Surgery* (New York: Romaine Pierson, 1934), 187–193. On paraffin, see John H. Harter, "Plastic Surgery of the Face," *Northwest Medicine* 28:4 (April 1929), 185–187; Noah E. Aronstam, "The Cosmetic Evil," *Medical Record* (New York) 146:7 (October 6, 1937), 313–314; "Dangers of Paraffined Beauty," *Literary Digest*, June 11, 1927, 22. George D. Wolf, "Paraffinoma of the Nose," *American Journal of Surgery* 55:1 (January 1942), 153, noted that paraffinomas were frequently encountered from 1900 to 1925 but rare by 1942. "Methods of Removing Superfluous Hair," *Hygeia*, June 1926, 335–336, warned that X-rays powerful enough to destroy the hair follicle would disfigure the skin.

Jerome P. Webster's files contain numerous examples of patients who came to him after undergoing such treatments, sometimes as much as twenty years previously (JPW/Melissa Carroll, Claire Conway, Ida Davis, Isabella Ruiz).

The new body consciousness of the 1920s also inspired a new preoccupation with dieting, which sparked unprecedented numbers of get-rich-quick schemes; see Arthur J. Cramp, "Swindling the Stylish Stout," *Hygeia*, September 1926, 511–512.

11. *New York Mirror*, December 1, 1924, p. 1 and ff.

12. *New York Times*, March 4, 1925, 21:6; Cole, "Lost and Found"; "Beauty Surgery for Busy Thugs," *Literary Digest*, April 7, 1934; Gretta Palmer, "When Plastic Surgery Is Justified," *Ladies Home Journal*, December 1939, 20–21.

13. John Cawelti, *Apostles of the Self-Made Man* (Chicago: University of Chicago Press, 1965), 48; Warren Susman, "'Personality' and the Making of Twentieth Century Culture," in *Culture as History: The Transformation of American Society in the Twentieth Century* (New York: Pantheon, 1984), 273–274.

14. Susman, "'Personality,'" esp. 277–280.

15. Sylvia of Hollywood [Sylvia Ullback], *Hollywood Undressed: Observations of Sylvia as Noted by Her Secretary* (New York: Brentano's, 1931), 87–88, 128–129; and *Pull Yourself Together, Baby!* (New York: McFadden Book Co., 1936), ix–xi.

16. Roland Marchand, *Advertising the American Dream: Making Way for Modernity, 1920–1940* (Berkeley: University of California Press, 1985), 209–212.

17. Ibid., 209–212.

18. Ibid., 210, 290; Lois Banner, *American Beauty* (Chicago: University of Chicago Press, 1983), 272; Thyra Samter Winslow, "Beauty for Sale," *New Republic*, November 25, 1931, 40–42.

19. As industries, both plastic surgery and advertising were relatively new, and it is not surprising that the parable their practitioners found most compelling was the one that bolstered their standing.

20. F. A. Booth, "Cosmetic Surgery of the Face, Neck and Breast," *Northwest Medicine* 21:6 (June 1922), 170–172; Jacques W. Maliniak, "Facts and Fallacies of Cosmetic Surgery," *Hygeia*, March 1934, 200–202; Schaeffer, "Plastic Surgery," 14; *New York Times*, May 16, 1927, VII 17:1.

21. Davis, "Art and Science," 203–210, esp. 206; H. Lyons Hunt, "The Task of the Plastic Surgeon," *American Medicine* 40 (September 1934), 361–362; *New York Times*, February 12, 1939, II 10:2.

22. In *The Damned and the Beautiful: American Youth in the 1920's* (New York: Oxford University Press, 1977), Paula Fass notes college students' emphasis on the "externals of appearance and the accessories of sociability," as well as their "scrupulous attention to grooming" (230, 243).

23. J. Eastman Sheehan, "Some Remarks on Plastic Surgery," *American Journal of Surgery* 39:4 (April 1925), 89; Joseph C. Beck, "Cosmetic Surgery of the Nose," *Hygeia*, July 1926, 393–394; *New York Times*, July 13, 1929, 32:4.

24. Robert McElvaine, *The Great Depression* (New York: Times Books, 1984), 3–24, 196–223; and Robert McElvaine, *Down and Out in the Great Depression: Letters from the Forgotten Man* (Chapel Hill: University of North Carolina Press, 1983), 7, 17, 25; Adalbert G. Bettman, "The Psychology of Appearances," *Northwest Medicine* 28:4 (April 1929), 182–185; H. O. Bames, "Esthetic Plastic Surgery," *California*

and Western Medicine 33:2 (August 1930), 588; George D. Wolf, "New Noses for Old," *Hygeia,* November 1931, 1005–1006; Clarence Straatsma, "Plastic Surgery: Its Uses and Limitations," *New York State Journal of Medicine* 32:5 (March 1, 1932), 254; Claire L. Straith, "Plastic Surgery: Its Psychological Aspects," *Journal of the Michigan State Medical Society* 31:1 (January 1932), 13–18; Maliniak, *Sculpture in the Living,* 69–70, 202–203.

25. Wolf, "New Noses"; James Stotter, *Beauty Unmasked* (New York: Raymond Press, 1936), introduction.

26. Marchand, *Advertising,* 213–217; T. J. Jackson Lears, "American Advertising and the Reconstruction of the Body," in *Fitness in American Culture: Images of Health, Sport, and the Body, 1830–1940,* ed. Kathryn Grover (Amherst: University of Massachusetts Press; Rochester, N.Y.: Margaret Woodbury Strong Museum, 1989), 62. Susan Reverby correctly observes that neither Lears nor Marchand takes gender into account, and there is clearly a difference in their concerns, with men's fears centering on jobs and women's on their prospects in the marriage market. For a fascinating comparative case, see Julia Rechter, "'The Glands of Destiny': Scientific, Medical, and Popular Views of the Sex Hormones in 1920s America" (Ph.D. diss., University of California at Berkeley, 1997).

27. JPW/Muriel Johnson; Richard Thomas; Lily Pells; Betty Hogan; Adela Captiva; Jean Swenson; Lucy Wolf; Jane Hatch.

28. Maliniak, *Sculpture in the Living,* 63; Joseph C. Beck and M. Reese Guttman, "Recent Advances in Plastic and Reconstructive Surgery of the Ear, Nose and Throat," *American Journal of the Medical Sciences* 196 (December 1938), 875–882; Blair, "Plastic Surgery of the Head, Face and Neck," 236–240; Albert D. Davis, "The Value and Limitations of Plastic Operative Procedures," *Medical Times* 67:4 (April 1939), 162–163.

29. See for example, *New York Times,* June 14, 1918, 6:2; January 16, 1916, IV 6:1; July 27, 1919, 12:1; M. F. Arbuckle, "Plastic Surgery of the Face: Its Recent Development and Its Relation to Civilian Practice," *JAMA* 75:2 (July 10, 1920), 102; Gustave Tieck, "New Intranasal Procedures for Correction of Deformities of the Nose Successfully Applied in Over 1,000 Cases during the Past Twelve Years," *American Journal of Surgery* 34:5 (May 1920), 117; Bettman, "The Psychology of Appearances," 182–185; see also Samuel Iglauer, "Correction of Outstanding and Cauliflower Ears," *Hygeia,* April 1926, 196.

30. *San Francisco Examiner,* July 13, 1921, 18:1; *New York Times,* April 8, 1927, 22:6. Dr. Carleton Simon, former deputy police commissioner and, according to the *Times,* an authority on criminology, spoke in support of such programs at the 1933 meeting of the Society of Plastic and Reconstructive Surgeons. Simon affirmed the importance of plastic surgery, noting that some Americans who might otherwise have led "law abiding lives" had turned to crime "because facial disfigurements had handicapped them and given them inferiority complexes." During the late 1930s, under police commissioner Austin H. MacCormick, an experiment was organized whereby New York surgeons, including Maxwell Maltz, operated on one hundred criminals selected from reform schools and prisons. Juvenile offenders were given first priority, as they were deemed more likely to benefit. The state of Illinois also experimented with plastic surgery in the 1930s with, according to Chicago surgeon

John F. Pick, "excellent psychologic and sociologic results." See *New York Times,* May 27, 1933, 15:8; Maxwell Maltz, *New Faces, New Futures: Rebuilding Character with Plastic Surgery* (New York: Richard R. Smith, 1936), 251–266, esp. 259–264; John F. Pick, "Ten Years of Plastic Surgery in a Penal Institution: Preliminary Report," *Journal of the International College of Surgeons* 11:3 (May/June 1948), 315–318.

    31. Cole, "Lost and Found."

    32. Nathan G. Hale Jr., *Freud and the Americans: The Beginnings of Psychoanalysis in the United States, 1876–1917* (New York: Oxford University Press, 1971), 432–433; Walter Bromberg, *Psychiatry between the Wars, 1918–1945: A Memoir* (Westport, Conn.: Greenwood Press, 1982), 126; Jill G. Morawski and Gail A. Hornstein, "Quandary of the Quacks: The Struggle for Expert Knowledge in American Psychology, 1890–1940," in *The Estate of Social Knowledge,* ed. JoAnne Brown and David K. van Keuren (Baltimore: Johns Hopkins University Press, 1991), 106–133.

    33. John C. Burnham, *How Superstition Won and Science Lost: Popularizing Science and Health in the United States* (New Brunswick, N.J.: Rutgers University Press, 1987), 85–95; John M. O'Donnell, *The Origins of Behaviorism: American Psychology, 1870–1920* (New York: New York University Press, 1985), 4, 38, 77, 217; Bromberg, *Psychiatry,* 12; Paul M. Dennis, "Psychology's First Publicist: H. Addington Bruce and the Popularization of the Subconscious and Power of Suggestion before World War I," *Psychological Reports* 68 (June 1991), 754–765; Maurice Green and R. W. Rieber, "The Assimilation of Psychoanalysis in America," in *Psychology: Theoretical-Historical Perspectives,* ed. R. W. Rieber and Kurt Salzinger (New York: Academic Press, 1980), 288. See also Fred Matthews, "The Americanization of Sigmund Freud: Adaptations of Psychoanalysis before 1917," *Journal of American Studies* 1 (1967), 39–62; and Ludy T. Benjamin Jr., "Why Don't They Understand Us? A History of Psychology's Public Image," *American Psychologist* 41:9 (September 1986), 941–946.

    34. Catherine Lucille Covert, "Freud on the Front Page: Transmission of Freudian Ideas in the American Newspaper of the 1920's" (Ph.D. diss., Syracuse University, 1975), 236; Marjorie Hope Nicolson, "Scholars and Ladies," *Yale Review* (Summer 1930), 784; Frederick J. Hoffman, *The Twenties: American Writing in the Postwar Decade* (New York: Viking, 1949, 1955), 89–90. Also see Roderick Nash, *The Nervous Generation: American Thought, 1917–1930* (Chicago: Ivan R. Dee/Elephant Paperbacks, 1990), 52; John C. Burnham, "The New Psychology: From Narcissism to Social Control," in *Paths into American Culture: Psychology, Medicine, and Morals* (Philadelphia: Temple University Press, 1988), 74–75, 85–86; Hale, *Freud,* 432–433; Bromberg, *Psychiatry,* 5, 15, 103, 126; William H. Burnham, *The Normal Mind: An Introduction to Mental Hygiene and the Hygiene of School Instruction* (New York: D. Appleton-Century Co., 1924), 246–267.

    35. Hale, *Freud,* 400–402, 434, 475; Bromberg, *Psychiatry,* 17, 61, 74; Harvey O. Higgins, "Your Other Self," *Outlook,* November 28, 1928, 1228; G. Lindzey, *Theories of Personality,* 2d ed. (New York: John Wiley & Sons, 1970), 127, in Heinz L. Ansbacher, "Alfred Adler: A Historical Perspective," *American Journal of Psychiatry* 127:6 (December 1970), 778; *New Yorker,* "Profiles," May 5, 1928, 29–31. According to Bromberg (*Psychiatry,* 90), at one point New York counted more Adlerian therapists than Jungian analysts. In *The Nervous Generation* (56), Nash suggests that

Freudian psychology, with its reliance on the subconscious, was particularly likely to find supporters in the early twentieth century. Freudian psychology portrayed man not as master of his fate but as driven by forces (albeit forces inside his head) that he neither fully understood nor controlled. Adler, conversely, appealed for opposite reasons.

36. Ansbacher, "Alfred Adler," 777–782; Edward Hoffman, *The Drive for Self: Alfred Adler and the Founding of Individual Psychology* (Reading, Mass.: Addison-Wesley, 1994), 196–209; Nathan Hale, personal communication, January 28, 1993. I am indebted to Professor Hale for many of the references in this chapter, as well as for his encouragement, which led me to pursue an avenue of inquiry I might otherwise have passed by.

Adler's work began to attract attention in the United States during the teens and twenties. Psychologist G. Stanley Hall used Adler's books in seminars and invited him to visit the United States, although the visit was delayed because of the outbreak of war. William Alanson White wrote the introduction to the English translation of Adler's *The Neurotic Constitution*, published in 1917; Smith Ely Jeliffe's translation of Adler's 1907 book on organ inferiority was published that same year.

Edward Hoffman offers the most recent take on Adler's life; see also Phyllis Bottome, *Alfred Adler: Apostle of Freedom* (London: Faber and Faber, 1939); Manès Sperber, *Masks of Loneliness: Alfred Adler in Perspective*, trans. Krishna Winston (New York: Macmillan, 1974); Gardner Murphy, "The Response to Freud," in *Historical Introduction to Modern Psychology* (New York: Harcourt Brace & Co., 1949), 331–348; A. A. Roback, *History of American Psychology* (New York: Collier, 1964), 330–331.

Adler was a prolific writer. A useful starting point is "Individual Psychology," the summary of his work he penned for inclusion as chapter 21 in *Psychologies of 1930*, ed. Carl Murchison (Worcester, Mass.: Clark University Press, 1930), 395–405. His popular publications included Lola Jean Simpson's "as told to" series in *Ladies Home Journal* ("First Comes Mother," February 1930, 26–27, 216–222; "Then Comes Father," November 1930, 36–37, 284–290; and "The Wide, Wide World," October 1931, 40–41, 269–274); "A Doctor Remakes Education," *Survey*, September 1, 1927, 490–495; "On Teaching Courage," *Survey*, November 15, 1928, 241–242; and "Are Americans Neurotic?" *Forum*, January 1936, 44–45. For summaries of his work, see Green and Rieber, "The Assimilation of Psychoanalysis in America," esp. 278–281; Kurt Adler, "The Relevance of Adler's Psychology to Present-Day Theory," *American Journal of Psychiatry* 127:6 (December 1970), 773; Ansbacher, "Alfred Adler," 778–779.

Many in the psychological field misunderstood Adler's work and criticized him for overemphasizing the sexual aspects of inferiority; for example, see William I. Thomas and Dorothy Swain Thomas, *The Child in America: Behavior Problems and Programs* (New York: Alfred A. Knopf, 1928), 26, 464–465. In *Masks of Loneliness* (20–21), Sperber notes: "The inferiority complex, an expression which was quickly to become famous and to make Adler himself famous, was frequently and improperly understood to be an extension and a mental reflection of inferior organs. This error was soon recognized even by laymen, for we all know that feelings of inferiority are not attributable to inadequate organs alone."

37. The genesis of the term is unclear, but the concept is clearly Adler's. Lorine Pruette, then a Clark University Ph.D. candidate, used the term *inferiority complex*

in "Some Applications of the Inferiority Complex to Pluralistic Behavior," *Psychoanalytic Review* 9 (1922), 28–39. Bernard Glueck, William Alanson White, and William Healy, the three psychiatrists upon whom Clarence Darrow called in the Leopold-Loeb case, were not Adlerians, but Leopold's "inferiority-superiority complex" was one of the factors to which they testified. Adler, in "Individual Psychologies" (198) estimated that popularization came around the publication date of *The Practice and Theory of Individual Psychology,* published simultaneously in Munich and New York in 1924, at which point "our great Stanley Hall turned away from Freud and ranged himself with the supporters of individual psychology, together with many other American scholars who popularized the 'inferiority and superiority complexes' throughout their whole country." In 1928 the *New Yorker* attributed "the contribution of the 'inferiority complex' idea" to Adler, but Harvey O. Higgins, in *Outlook,* as clearly attributed it to Freud: see "Profiles," *New Yorker,* May 5, 1928, 29–31 and Higgins, "Your Other Self," 1229. Ira S. Wile, in a review of Adler's late work *What Life Should Mean to You* (*Mental Hygiene* 16:1 [January 1932], 139), credits Adler with inventing the inferiority complex.

In *Spectacle of a Man* (New York: Jefferson House, 1937), by John Coignard (pseud.), one of the first novels to build a plot around Freudian psychoanalysis, discussions of inferiority feelings (39, 148–149) are sprinkled freely among the more Freudian topics. See also George K. Pratt, "Wives Who Help Their Husbands to Fail" (96–97) and "Day-Dreamers and Bluffers" (184–189) and Karl Menninger, "Depressions" (194), in *Why Men Fail,* ed. Morris Fishbein (New York: New York Tribune, 1927). In child guidance literature, see Burnham, *The Normal Mind,* 400, 451–487, 537; Smiley Blanton and Margaret Blanton, *Child Guidance* (New York: Century Co., 1927), 231–232; Thomas and Thomas, *The Child in America,* 26, 464–465; William E. Carter, "Physical Findings in Problem Children," *Mental Hygiene* 10:1 (January 1926), 75–84; Lawson G. Lowrey, "Competitions and the Conflict over Difference: The Inferiority Complex in the Psychopathology of Childhood," *Mental Hygiene* 12:2 (April 1928), 316–330; and Edward A. Strecker, "Everyday Psychology of the Normal Child," *Mental Hygiene* 17:1 (January 1933), 76.

38. Douglas A. Thom, "Mental Hygiene and the Depression," *Mental Hygiene* 16:4 (October 1932), 564–576; "Report of Subcommittee V, the Committee on Mental Hygiene of the Steering Committee on Social Planning, Rochester Council of Social Agencies, Organizing a Community for Mental Hygiene," *Mental Hygiene* 17:3 (July 1933), 424–450; Donald A. Laird, "Why Do We Buy?" *Review of Reviews,* January 1935, 32–35, 76; Marchand, *Advertising,* 210, 290.

I am indebted to Heinz Ansbacher (personal communication, June 11, 1996) for a story that suggests that this concept's popularity crossed national borders. In the early 1940s a young woman in Germany apologized to her service garage for her old Model A Ford; the mechanic asked, "What's the matter? You have an inferiority complex?" In Germany the cumbersome *Minderwertigkeitskomplex* was, in popular parlance, abbreviated into the chummy *"Min-ko."*

39. Dana Burnet, "The Inferiority Complex," *Collier's,* January 26, 1924, 3–4, 28–31; Allan Harding, "The Four Commonest Complexes and How to Get Rid of Them," *American Magazine,* April 1924, 38–39, 149–157; Winthrop D. Lane, "Your Child and That Fashionable Complex," *Delineator,* October 1927, 16, 62; Edouard Claparède,

"Inferiority Complex," *Review of Reviews*, September 1930, 76–77; Neal O'Hara, "Great American Worm," *American Magazine*, December 1930, 16–17; "Differences May Cause Inferiority Complex," *Hygeia*, April 1931, 387; "Fighting Our Inferiority Complex," *Literary Digest*, June 11, 1932, 28; Paul Popenoe, "Your Inferiority Complex," *Scientific American*, May 1939, 288–290.

40. Stanley P. Davies, "Education of the Public in Mental Hygiene," *Mental Hygiene* 16:2 (April 1932), 238, 240–241; "How's Your Old I.C.?" *Collier's*, December 16, 1939, 70; Nash, *The Nervous Generation*, 52.

41. Vilray P. Blair, "Operations for Relief of Hare Lip and Cleft Palate," *Hygeia*, June 1926, 325–326; William Wesley Carter, "The Importance of Nasal Plastic Surgery," *Laryngoscope* 40:7 (July 1930), 502; George Warren Pierce, "Comment," in Bames, "Esthetic Plastic Surgery," 591; Straatsma, "Plastic Surgery" 254.

42. Jacques W. Maliniak, "American Society of Plastic and Reconstructive Surgery: Its Beginning, Objectives, and Progress, 1932–1947," *PRS* 2:6 (November 1947), 518.

43. Maliniak, *Sculpture in the Living*, 27, 65, 70, 193; "Your Child's Face and Future," *Hygeia*, May 1935, 410–413; see also Iglauer, "Correction of Outstanding and Cauliflower Ears"; Wolf, "New Noses"; Arthur H. Bulbulian, "Artificial Ears and Noses," *Hygeia*, November 1940, 981.

44. *New York Times*, May 16, 1927, VII 17:1; Maltz, *New Faces, New Futures*, introduction by Alfred Adler, ix, also 9, 162, 194–195, 295, 303.

45. Henry Junius Schireson, *As Others See You: The Story of Plastic Surgery* (New York: Macaulay Co., 1938), 112; Stotter, *Beauty Unmasked*, 80.

46. Iago Galdston to Jerome P. Webster, February 5, 1940 (JPW/Sarah Miller); Estella Strayer to Jerome P. Webster, February 10, 1945 (JPW/S-General through 1950). Webster used the term more often in discussing women than men, but the fact that he saw so many more women than men seems to account for this.

47. JPW/Alicia Martin; Diane Davis.

48. Maliniak, *Sculpture in the Living*, 26.

49. Carter, "Physical Findings," 75–84; Thomas and Thomas, *The Child in America*, 26, 464–465; Lowrey, "Competitions," 316–330; Strecker, "Everyday Psychology," 65–81; Karl Menninger, *The Human Mind* (New York: Alfred A. Knopf, 1937), 73–74; Bromberg, *Psychiatry*, 61.

50. Thomas and Thomas, *The Child in America*, 464–465; Lowrey, "Competitions," 316–330. In his memoirs, psychoanalyst Walter Bromberg noted that the animosity between Freud and Adler was real, resulting in public name-calling. In the United States, followers of the various schools adopted similar attitudes: "The cleavages between the Freudians, Jungians, Rankians, and Adlerians . . . almost amounted to religious wars" (Bromberg, *Psychiatry*, 76, 90–92). Davies, "Education of the Public in Mental Hygiene," *Mental Hygiene* 238, 240–241; Bromberg, *Psychiatry*, 74; Menninger, "Depressions" and *The Human Mind*, 70–71.

51. Bloodgood, "Possibilities and Dangers"; Everett S. McCalland, "Minor Plastic Surgery and Its Relation to the Inferiority Complex," *Medical Record* (New York) 146:10 (November 17, 1937), 419–424; see also Joseph C. Beck, "Present Status of Plastic Surgery about the Ear, Face and Neck," *Laryngoscope* 30:5 (May 1920), 282, "A Resume," *Journal of the Indiana State Medical Association* 18:5 (May 1925),

167, and "Cosmetic Surgery of the Nose"; H. Lyons Hunt, "The Treatment of Facial Scars with Remarks on Their Psychological Aspects," *American Journal of Surgery* 4:3 (March 1928), 314–315; Jacques W. Maliniak, "Problems Confronting Plastic Surgery," *Journal of the Medical Society of New Jersey* 30 (June 1933), 439–441 and *Sculpture in the Living*, 26–27, 68, 126.

52. Sperber, *Masks of Loneliness*, 77.

53. Such lists are exceedingly common in the literature of this period. See, for example, Jacob Sarnoff, "What to Expect of Plastic Surgery," *Medical Record* 144:2 (July 15, 1936), 58–61; Claire L. Straith, "Reconstructions about the Nasal Tip," *American Journal of Surgery* 43:2 (February 1939), 223–236; Davis, "The Value and Limitations," 162.

54. M. Reese Guttman, "Modern Changes in Plastic and Reconstructive Surgery of the Face and Neck," *Illinois Medical Journal* 76:4 (October 1939), 349; Lois Mattox Miller, "Surgery's Cinderella," *Independent Woman*, July 1939, 201, 222–223; also see A. M. Berman, "Comment," in Joseph C. Beck, "Plastic and Reconstructive Surgery about the Face and Neck—Then and Now," *Illinois Medical Journal* 76:3 (September 1939), 240; Douglas A. Macomber, "Recent Developments in Plastic Surgery," *Rocky Mountain Medical Journal* 35(July 1938), 532.

55. Schaeffer, "Plastic Surgery," 11; William Kiskadden, "Comment," in Bames, "Esthetic Plastic Surgery," 591; John F. Pick, "Present Status of Plastic Surgery," *Illinois Medical Journal* 72:2 (August 1937), 178; A. M. Berman in Beck, "Plastic and Reconstructive Surgery," 238.

56. Bettman, "The Psychology of Appearances"; Schireson, *As Others See You*, 89; John Van Duyn, "Psyche and Plastic Surgery," *Southern Medical Journal* 58:10 (October 1965), 1255–1257.

57. "New Noses in 40 Minutes," *Popular Science Monthly*, November 1937, 34–35; *Science News Letter*, September 11, 1938, 185; Miller, "Surgery's Cinderella"; *Science News Letter*, September 17, 1938, 185 and November 11, 1939, 312.

58. Ruth Murrin, "A New Nose in a Week," *Good Housekeeping*, November 1940, 82–83.

59. Palmer, "When Plastic Surgery Is Justified"; Murrin, "A New Nose in a Week."

FOUR   *The Lifting of the Middle Class*

1. "Elizabeth Taylor's Astonishing Lift" (anonymous, circa 1973, NAPS, HMS c84 #25); *Ash Wednesday* (Paramount, 1973); Ellen Goodman, "Aging Gracefully," *San Francisco Chronicle*, November 19, 1992, A25.

2. *New York Times*, December 8, 1944, 14:6 (see also July 2, 1944, IV 9:6; October 1, 1944, IV 11:6).

On preparing for war, see Jacques Maliniac, "Plastic Surgery in War: Preparedness of the Profession at Large," *Medical Record* (New York) 154:9 (November 5, 1941), 325–327; Robert H. Ivy, "Plastic and Maxillofacial Surgery," *Surgical Clinics of North America* 21:6 (December 1941), 1583; Captain H. L. D. Kirkham, Commander James T. Mills, and Lt. Commander L. E. Potter, Medical Corps, U.S. Navy Reserve,

"Plastic Surgery as Related to War Surgery," *Surgical Clinics of North America* 23:6 (December 1943), 1603–1611.

For popular coverage, see Albert Q. Maisel, "New Faces for New Men," *Science Digest*, April 1943, 28–32 ; Marie Beynon Ray, "Saving His Face," *Woman's Home Companion*, September 1944, 25, 56, 58; Beulah Schacht, "Giving the Boy a New Face," *St. Louis Globe-Democrat*, March 10, 1946, E1. See also Quentin Reynolds, "New Bodies for Old," *Collier's*, October 24, 1942, 20–21, 62; "War Surgery for Sex," *Newsweek*, February 8, 1943, 78; Jane Stafford, "Guarding Army Health," *Science News Letter*, May 8, 1943, 294–295; "Study Plastic Surgery," *Science News Letter*, December 11, 1943, 383; David Brown and Radford Lumsden, "Surgery Heals the Scars of War," *Hygeia*, January 1944, 26–27, 50; "Plastic Surgery between Wars," *Science Digest*, September 1944, 90–91; "A Wounded Veteran Gets a New Face," *Life*, November 6, 1944, 79–80, 82; Kyle Crighton, "New Faith at Valley Forge," *Collier's*, December 16, 1944, 20–21, 80; "New Methods of Plastic Surgery," *Science Digest*, December 1944, 76; "New Faces for Heroes," *Newsweek*, April 16, 1945, 65; Maxine Davis, "The New Plastic Surgery," *Good Housekeeping*, July 1945, 42, 178; "Plastic Miracles," *Newsweek*, February 17, 1947, 57; "The Man Who Makes Faces," *Time*, September 27, 1948; Katharine Best and Katharine Hillyer, "The Club Nobody Wants to Join," *Coronet*, January 1949, 99–102.

Writer Geri Trotta, in "The Face Plastic Surgery Can Build You" (*Look*, April 3, 1948, 78) called *Dark Passage* "near witchery . . . absurd," but Americans loved it.

3. Elaine Tyler May, *Homeward Bound: American Families in the Cold War Era* (New York: Basic Books, 1988), 14, 27; Susan Douglas, *Where the Girls Are: Growing Up Female with the Mass Media* (New York: Times Books/Random House, 1994), 245–268.

On the historical, scientific, and cultural meanings of aging in America, see David Hackett Fischer, *Growing Old in America* (New York: Oxford University Press, 1977); W. Andrew Achenbaum, *Old Age in the New Land: The American Experience since 1790* (Baltimore: Johns Hopkins University Press, 1978); and William Graebner, *A History of Retirement: The Meaning and Function of an American Institution* (New Haven: Yale University Press, 1980), the acknowledged classics in this field. More recently, Thomas Cole, in *The Journey of Life: A Cultural History of Aging in America* (New York: Cambridge University Press, 1992), suggests that postmodern culture offers opportunities to interpret aging in a more complex and positive light. In *Mirror, Mirror: The Terror of Not Being Young* (New York: Linden Press/Simon & Schuster, 1983), psychologist Elissa Melamed addresses the double standard as it relates to women and aging. Lois Banner's *In Full Flower: Aging Women, Power, and Sexuality* (New York: Alfred A. Knopf, 1992) offers a challenging treatment of this topic.

4. Paul Starr, *The Social Transformation of American Medicine* (New York: Basic Books, 1982), 335–337; Arnold S. Relman, "The Future of Medical Practice," in *In Search of the Modern Hippocrates*, ed. Roger J. Bulger (Iowa City: University of Iowa Press, 1987), 199–205.

5. Paul W. Greeley, "Progress," *PRS* 9:2 (February 1952), 89; Secretary-Treasurer's Report, May 1960 (NAPS, ABPS #406); Frederick A. Figi, "Presidential Address," *PRS* 10:1 (January 1957), 2; T. R. McCoy, "Beauty Can Be Bought,"

American Weekly, April 26, 1959, 8–9; *New York Times,* July 14, 1959, 30:1; Herbert Conway, "Distribution of Plastic Surgeons in the United States," *PRS* 35:2 (February 1965), 183. See also Gustave Aufricht, "The Development of Plastic Surgery in the United States," *Transactions of the American Society of Plastic and Reconstructive Surgeons 13th Annual Meeting* (1944), 9–32.

      6. Robert Potter, "Farewell to Ugliness," *American Weekly,* March 31, 1946; April 7, 1946; April 14, 1946. Given the hyperbole in which Potter indulged, Fishbein's enthusiasm is curious. Perhaps he believed the articles were balanced and realistic, or maybe he was simply relieved that they were less unbalanced than he had expected. At any rate, his endorsement, which carried his name and title in large type, seemed to indicate that the series had been approved by the AMA; it would have increased, rather than limited, readers' expectations.

      The *American Weekly* began its journalistic climb when it became a tabloid in 1944. By 1955, it had annual revenues of $18 million and a circulation of 10 million, 25 percent of the U.S. adult population. The magazine ceased publication on September 7, 1963, at which point its circulation had fallen to 3.5 million. See Glen W. Peters, "The American Weekly," *Journalism Quarterly* 48:3 (Autumn 1971), 467–471.

      7. Leon Sutton to ASPRS members (no date, probably 1952) in JPW/ASPRS 1950–1960.

      8. William Milton Adams, "Problems and Opportunities in the Field of Plastic Surgery," *PRS* 15:1 (January 1955), 1–2; Michael Gurdin and George F. Crikelair, "Public Relations Is Everybody's Business," *PRS* 33:6 (June 1964), 575. See also Greeley, "Progress," 92; Francis X. Paletta, "History of the American Society of Plastic and Reconstructive Surgeons, Inc., 1931–1981: Its Growth, Change, Unity," *PRS* 68:3 (September 1981), 110; Leon E. Sutton, "Plastic Surgery and the Public," *PRS* 7:1 (January 1951), 1. Pam Hait, "History of the American Society of Plastic and Reconstructive Surgeons," *PRS* 94:4 (September 1994), 1A–100A, is an indispensable source on the press and public relations, as well as on the specialty's overall history. Surgeon Truman G. Blocker, in "Plastic Surgery in America: A Progress Report," *PRS* 18:3 (September 1956), 159–160, also noted progress, as demonstrated by an increase in magazine and television publicity and a "decrease in sensational newspaper publicity." Simona Morini, *Body Sculpture* (New York: Delacorte, 1972), 175.

      9. Gurdin and Crikelair, "Public Relations Is Everybody's Business," 575; John L. Bach, "Dr., Meet the Press," *JAMA* 149:12 (July 19, 1952), 1137–1141. See also Irvine H. Page, "The Creation of Our Public Image," *Modern Medicine* (March 30, 1964) (NAPS, Tamerin #9).

      10. Ethel Lloyd Patterson, "Why Grow Old?" *Ladies Home Journal,* September 1922, 28, 159.

      11. Walter C. Alvarez, "Face-Lifting: For What, For Whom, For How Much?" *Good Housekeeping,* September 1957, 86–87, 186–189; Anonymous, "Diary of a Face Lift," *Ladies Home Journal,* May 1962, 28, 30, 32, 101.

      12. E. Hoyt de Kleine, "The Crossroads of Cosmetic Surgery," *PRS* 16:2 (August 1955), 145–149. Frederick A. Figi, in his 1957 Presidential Address, also warned against overpricing as one of the practices "that tend to discredit one or one's colleagues"; see *PRS* 10:1 (January 1957), 1.

13. De Kleine, "The Crossroads," 2; see also Adams, "Problems and Opportunities," 2. Douglas W. Macomber, in response to de Kleine's article, warned his colleagues that placing their faith in cosmetic surgery would lead to trouble when the "fabulous and unnatural economic period" they were now enjoying ended. See "Our Specialty at the Crossroads?" *PRS* 17:3 (March 1956), 258–260.

14. Secretary's Report, 1939 (NAPS, c86 #8); John Staige Davis to Vilray P. Blair, December 16, 1939 (NAPS, ABPS #238).

15. Minutes, American Board of Plastic Surgery, June 2, 1946 (NAPS, ABPS #24); James Barrett Brown to American Board of Plastic Surgery, May 27, 1948 (NAPS, ABPS #188); Bradford Cannon, secretary, ABPS to Leon Sutton, chairman, ASPRS Public Relations Committee, May 18, 1953 (NAPS, ABPS #294); Mrs. B.H. to Miss Maxine Davis (no date, evidently 1949), Maxine Davis (McHugh) to JPW, April 29, 1949, JPW to Mrs. James McHugh, May 18, 1949 in JPW/M-General, 1931–1949.

16. Estelle E. Hillerich, corresponding secretary, ABPS, to Alice Lake, public information officer and press representative, ASPRS, June 17 and July 26, 1960 (NAPS, ABPS #294); Estelle E. Hillerich to Frank McDowell, August 18, 1961 (NAPS, ABPS #297). See Reed O. Dingman to Dorothea Zak Hanle, ed., *Make-up and Beauty Guide* (no date) for an example of how the Board attempted to prevent use of its name (NAPS, ABPS #297).

17. James Barrett Brown to American Board of Plastic Surgery, May 27, 1948 (NAPS, ABPS #188); Mrs. E.Y. to American Board of Plastic Surgery, July 20, 1949 (NAPS, ABPS #313).

18. Geri Trotta, "The Wish to Be Beautiful," *Harper's Bazaar*, June 1960, 101, 126; Frank McDowell, "Confidential Report to the Executive Committee of the American Society of Plastic and Reconstructive Surgeons and the American Association of Plastic Surgeons" (undated, probably 1961; NAPS, ABPS #295); unsigned notation on number of cards sent (NAPS, ABPS #302); see also Estelle E. Hillerich to Frank McDowell, August 18, 1961 (NAPS, ABPS #297); Alice Lake to Kenneth Pickerell, August 16, 1960 (NAPS, ABPS #294).

19. Frank McDowell to Paul R. Hawley, director, American College of Surgeons (NAPS, ABPS #295); Clarence W. Monroe, "A Plea for Balance," *PRS* 52:5 (November 1973), 471–473. In addition to generally wanting to curb sensational publicity, many surgeons were troubled by an increasing tendency among journalists to quote surgeons by name. In May 1964, for example, the public relations committee of the Regional Society of Plastic and Reconstructive Surgery in New York adopted the following policy: "We will help verify articles about and pertaining to Plastic Surgery which specifically mention no names of practicing plastic surgeons unless a contribution is so newsworthy or timely as to warrant this." "Report of the Public Relations Committee of the Regional Society of Plastic and Reconstructive Surgery" (New York), May 7, 1964 (NAPS, HMSc84 Tamerin #8). On the 1973 resumption, see Paletta, "History of the ASPRS," 292–369, esp. 320–322.

20. *New York Times,* June 24, 1944, 17:2.

21. Lois Banner, *American Beauty* (Chicago: University of Chicago Press, 1983), 271–286; Beth Bailey, *From Front Porch to Back Seat: Courtship in Twentieth-Century America* (Baltimore: Johns Hopkins University Press, 1988), 70–72; also see

Susan Bordo, *Unbearable Weight: Feminism, Western Culture, and the Body* (Berkeley: University of California Press, 1993), 25.

22. Lily Daché, *Lily Daché's Glamour Book,* ed. Dorothy Roe Lewis (Philadelphia: J. B. Lippincott, 1956), 30–31; Potter, "Farewell to Ugliness," April 7, 1946; April 14, 1946.

23. Minutes, American Board of Plastic Surgery, June 2, 1946 (NAPS, ABPS #24); James Barrett Brown to ABPS, May 27, 1948 (NAPS, ABPS #188); Olga Kahler, "I'm Glad I Had My Face Lifted," *Your Life,* December 1948, 80–84.

24. See Maxwell Maltz, *New Faces, New Futures: Rebuilding Character with Plastic Surgery* (New York: Richard R. Smith, 1936), 125; James Stotter, *Beauty Unmasked* (New York: Raymond Press, 1936), 20, 58; Robert O. Renie, "Economic Considerations of Cosmetic Surgery," *American Journal of Surgery* 55:1 (January 1942), 126; Joseph Safian, "Ethical Plastic Surgery vs. the Quack Beauty Doctor," radio lecture, WEAF, New York City, June 30, 1926 (NAPS, Safian correspondence); Murray Berger, *A Nose to Fit Your Face: How the Skill of a Surgeon Can Restore and Create Beauty* (Garden City, N.Y.: Country Life Press/Doubleday, 1952), 98–99, 104; Gayelord Hauser, *Look Younger, Live Longer* (New York: Farrar, Straus and Young, 1951), 139; Adolph Abraham Apton, *Your Mind and Appearance: A Psychological Approach to Plastic Surgery* (New York: Citadel Press, 1951), 135.

25. Eugenia Harris, "9 Myths about Face-Lifting," *McCalls,* June 1961, 78–79, 182; Ramona Leigh, "Trade Your Face," *Popular Medicine,* January 1962, 49–53; Arthur J. Snider, "Report on Plastic Surgery," *Science Digest,* December 1964, 18–19.

26. Morris Fishbein, M.D., "New Faces for Old," *This Week* (*New York Herald Tribune Magazine*) August 14, 1938, in JPW/Morgue 3.

27. James Buford Johnson, "The Problem of the Aging Face," *PRS* 15:1 (January 1955), 117; Lawrence Galton, "What Plastic Surgery Does for the Stars," *Cosmopolitan,* November 1959, 22–23; Elizabeth Byrd, "Mirror, Mirror on the Wall," *McCalls,* February 1967, 76, 168–171.

28. Dixie Dean Harris, "Now You Can Have . . . ," *Esquire,* November 1965, 134–136, 189–192; Josephine Lowman, "Why Grow Old?" *Oakland Tribune,* April 27, 1953, 18:6.

29. McCoy, "Beauty Can Be Bought"; Leigh, "Trade Your Face"; Anon., "Diary of a Face Lift"; *San Francisco Chronicle,* December 9, 1969, 26; D. McCullagh Mayer and Wilson A. Swanker, "Rhytidoplasty," *PRS* 6:4 (October 1950), 255; Martin Abramson, "The Amazing Dr. Beauty," *Houston Chronicle,* April 23, 1972 (NAPS, Tamerin #24).

30. "The Imagined Image," *Vogue,* September 15, 1961, 173, 213, 217; Harris, "9 Myths"; Anonymous, "Why I Had My Face Lifted," *Harper's Bazaar,* January 1969, 134–135, 152.

31. Kahler, "I'm Glad"; Elizabeth Honor, "Beauty Can Be Bought," *Cosmopolitan,* June 1958, 70–73; Edith Meiser, "Stranger in My Mirror," *Ladies Home Journal,* July 1959, 66, 132–134, 136.

32. Berger, *A Nose to Fit Your Face,* 102; John Conley, *Face-Lift Operation* (Springfield, Ill.: Charles C. Thomas, 1968), 120–122; Sylvia Rosenthal, *Cosmetic Surgery: A Consumer's Guide* (Philadelphia and New York: Tree Communications/J. B. Lippincott, 1977), 26.

33. "Surgery for Wrinkles," *Hygeia*, September 1948, 612; "Imagined Image"; Enrique C. Sabbagh, Jack Hipps, and Richard E. Straith, "Blepharoplasty: Social, Economic, and Technical Aspects," *Postgraduate Medicine* 36:1 (July 1964), 23–27; Wilmer C. Hansen, "What Plastic Surgery Can Do," *Science Digest*, June 1957, 16, 20; *San Francisco Chronicle*, August 28, 1960, IIs.

34. "Imagined Image"; Harris, "9 Myths"; Anon., "Why I Had My Face Lifted."

35. Anonymous, "Choosing the Right Plastic Surgeon: A Personal History," *Harper's Bazaar*, October 1967, 316–317, 258; Amy Vanderbilt, "My New Face," *Ladies Home Journal*, April 1971, 52–54, 57, 140.

36. "Imagined Image"; Harris, "Now You Can Have"; Anon., "Choosing"; Anon., "Why I Had My Face Lifted"; Anon., "Diary of a Face Lift."

37. "Imagined Image"; Anon., "Diary of a Face Lift"; Anon., "Why I Had My Face Lifted"; "New Wrinkles for Old Age," *Newsweek*, April 28, 1969, 70.

38. Milton T. Edgerton, William L. Webb Jr., Regina Slaughter, and Eugene Meyer, "Surgical Results and Psychosocial Changes Following Rhytidectomy," *PRS* 33:6 (June 1964), 503–514; see also *New York Times*, April 8, 1969, 49:7; May 29, 1972, 22:1. On a similar seminar sponsored by Bloomingdale's in Manhasset, see the clipping in NAPS, HMSc84 Tamerin #24. San Francisco's Cathedral Hill Medical Center formed a nonprofit consulting service in 1974 to fulfill what it described as the public's "insatiable" appetite for information on cosmetic surgery; see *San Francisco Chronicle*, April 24, 1974, 5:8.

39. Harris, "Now You Can Have"; "New Wrinkles"; "Cosmetic Surgery Comes of Age," *McCalls*, April 1970, 74, 77, 130–133; T. J. Jackson Lears, "American Advertising and the Reconstruction of the Body," in *Fitness in American Culture: Images of Health, Sport, and the Body, 1830–1940*, ed. Kathryn Grover (Amherst: University of Massachusetts Press; Rochester, N.Y.: Margaret Woodbury Strong Museum, 1989), 47–66, esp. 48–49, 62.

40. Henry Junius Schireson, *As Others See You: The Story of Plastic Surgery* (New York: Macaulay Co., 1938), 23; Maltz, *New Faces, New Futures*, 76, 192; Stotter, *Beauty Unmasked*, 52, 132–133; Renie, "Economic Considerations," 126.

41. Ivor and Sally Davis, "The Great Male Face Race," *LA Magazine*, February 1975, 63, 103–104; Alvarez, "Face-Lifting"; *New York Times*, November 9, 1967, 51:1; *San Francisco Examiner*, August 4, 1972, 26; "New Wrinkles"; see also *New York Times*, April 8, 1969, 49:7.

42. "Plastic Surgery for Men," *Coronet*, May 1961, 100–104.

43. *New York Times*, April 8, 1969, 49:7; Patrick M. McGrady Jr., "The Art of Manly Face-Lifting," *Vogue*, June 1969, 117, 168–169; Everett R. Holles, "Face-Lifting Erases Age in Men, Too," *New York Times*, June 28, 1971, 26:1.

44. Thomas J. Baker and Howard L. Gordon, "Rhytidectomy in Males," *PRS* 44:3 (September 1969), 219.

45. Holles, "Face-Lifting Erases Age."

46. *San Francisco Chronicle*, July 15, 1971, 21; *San Francisco Chronicle*, September 19, 1973, 38; *New York Times*, July 25, 1974, 34:1.

47. *San Francisco Chronicle*, September 20, 1973, 23; James Kelly, "Cosmetic Lib for Men," *New York Times Magazine*, September 25, 1977, 119; John M.

Hamilton, "Rhytidectomy in the Male," *PRS* 53:6 (June 1974), 629–633; Davis and Davis, "Great Male Face Race." Beauty writer Harriet LaBarre, in *Plastic Surgery: Beauty You Can Buy* (New York: Holt, Rinehart & Winston, 1970), 177, similarly observed that embarrassment made men more vulnerable to quacks.

48. David Lilienthal (pseud. Ely), *Seconds* (New York: Pantheon Books, 1963), 64–65.

49. *San Francisco Chronicle*, December 21, 1971, 22; Daniel C. Baker, Sherrel J. Aston, Cary L. Guy, and Thomas D. Rees, "The Male Rhytidectomy," *PRS* 60:4 (October 1977), 519; Gertrude Lang, "Facing the Facts about Face-Lifts," *Retirement Living*, February 1978, 23–25.

50. Russell Baker, "Face Lift," *New York Times Magazine*, December 3, 1978, 18; Dr. Norman Pastorek, quoted in Victoria Secunda, *By Youth Possessed: The Denial of Age in America* (Indianapolis: Bobbs-Merrill Co., 1984), 199; "What Cosmetic Surgery Can and Can't Do," *Business Week*, January 21, 1980, 104–105, 108; "Put on a Successful Face," *Psychology Today*, December 1983, 70; Josleen Wilson, *The American Society of Plastic and Reconstructive Surgeons' Guide to Cosmetic Surgery* (New York: Simon and Schuster, 1992), 13, 26, 191, 199; *New York Times*, June 9, 1996, 1, 8, 9.

On the new frontiers, see, for example, Adrien E. Aiache, "Surgical Treatment of Gynecomastia in the Body Builder," *PRS* 83:1 (January 1989), 61–66; "Calf Implantation," *PRS* 83:3 (March 1989), 488–492; and "Male Chest Correction: Pectoral Implants and Gynecomastia," *Clinics in Plastic Surgery* 18:4 (October 1991), 823–828; Edward Tenno, "Implants for Male Aesthetic Surgery," *Clinics in Plastic Surgery* 18:4 (October 1991), 731–749; and Brian H. Novack, "Alloplastic Implants for Men," *Clinics in Plastic Surgery* 18:4 (October 1991), 829–856; Elisabeth Rosenthal, "Cosmetic Surgeons Seek New Frontiers," *New York Times*, September 14, 1991, B5–B6; Lisa Bannon, "How a Risky Surgery Became Profit Center in Los Angeles," *Wall Street Journal*, June 6, 1996 (interactive edition).

51. Wilson, *ASPRS Guide*, 13–15.

52. Kahler, "I'm Glad"; Meiser, "Stranger"; Toni Kosover, "When the Lady Needs a Lift, She Gets One," *W*, November 14, 1969, 18; Vanderbilt, "My New Face"; "Phyllis Diller Tells One about a Face-Lift—Hers," *Life*, February 11, 1972, 73.

53. Alvarez, "Face-Lifting"; Harris, "9 Myths"; Anon., "Why I Had My Face Lifted."

54. Irving B. Goldman, ed., "Religious Views on Cosmetic Surgery," *Eye, Ear, Nose, and Throat Monthly* 40:12 (December 1961), 856–858; 41:1 (January 1962), 61–63; 41:2 (February 1962), 133–134; 41:3 (March 1962), 220–221.

55. Ibid., 41:2 (February 1962), 133–134; 41:3 (March 1962), 220–221.

56. Ibid.

57. Albert P. Seltzer, "Religion and Cosmetic Surgery," *Journal of the National Medical Association* 57:3 (May 1965), 205–207; Reuven K. Snyderman, "Jewish Law and Cosmetic Surgery," *PRS* 78:2 (August 1986), 259.

58. *San Francisco Chronicle*, July 20, 1971, 33; *San Francisco Examiner and Chronicle*, November 24, 1974, A18.

59. *San Francisco Examiner*, October 2, 1978, 1, 6; October 3, 1978, 3.

60. *San Francisco Examiner*, March 23, 1979, 7; March 25, 1979, A2; *New York Times*, March 25, 1979, 18:3.

61. Anonymous, "The Face Lift That Flopped," *Good Housekeeping*, March 1978, 27–28, 30–34.

62. Ann Scheiner, "My Face-Lift: A Cautionary Tale," *Ms.*, November 1986, 58. See also Paula Bernstein, "Second Thoughts on Your First Face-Lift," *Harper's Bazaar*, August 1985, 197, 225; and Shay McConnell, "Will Your Face-Lift Be a Letdown?" *Harper's Bazaar*, August 1987, 97, 106, 185–186.

63. *New York Times*, July 20, 1976, 36:1; Anon., "Diary of a Face Lift"; Anonymous, "The Lift That Left Me Low," *Harper's Bazaar*, September 1981, 158, 166, 168, 184.

64. Douglas, *Where the Girls Are*, 245–294.

65. See Richard B. Aronsohn and Richard A. Epstein, *The Miracle of Cosmetic Plastic Surgery* (Los Angeles: Sherbourne Press, 1970), 62–65, 69, 141–145; Conley, *Face-Lift Operation*, v; Rosenthal, *Cosmetic Surgery*, 20; *San Francisco Chronicle*, April 25, 1979, 17 and April 26, 1979, 25; May 8, 1983, 8; Richard Ellenbogen and Jan V. Karlin, "Visual Criteria for Success in Restoring the Youthful Neck," *PRS* 66:6 (December 1980), 826–837; John Q. Owsley Jr., "Update: SMAS-Platysma Face Lift," *PRS* 71:4 (April 1983), 573–574; Lawrence B. Robbins and Kevin E. Shaw, "En Bloc Cervical Lipectomy for Treatment of the Problem Neck in Facial Rejuvenation Surgery," *PRS* 83:1 (January 1989), 53–60; Moynihan quoted in *New York Times*, February 5, 1989, 3:1.

66. Robert M. Goldwyn, "Saying 'No' to Your Hospital," *PRS* 79:4 (April 1987), 621; "Malpractice Insurance: Taxation without Representation," *PRS* 81:5 (May 1988), 768–769.

67. Mary Carpenter, "Can a Face-Lift Make You Look Worse?" *Harper's Bazaar*, September 1981, 112, 140, 152; Mark Gorney, "Who Is Responsible?" *PRS* 84:5 (November 1989), 800–801; see also "Mirror Mirror on the Wall," *PRS* 74:1 (July 1984), 117–122 and *San Francisco Chronicle*, February 14, 1977, 1.

68. On the mini- and forehead (or eyebrow) lift, see Kathryn L. Stephenson, "The 'Mini-Lift': An Old Wrinkle in Face Lifting," *PRS* 46:3 (September 1970), 226–235; Thomas J. Baker and Howard L. Gordon, "The Temporal Face Lift ('Mini-Lift')," *PRS* 47:4 (April 1971), 313; Bernard L. Kaye, "The Forehead Lift," *PRS* 60:2 (August 1977), 161–171; and LaBarre, *Beauty You Can Buy*, 44–45. On the controversy over doing face-lifts at younger ages, see *San Francisco Chronicle*, October 28, 1974, 21 and *New York Times*, December 23, 1984, III 13:2. On chemical face peeling, see Howard J. Brody, *Chemical Peeling* (St. Louis: Mosby Year Book, 1992) and Robert Kotler (with contributions by Willard L. Marmelzat, Richard G. Glogan, and Thomas J. Baker), *Chemical Rejuvenation of the Face* (St. Louis: Mosby Year Book, 1992), especially Marmelzat, "Bits of History, Bits of Mystery—A Historical Review of Chemical Rejuvenation of the Face," 1–40. I am indebted to Dr. Marmelzat for bringing this to my attention. Several folders in the American Board of Plastic Surgery archive contain relevant materials; see NAPS, ABPS #203 and #403. Los Angeles plastic surgeon Herbert Otto Bames discussed face peeling in the 1920s: see "Truth and Fallacies about Face Peeling and Face Lifting," *Medical Journal and Record* 126:2 (July 20, 1927), 86. In "Chemical Face Lifting," *PRS* 29:4 (April 1962), 371, Clyde Litton introduced the technique to modern-day plastic surgeons with the observation, "I must admit from the start that it took a lot of courage to apply this solution to the patient's face for the first time." See also "New

Wrinkles" and Sally Ogle Davis, "Just Peel the Wrinkles Away," *LA Magazine,* January 1980, 166.

69. Sarah Stage, personal communication, May 1, 1993; Berger, *A Nose to Fit Your Face,* 97–98.

70. Kahler, "I'm Glad"; "Imagined Image"; Goodman, "Aging Gracefully."

FIVE   *The Michael Jackson Factor*

1. Michael Goldberg and David Handelman, "Is Michael Jackson for Real?" *Rolling Stone,* September 24, 1987, 50–56, 87.

2. Frances Cooke Macgregor, *Transformation and Identity: The Face and Plastic Surgery* (New York: Quadrangle Press/New York Times Book Co., 1974), 97.

3. Sam Emerson, "The Last Word on Michael," *People,* special issue, "All about Michael," November/December 1984, 78.

4. Popular press coverage of Jackson is extensive; only select articles are listed here. Generally, articles in African American magazines like *Jet* and *Ebony* have tended to focus on Jackson's music rather than on his face; see *Ebony*: "Michael," December 1982, 126–130; "Diana and Michael," November 1983, 29–30; "The Michael Jackson Nobody Knows," December 1984, 155–158; "New and Revealing Look," June 1988, 176; "Biggest Brother Sister Stars," August 1991, 40; *Jet*: R. E. Johnson, "The Jackson Family Talk," March 26, 1984, 56–60; R. E. Johnson, "Michael Jackson," March 21, 1988, 56–63. See also Carin Rubenstein, "The Michael Jackson Syndrome," *Discover,* September 1984, 68–70; Albert Goldman, "Analyzing the Magic," *People,* special issue, "All About Michael," November/December 1984, 73–77; Todd Gold, "Living with Michael Jackson," *McCalls,* February 1985, 28, 30–33; Jon Pareles, "The Trouble with Michael Jackson," *Mademoiselle,* March 1987, 87, 110; C. Durkee, "Unlike Anyone Else," *People,* September 14, 1987, 86–87, 93–98; Mikal Gilmore, "The Invisible Man Returns," *Rolling Stone,* May 19, 1988, 35–37; Todd Gold, "The Score on Michael Jackson," *McCalls,* August 1988, 66–70. On his plastic surgery and the reaction to it, see J. Randy Taraborrelli, *Michael Jackson: The Magic and the Madness* (New York: Birch Lane Press/Carol Publishing Group, 1991), 256–257, 259, 261, 349, 357–358, 364, 398–399, 403, 419–424, 474, 533–537.

5. Not all plastic surgeons suffer from what sociologist Frances Cooke Macgregor calls the "Pygmalion complex," but the image of the plastic surgeon as artist is strikingly common. An early example is H. O. Bames, "Esthetic Plastic Surgery," *California and Western Medicine* 33:2 (August 1930), 588; the quintessential example is Maxwell Maltz, *Dr. Pygmalion: The Autobiography of a Plastic Surgeon* (New York: Thomas Y. Crowell Co., 1953); more recent examples include Donald T. Moynihan and Shirley Hartman, *Skin Deep: The Making of a Plastic Surgeon* (Boston: Little, Brown, 1979), 175, and Elizabeth Morgan, *Solo Practice: A Woman Surgeon's Story* (Boston: Little, Brown, 1982), 36.

Earlier in the century, surgeons sometimes offered numerical prescriptions or geometric relationships for facial attractiveness. Detroit surgeon Claire L. Straith even invented an instrument he called the Profilometer to help surgeons create beautiful profiles; see "Reconstructions about the Nasal Tip," *American Journal of Surgery* 43:2 (February 1939), 223–236. See also M. Reese Guttman, "Modern Changes in Plastic and Reconstructive Surgery of the Face and Neck," *Illinois Medical Journal* 76:4 (October 1939), 349, and Lester W. Eisenstadt, "Surgical Correction of Chin Malformations," *American Journal of Surgery* 71:4 (April 1946), 491, which offer ideal angles for male and female noses and for Caucasian lips. For an example of how ethnic and racial considerations are translated into artistic and geometric (although not numeric) terms, see R. C. Pearlman, "Nasal Plastic Operation," *American Journal of Surgery* 64:2 (August 1947), 151–162. Today, numerical measurements are largely out of fashion, but some surgeons continue to rely on them; see Leslie G. Farkas and John C. Kolar, "Anthropometrics and Art in the Aesthetics of Women's Faces," *Clinics in Plastic Surgery* 14:4 (October 1987), 599–616.

6. Race and ethnicity are often described in coded terms when the topic is beauty. For an example, see Jean Teague, "Girl with a New Nose," *Mademoiselle,* June 1958, 56, in which she explains that her nose had "much more character than I wanted." Sander Gilman has explored the connection between race, ethnicity, and plastic surgery in "The Jewish Nose: Are Jews White? Or, the History of the Nose Job," in *The Jew's Body* (New York: Routledge, 1991).

7. On immigration and American reaction to it, see Alan Kraut, *Silent Travelers: Germs, Genes, and the Immigrant Menace* (New York: Basic Books, 1994), and John Higham's classic *Strangers in the Land: Patterns of American Nativism, 1860–1925* (New York: Atheneum, 1963, 1973).

8. Lois W. Banner, *American Beauty* (Chicago: University of Chicago Press, 1983), 41, 50; Kraut, *Silent Travelers,* 256.

9. On working-class whiteness and blackness, see Eric Arnesen, "'Like Banquo's Ghost It Will Not Down': The Race Question and the American Railroad Brotherhoods, 1880–1920," *American Historical Review* 99:5 (December 1994), 1601–1633; on the construction of whiteness, see David Roediger, *The Wages of Whiteness: Race and the Making of the American Working Class* (London: Verso, 1991) and *Towards the Abolition of Whiteness: Essays on Race, Politics, and Working Class History* (London: Verso, 1994); and, most recently, Mike Hill, ed., *Whiteness: A Critical Reader* (New York: New York University Press, 1997); Noel Ignatiev's *How the Irish Became White* (New York: Routledge, 1995) is a fascinating case study; Peggy Pascoe's "Miscegenation Law, Court Cases, and Ideologies of 'Race' in Twentieth-Century America," *Journal of American History* 83:1 (June 1996), 44–69, focuses not on whiteness (or lack thereof) but on the changing cultural and biological definitions of race and traces the emergence of new racial ideologies that are no less complex than those that held sway in the nineteenth century.

10. Higham, *Strangers,* 150–153; Daniel J. Kevles, *In the Name of Eugenics: Genetics and the Uses of Human Heredity* (Berkeley: University of California Press, 1990).

11. Higham, *Strangers,* 153–157.

12. Banner, *American Beauty,* 206.

13. Knight V. Dunlap, *Personal Beauty and Racial Betterment* (St. Louis: C. V. Mosby Co., 1920), 17–19; Roy M. Dorcus, "Knight Dunlap," *American Journal of Psychology* 63:1 (January 1950), 114–119. Also see Gilman, "The Jewish Nose."

14. Higham, *Strangers,* 160.

15. For a different reading of Jackson, see David Yuan, "The Celebrity Freak: Michael Jackson's 'Grotesque Glory,'" in *Freakery: Cultural Spectacles of the*

Extraordinary Body, ed. Rosemarie Garland Thomson (New York: New York University Press, 1996), 368–384.

16. Norman Katkov, *The Fabulous Fanny* (New York: Alfred A. Knopf, 1953), 141; Herbert G. Goldman, *Fanny Brice: The Original Funny Girl* (New York: Oxford University Press, 1992), 112; and Barbara W. Grossman, *Funny Woman: The Life and Times of Fanny Brice* (Bloomington: Indiana University Press, 1991), 147–151; Ethel E. Sanders, "Semitic Silhouettes," *Opinion: A Journal of Jewish Life and Letters,* December 1932, 24–26. See also Fanny Brice (as told to Palma Wayne), "Fanny of the Follies," *Hearst's International—Cosmopolitan,* February 1936, 20–23, 138–139; Hettie Jithian Cattell, "Fanny Brice: Her Own Story," *Panorama: New York's Illustrated News Weekly,* October 1, 1928, 12–13; October 6, 1928, 10; October 13, 1928, 8; Eve Bernstein, "Fanny Brice Tells Her Story," *Jewish Tribune,* December 28, 1928, 4.

17. Grossman, *Funny Woman,* 148; see also *New York Times,* August 15, 1923, 10:3 and August 16, 1923, 14:4.

18. John B. Roberts, "The Cosmetic Surgery of the Nose," *JAMA* 19:8 (August 20, 1892), 231–233; Maurice H. Cottle, "John Orlando Roe, Pioneer in Modern Rhinoplasty," *Archives of Otolaryngology* 80 (July 1964), 22–23.

19. Hazel Rawson Cades, *Any Girl Can Be Good-Looking* (New York: D. Appleton-Century Co., 1927), 16; William Wesley Carter, "The Importance of Nasal Plastic Surgery," *Laryngoscope* 40:7 (July 1930), 504; Vilray P. Blair, "Plastic Surgery of the Head, Face, and Neck," *Journal of the American Dental Association* 23 (February 1936), 236–240.

20. Kraut, *Silent Travelers,* 256. For examples of psychological readings of plastic surgery in the postwar years, see Arthur J. Barsky, "Psychology of the Patient Undergoing Plastic Surgery," *American Journal of Surgery* 65:2 (August 1944), 238–243; Alma Dei Morani, "Indications for Plastic Surgery," *Medical Women's Journal* 52:2 (February 1945), 22; Gordon B. New and John B. Erich, "Retruded Chins: Correction by Plastic Operation," *JAMA* 115:3 (July 20, 1946), 187; Gerald Hill and A. Gilbert Silver, "Psychodynamic and Esthetic Motivations for Plastic Surgery," *Psychosomatic Medicine* 12:6 (November/December 1950), 345–355; Albert P. Seltzer, "Esthetic (Cosmetic) Surgery of the Face and Neck: Where Shall the EN&T Specialist Stand on the Question?" *Archives of Otolaryngology* 63 (1956), 580–583; David M. C. Ju, "The Psychological Effect of Protruding Ears," *PRS* 31:5 (May 1963), 424–426; George V. Webster, "Random Reflections on Rhinoplasty," *PRS* 39:2 (February 1967), 147; Milton T. Edgerton, "The Plastic Surgeon's Obligations to the Emotionally Disturbed Patient," *PRS* 55:1 (January 1975), 81–83; Macgregor, *Transformation,* 174.

21. Macgregor, *Transformation,* 76, 88–89.

22. In this section, I rely on data provided by the patient records of Jerome Pierce Webster, primarily between 1930 and 1950. Two studies published by sociologist Frances Cooke Macgregor—*Facial Deformities and Plastic Surgery: A Psychosocial Study* (Springfield, Ill.: Charles C. Thomas, 1953) and *Transformation and Identity: The Face and Plastic Surgery* (New York: Quadrangle Press/New York Times Book Co., 1974)—both of which include data collected between 1946 and 1954 at the New York University School of Medicine, the Manhattan Ear, Eye, and Throat Hospital, and the Institute of Reconstructive Plastic Surgery at the New York University

Medical Center, also deserve mention. Günter B. Risse and John Harley Warner's "Reconstructing Clinical Activities: Patient Records in Medical History," *Social History of Medicine* 5 (1992), 1–23, was invaluable as I attempted to evaluate the data.

23. The knowledge and personal perspective provided by my father, Matt Haiken, enabled me to equate (tentatively, in some cases) occupation with social class.

24. Names given here are pseudonyms referencing patient records held in the Jerome Webster Papers, Special Collections, Columbia University Health Sciences Library, New York, New York. The key is held by the archivist.

25. Macgregor, *Transformation*, 89–91.

26. See also: JPW/Christina Hughes, Theodore Lesch, Francesco Pesci, Madeline Ross, Betty Rosenberg.

27. Macgregor, *Transformation*, 89–90.

28. Ibid., 99.

29. Ibid., 103–105.

30. Adolph Abraham Apton, *Your Mind and Appearance: A Psychological Approach to Plastic Surgery* (New York: Citadel Press, 1951), 49; Gilbert L. Hyroop, "Nasal Surgery—Economic and Psychological Aspects," *Journal of the International College of Surgeons* 43:4 (April 1965), 425–427.

31. Lewis Linn and Irving B. Goldman, "Psychiatric Observations concerning Rhinoplasty," *Psychosomatic Medicine* 11:5 (September/October 1949), 307–314.

32. Hill and Silver, "Psychodynamic and Esthetic Motivations," 354; Eugene Meyer, Wayne E. Jacobson, Milton T. Edgerton, and Arthur Canter, "Motivational Patterns in Patients Seeking Elective Plastic Surgery," *Psychosomatic Medicine* 22:3 (June/July 1960), 193–201; Wayne E. Jacobson, Milton T. Edgerton, Eugene Meyer, Arthur Canter, and Regina Slaughter, "Psychiatric Evaluation of Male Patients Seeking Cosmetic Surgery," *PRS* 26:4 (October 1960), 366; Wayne E. Jacobson, E. Meyer, M. T. Edgerton, A. Canter, and R. Slaughter, "Screening of Rhinoplasty Patients from the Psychologic Point of View," *PRS* 28:3 (September 1961), 279–280; Greer Ricketson, "Basis for Cosmetic Surgery," *Southern Medical Journal* 55:3 (March 1962), 271.

33. Joost A. M. Meerloo, "The Fate of One's Face with Some Remarks on the Implications of Plastic Surgery," *Psychiatric Quarterly* 30:1 (1956), 31–37.

34. *Photoplay*, February 1923, 113 and April 1923, 118; Geri Trotta, "Woman's New Ally: Cosmetic Surgery," *Harper's Bazaar*, July 1954, 35; Elizabeth Honor, "Cosmetic Surgery," *Cosmopolitan*, August 1956, 28–31; "What Cosmetic Surgery Can Solve," Make Up and Beauty Guide 48 (Dell 1000 Hints, no date [probably mid-1950s], in NAPS, C87 #403); Carlson Wade, "Instant Beauty through Plastic Surgery," *Lady's Circle*, April 1965, 19 (NAPS, C87 #403).

35. T. R. McCoy, "Beauty Can Be Bought," *American Weekly*, April 26, 1959, 8–9; "A New Nose Means a New Personality," *Look*, August 2, 1960, 74–77; Terry Morris, "Your Trouble May Be as Plain as the Nose on Your Face," *Family Weekly*, August 13, 1961, 4–5, 13.

36. Popular press coverage of Streisand is extensive—more than fifty articles in national magazines from 1963 to 1970. For a sampling, see C. Brossard, "Barbra Streisand: New Singing Sensation," *Look*, November 9, 1963, 12; S. Alexander,

"Barbra," *Life,* May 22, 1964, 51–52; L. Lerman, "Barbra Streisand Show," *Mademoiselle,* May 1964, 158–159; J. Wilson, "Kook from Madagascar," *HiFi,* May 1964, 43–45; "Wonderful Year of Barbra Streisand," *Vogue,* December 1964, 220–221; C. Taylor, "Follow a Star," *Seventeen,* January 1965, 76, 186; "Tears of Barbra Streisand," *Life,* March 18, 1966, 95–96; "Super Barbra," *Look,* April 5, 1966, 54–61; "Her Name Is . . . ," *Redbook,* January 1968, 54–55; "Her Name Is . . . ," *Saturday Review,* January 11, 1969, 108–109; "Her Name Is . . . ," *Life,* January 9, 1970, 90–92.

37. "Looming Star," *New Yorker,* May 19, 1962, 34–35; "Bea, B & B," *Newsweek,* June 3, 1963, 79; Pete Hamill, "Goodbye Brooklyn, Hello Fame," *Saturday Evening Post,* July 27, 1963, 22–23; "Success Is a Baked Potato," *Life,* September 20, 1963, 112.

38. Harriet LaBarre, *Plastic Surgery: Beauty You Can Buy* (New York: Holt, Rinehart and Winston, 1970), 2.

39. Tony Green, "Dr. Nose," *Philadelphia Magazine,* February 1978, 97–99, 144–147; Morris, "Your Trouble"; *San Francisco Chronicle,* February 5, 1972, 4; Patricia Morrisroe, "Forever Young," *New York Magazine,* June 9, 1986, 42–49.

40. Shana Alexander, "Barbra," *Life,* May 22, 1964, 51–52; James Spada, *Barbra: The First Decade* (Secaucus, N.J.: Citadel Press, 1977), 25; "What's Up Front . . . ," *Newsweek,* May 30, 1966, 91–92.

41. "What's Up Front"; Barbara Wagner, "Can a Nose Job Change Your Life?" *Seventeen,* November 1971, 136, 150.

42. *New York Times,* March 8, 1926, 35:4.

43. According to surgeon Henry Junius Schireson, some twenty thousand Japanese had had eyelid surgery by 1938. He asserted that Japanese women were motivated by aesthetics, men by function: the "obliquity" of the "Mongolian eye" was aesthetically unpleasant and an impediment to vision, which explained "why the Japanese are reputedly such poor marksmen, why this highly intelligent race has so high a percentage of airplane crashes." Schireson's claim was probably exaggerated and may have been entirely false. The man later dubbed the "King of Quacks" was an imaginative and adventurous surgeon, and his claim is not supported by other physicians. See *As Others See You: The Story of Plastic Surgery* (New York: Macaulay Co., 1938), 140–141.

44. Moynihan and Hartman, *Skin Deep,* 234–235.

45. D. Ralph Millard Jr., "The Oriental Eyelid and Its Surgical Revision," *American Journal of Opthalmology* 57 (1964), 646–649; see also D. Ralph Millard Jr., "Oriental Peregrinations," *PRS* 16:5 (November 1955), 319.

46. Leabert R. Fernandez, "Double Eyelid Operation in the Oriental in Hawaii," *PRS* 25:3 (March 1960), 257–264; George V. Webster, "Comment on Drs. Ohmori, Tange, Fukuoda, Kurata, Soeda and Hirayama, Modern Trends in Plastic Surgery in Japan," *PRS* 32:3 (September 1963), 309.

47. Khoo Boo-Chai, "Plastic Construction of the Superior Palpebral Fold," *PRS* 31:1 (January 1963), 74.

48. *New York Times,* July 13, 1965, 24:7; "Gaining Face in Japan," *Time,* November 4, 1957, 88; "Asia—New Angles," *Time,* December 23, 1966, 24–25. See also Khoo Boo-Chai, "Augmentation Rhinoplasty in the Orientals," *PRS* 34:1 (July 1964), 81; Khoo Boo-Chai, "The Facial Dimple—Clinical Study and Operative Technique," *PRS* 30:2 (August 1962), 281.

49. For a fascinating account of how contact may challenge and alter race- and ethnicity-specific standards of beauty, see Beth Bailey and David Farber, *The First Strange Place: Race and Sex in World War II Hawaii* (Baltimore: Johns Hopkins University Press, 1994), 167–209; for a broader treatment of gender's role in international affairs, see Cynthia Enloe, *Bananas, Beaches, and Bases: Making Feminist Sense of International Politics* (Berkeley: University of California Press, 1990).

50. "Asia—New Angles"; Tom Fox, "Operation Uplift in Vietnam," *Commonweal*, August 22, 1969, 502–503; *San Francisco Chronicle*, March 12, 1972 (Sunday Punch), 2; *New York Times*, May 21, 1973, 38:1.

51. *New York Times*, May 21, 1973, 38:1.

52. *San Francisco Chronicle*, December 19, 1970, 15; Victor Lipman, "Sculpting Skin with a Scalpel," *Honolulu*, March 1985, 44–46; see also *Miami Herald*, October 21, 1959, 19-A in JPW/Morgue 4.

53. Elaine Kim, "Beyond Railroads and Internment: Comments on the Past, Present, and Future of Asian American Studies," in Gary Y. Okihiro et al., *Privileging Positions: The Sites of Asian American Studies* (Pullman: Washington State University Press, 1995), 11; Beth Bailey, *From Front Porch to Back Seat: Courtship in Twentieth-Century America* (Baltimore: Johns Hopkins University Press, 1988), 57–58; see also Gin Yong Pang, "Attitudes toward Interracial and Interethnic Relationships and Intermarriage among Korean Americans: The Intersections of Race, Gender, and Class Inequality," in *New Visions in Asian American Studies: Diversity, Community, Power*, ed. Franklin Ng et al. (Pullman: Washington State University Press, 1994), 111–123.

54. Daniel Okimoto, *American in Disguise* (New York: Walker/Weatherhill, 1971), 200–201; Jeanne Wakatsuki Houston, *Farewell to Manzanar* (New York: Bantam, 1974), 123.

55. Kesaya E. Noda, "Growing Up Asian in America," in *Making Waves: An Anthology of Writings by and about Asian American Women*, ed. Asian Women United in California (Boston: Beacon Press, 1989), 244; Felicia Lowe, "Asian American Women in Broadcasting," ibid., 176; Todd Gitlin, *The Twilight of Common Dreams: Why America Is Wracked by Culture Wars* (New York: Metropolitan/Henry Holt, 1995), 115, 135, 141.

56. Judy Wu, "'Loveliest Daughter of Our Ancient Cathay': Representations of Ethnic and Gender Identity in the Miss Chinatown, U.S.A. Beauty Pageant," paper presented at Pacific Coast Branch, American Historical Association, San Francisco, August 1996.

57. Ibid., and Judy Wu, personal communication, September 13, 1996; Joanne Chen, "Before and After," *A Magazine* 2:1, 15 (I thank Judy Yung for this article and for those by Chang and McNulty cited in n. 59).

58. Edward Falces, David Wesser, and Mark Gorney, "Cosmetic Surgery of the Non-Caucasian Nose," *PRS* 45:4 (April 1970), 317–324; *New York Times*, April 29, 1987, III 4:3; Se-Min Baek, Soo-Shin Kim, Shinsuke Tokunaga, and Alan Bindinger, "Oriental Blepharoplasty: Single-Stitch, Non-Incision Technique," *PRS* 83:2 (February 1989), 236–242. See also Eugenia Kaw, "Medicalization of Racial Features: Asian American Women and Cosmetic Surgery," *Medical Anthropology Quarterly* 7:1 (March 1993), 74–89.

59. Kaw, "Medicalization," 79, 81; Chen, "Before and After," 16–18, 64–65; see also Irene Chang, "For Asians in U.S. . . . ," *Los Angeles Times,* August 22, 1989, V:1 and Sheila McNulty, "Asians Bear the Knife for Western Look," *San Jose Mercury News,* February 21, 1995.

60. Richard B. Aronsohn and Richard A. Epstein, in *The Miracle of Cosmetic Plastic Surgery* (Los Angeles: Sherbourne Press, 1970), note that blacks wrinkle less than whites do and that Negro culture has a "more tolerant viewpoint . . . toward the simulacra of aging" (71); see also Midge Wilson and Kathy Russell, *Divided Sisters: Bridging the Gap between Black Women and White Women* (New York: Anchor/Doubleday, 1996), 77. The tendency in blacks to formation of hypertrophic or keloid scars is widely noted in both medical and popular literature; see, for example, Ferdinand A. Ofodile, Deodatta Bendre, and James E. Norris, "Cosmetic and Reconstructive Breast Surgery in Blacks," *PRS* 76:5 (November 1985), 708–712; Michele Bergen, "Plastic Surgery: A Lift for the Face, Figure and Spirit," *Ebony,* January 1977, 40–42; Elin Jones, "Cosmetic Surgery: Facing the Facts about Changing Our Looks," *Essence,* April 1986, 36–41; Lawrence Otis Graham, *Member of the Club: Reflections on Life in a Racially Polarized World* (New York: HarperCollins, 1995), 228.

61. Ronald Takaki, *Strangers from a Different Shore: A History of Asian Americans* (New York: Penguin, 1989), 101–102, 330–331; Marlon Riggs's pioneering documentary *Ethnic Notions* (San Francisco: California Newsreel, 1986) remains a compelling source.

62. There is a rich and growing literature on the hierarchy of color. Carlainya Templeton, "Beauty, Color and Black America," unpublished senior history thesis, University of California at Berkeley, 1991, started me off; Paula Giddings, *When and Where I Enter: The Impact of Black Women on Race and Sex in America* (New York: William Morrow, 1984) remains an important source (see 115, 178, 185–187), as does Jacqueline Jones, *Labor of Love, Labor of Sorrow: Black Women, Work, and the Family from Slavery to the Present* (New York: Basic Books, 1985), 38; Kathy Russell, Midge Wilson, and Ronald Hall, *The Color Complex* (New York: Harcourt Brace Jovanovich, 1992) is invaluable, as is Wilson and Russell, *Divided Sisters* (73–75); Spike Lee's *School Daze* (1988) offers a humorous take; Lisa Page, "High Yellow White Trash," in *Skin Deep: Black Women and White Women Write about Race,* ed. Marita Golden and Susan Richards Shreve (New York: Nan A. Talese/Doubleday, 1995), is a personal account; the essays in Robert Chrisman and Robert L. Allen, eds., *Court of Appeal: The Black Community Speaks Out on the Racial and Sexual Politics of Clarence Thomas vs. Anita Hill* (New York: Ballantine, 1992) demonstrate how long are the half-lives of these ideas and how significantly they continue to shape our national life.

63. Adalbert G. Bettman, "The Psychology of Appearances," *Northwest Medicine* 28:4 (April 1929), 782; Jacques W. Maliniak, *Sculpture in the Living: Rebuilding the Face and Form by Plastic Surgery* (New York: Romaine Pierson, 1934), 55, 92.

64. Schireson, *As Others See You,* 164–165, 276.

65. Richard G. Druss, Francis C. Symonds, and George F. Crikelair, "The Problem of Somatic Delusions in Patients Seeking Cosmetic Surgery," *PRS* 48:3 (September 1971), 246; JPW/Samantha Burr, Elizabeth Cole.

66. Charles M. MacKenzie, "Facial Deformity and Change in Personality Fol-

lowing Corrective Surgery," *Northwest Medicine* 43:8 (August 1944), 230–231; Charles Firestone, "Cosmetic Reduction of Full, Everted Lower Lip," *Northwest Medicine* 45:7 (July 1946), 499–501.

67. Milton Tuerk, "Cosmetic Repair of a Facial Type of Lip Deformity," *PRS* 25:4 (April 1960), 376–378.

68. Moynihan and Hartman, *Skin Deep*, 184.

69. Macgregor, *Transformation*, 92; see also Frances Cooke Macgregor and Bertram Schaffner, "Screening Patients for Nasal Plastic Operations," *Psychosomatic Medicine* 12:4 (September/October 1950), 277–280; Gilbert B. Snyder, "Rhinoplasty in the Negro," *PRS* 47:6 (June 1971), 572–575.

70. Bergen, "Plastic Surgery: A Lift"; Graham, *Member of the Club*, 222–231.

71. Wilson and Russell, *Divided Sisters*, 90–93(Washington quote, 93).

72. Thomas D. Rees, "Nasal Plastic Surgery in the Negro," *PRS* 43:1 (January 1969), 13; Ferdinand A. Ofodile, "Letter to the Editor," *PRS* 74:6 (December 1984), 846; Joshafphat Shulman and Melvyn Westreich, "Rhinoplasty Update: Preoperative Evaluation of 4,040 Cases," *Aesthetic Plastic Surgery* 7 (1983), 232.

73. W. Earle Matory Jr. and Edward Falces, "Non-Caucasian Rhinoplasty: A 16-Year Experience, *PRS* 77:2 (February 1986), 239; Thomas D. Rees, "Discussion of W. Earle Matory Jr. and Edward Falces, 'Non-Caucasian Rhinoplasty,' " *PRS* 77:2 (February 1986), 252.

74. Edmund A. Zingaro and Edward Falces, "Aesthetic Anatomy of the Non-Caucasian Nose," *Clinics in Plastic Surgery* 14:4 (October 1987), 749–765. See also Falces, David Wesser, and Mark Gorney, "Cosmetic Surgery of the Non-Caucasian Nose," *PRS* 45(April 1970), 317; Gilbert B. Snyder, "Rhinoplasty in the Negro," *PRS* 47 (June 1971), 572; Robert S. Flowers, "The Surgical Correction of the Non-Caucasian Nose," *Clinics in Plastic Surgery* 4 (January 1977), 69.

75. Taraborrelli, *Michael Jackson*, 256–257, 259, 261, 349, 357–358, 364, 398–399, 403, 419–424, 474, 533–537.

76. Ibid., 79, 91, 220–221.

77. Susan Bordo, *Unbearable Weight: Feminism, Western Culture, and the Body* (Berkeley: University of California Press, 1993), 246–265.

78. *Oprah Winfrey Show*, October 7, 1996.

79. "A Nose Is a Nose Is a Nose," *Time*, October 8, 1945, 69–70; Simona Morini, "The Importance of Noses," *Vogue*, October 1, 1970, 138–139, 213, 215; Kelli Pryor, "Nose by Nefertiti," *Art News*, February 1984, 15–16.

80. Jane Fort, "A New Nose, A New Identity?" *Teen*, February 1980, 64–65, 81.

81. Diana Stephens, "On Having a Nose Job—And Why I'm Sorry That I Did," *Mademoiselle*, February 1978, 34, 36.

82. Samuel M. Bloom, "Rhinoplasty in Adolescents," *Archives of Otolaryngology* 92:1 (July 1970), 66; "New Bodies for Sale," *Newsweek*, May 27, 1985, 64–69; Paula Dranov, "Vanity Fair," *Health*, May 1987, 65–69.

83. "New Bodies"; Dranov, "Vanity Fair"; Pryor, "Nose by Nefertiti."

84. *San Francisco Chronicle*, September 21, 1974, 11; April 26, 1979, 24; M.G. Lord, *Forever Barbie: The Unauthorized Biography of a Real Doll* (New York: William Morrow, 1994), 162–163.

85. Eve Scott, "Staying Well: Plain Facts about Plastic Surgery," *Seventeen*, April 1980, 34, 38; Francene Sabin, "A Teen's Guide to Cosmetic Surgery," *Seventeen*, March 1984, 253–254, 266–268; Wilson and Russell, *Divided Sisters*, 110.

86. Julie Smith, "Don't Call Me Barbra!" *Seventeen*, September 1976, 192; Kathleen Rockwell Lawrence, "The Nose Job," *Glamour*, September 1990, 338, 349–350; Green, "Dr. Nose."

87. Jane Brody, "Personal Health," *New York Times*, February 9, 1989, II 17:1.

88. Margaret Mead, introduction to Macgregor, *Transformation*, xiii–xiv; Ronald P. Strauss, "Ethical and Social Concerns in Facial Surgical Decision Making," *PRS* 72:5 (November 1983), 727–730.

89. Lord, *Forever Barbie*, 177.

90. Marita Golden, "Introduction," in Golden and Shreve, *Skin Deep*, 3.

SIX   *Beauty and the Breast*

1. *New York Times*, November 14, 1991, 1; November 15, 1991, A8. For a concise review of the controversy, see Nancy Bruning, *Breast Implants: Everything You Need to Know* (Alameda, Calif.: Hunter House, 1992), 5–21, and Pam Hait, "History of the ASPRS," *PRS* 94:4 (September 1994), 91A–99A. See also Marcia Angell, M.D., *Science on Trial: The Clash of Medical Evidence and the Law in the Breast Implant Case* (New York: Norton, 1996).

2. *New York Times*, January 16, 1992; January 29, 1992, C1; *San Francisco Chronicle*, February 11, 1992, 1.

3. For articles that address specifically the issue of silicone breast implants, see, for example, Sandra Blakeslee, "The True Story behind Breast Implants," *Glamour*, August 1991, 186–189, 230–231; "The Price of Beauty," *Economist*, January 11, 1992, 25–26; "On the Cutting Edge," *People*, January 27, 1992, 60; Nicholas Regush, "Toxic Breasts," *Mother Jones*, January/February 1992, 25–31; "The Implant Panic," *Vogue*, May 1992, 166, 168, 170; "Breastworks," *Elle*, July 1992, 96. The broader conspiracy argument reached its widest audience with Naomi Wolf's *The Beauty Myth: How Images of Beauty are Used against Women* (New York: William Morrow, 1991) and coincidentally was given credence by Susan Faludi's enormously popular *Backlash: The Undeclared War against American Women* (New York: Crown, 1991). See also Helen S. Edelman, "Why Is Dolly Crying? An Analysis of Silicone Breast Implants in America as an Example of Medicalization," *Journal of Popular Culture* 28:3 (Winter 1994), 19–32.

4. Nancy Bruning, who received a silicone implant after a mastectomy in 1980, offers the most cogent summary of the various versions in the introduction and chapter 1 of *Breast Implants*.

5. Anna Quindlen, "Not about Breasts," *New York Times*, January 19, 1992; Bruning, *Breast Implants*, 11–12.

6. Two studies suggesting no connection have been published to date in the *New England Journal of Medicine*: S. E. Gabriel et al., "Risk of Connective-Tissue Diseases and Other Disorders after Breast Implantation," 330 (1994), 1697–1702 and J. Sanchez-Guerrero et al., "Silicone Breast Implants and the Risk of Connective Tissue Diseases and Symptoms," 332 (1995), 1666–1670. A third study suggesting only

a slight (and questionable) connection is C. H. Hennekens et al., "Self-Reported Breast Implants and Connective Tissue Diseases and Symptoms," *JAMA* 275 (1996), 616–621. The modern history of "contested" diseases ranges from the debate over Agent Orange through Downwinders' accounts of nuclear testing to Gulf War Syndrome. See Elaine Showalter, *Hystories: Hysterical Epidemics and Modern Culture* (New York: Columbia University Press, 1997); Steve Kroll-Smith and H. Hugh Floyd, *Bodies in Protest: Environmental Illness and the Struggle over Medical Knowledge* (New York: New York University Press, 1997); and Chris Thompson, "The Gulf War Comes Home," *East Bay Express,* April 4, 1997, 1, 10–11, 14, 16–17, and April 11, 1997, 1, 6–8, 10.

7. Josleen Wilson, *The American Society of Plastic and Reconstructive Surgeons' Guide to Cosmetic Surgery* (New York: Simon and Schuster, 1992), 252–258. Accounts of risks and benefits, of course, differ. For an example of a more optimistic account, see Geri Trotta, "Woman's New Ally: Cosmetic Surgery," *Harper's Bazaar,* July 1954, 35, which asserts that "young girls, confronted with this problem (and it can be devastating psychologically and socially) are enabled by corrective operation, which does leave some slight fine-line scars, to look natural and also after childbirth, if they choose, to function as nursing mothers." Although some restrictions may apply, because reduction is generally considered to be reconstructive rather than cosmetic surgery—in other words, is justified by medical concerns—it is usually covered by insurance.

8. Maxwell Maltz, *New Faces, New Futures: Rebuilding Character with Plastic Surgery* (New York: Richard R. Smith, 1936); Maxine Davis, "Does Plastic Surgery Work?" *Pictorial Review,* December 1937, 18.

9. Hans May, "Scope and Problems of Plastic Surgery," *Pennsylvania Medical Journal* 42 (September 1939), 1457–1458; Lois Mattox Miller, "Surgery's Cinderella," *Independent Woman,* July 1939, 201.

10. Constance J. Foster, "Reconstructive Surgery," *Parents' Magazine,* November 1943, 28; Marguerite Clark, "Breast Surgery," *McCalls,* April 1948, 2.

11. Elizabeth Honor, "Cosmetic Surgery," *Cosmopolitan,* August 1956, 28–31; Ginny Evans, "The Operation That Changed My Life," *Good Housekeeping,* November 1976, 96; see also Jillian Frank, "I Had Breast-Reduction Surgery," *Cosmopolitan,* July 1982, 114.

12. "Breast Reduction: Is It for You?" *Women's Sports and Fitness,* July 1986, 56; "Now I Can Be Free," *People,* April 26, 1993, 83.

13. Some surgeons, most neither members of the plastic surgical societies nor certified by the American Board of Plastic Surgery, did claim early successes in surgically treating small breasts. Henry Junius Schireson was one of these; in his 1938 book *As Others See You: The Story of Plastic Surgery* (New York: Macaulay Co.), 218–226, he reported successful breast augmentation using a "pedical flap/fat-fascia graft." Adolph M. Broom, "Prosthetic Restorations for the Breast," *Archives of Surgery* 48:5 (May 1944), 388; Deborah N. Schalk, "The History of Augmentation Mammaplasty," *Plastic Surgical Nursing* 8:3 (Fall 1988), 88; Clark, "Breast Surgery." The history of paraffin is addressed in Chapter 1.

14. H. O. Bames, "Breast Malformations and a New Approach to the Problem of the Small Breast," *PRS* 5:6 (June 1950), 499; H. O. Bames, "Augmentation

Mammaplasty by Lipo-Transplant," *PRS* 11:5 (May 1953), 404; Schalk, "History of Augmentation Mammaplasty," 88. This operation has been "rediscovered" several times. In 1960, Dr. Morton I. Berson of New York recommended a "new derma-fat-fascia graft" at a congress in Mexico City. See *San Francisco Chronicle,* May 7, 1960, 18.

15. "The Business of Bolstering Bosoms," *JAMA* 153:13 (November 28, 1953), 1200–1201.

16. Robert Alan Franklyn, *Beauty Surgeon* (Long Beach, Calif.: Whitehorn, 1960), 15–22.

17. "Business of Bolstering."

18. *Los Angeles Times,* January 11, 1954, 17:1; William S. Kiskadden, "Operations on Bosoms Dangerous," *PRS* 15:1 (January 1955), 79; Herbert Conway and James Smith, "Breast Plastic Surgery," *PRS* 21:1 (January 1958), 13–14; Franklyn, *Beauty Surgeon,* 27–30; Schalk, "History," 88–89. In 1975 a Los Angeles plastic surgeon remembered Franklyn as having been one of "the ones everyone loved to hate." See Ivor and Sally Davis, "The Great Male Face Race," *LA Magazine,* February 1975, 63, 103–104.

19. Beth Bailey, *From Front Porch to Back Seat: Courtship in Twentieth-Century America* (Baltimore: Johns Hopkins University Press, 1988), 73–74; Franklyn, *Beauty Surgeon,* 27–30.

20. Honor, "Cosmetic Surgery"; Carlson Wade, "Instant Beauty through Plastic Surgery," *Lady's Circle,* April 1965, 19 (NAPS, HMS C87 #403).

21. M. T. Edgerton and A. R. McClary, "Augmentation Mammaplasty: Psychiatric Implications and Surgical Indications," *PRS* 21:4 (April 1958), 279–300.

22. Ibid.

23. M. T. Edgerton, E. Meyer, and W. E. Jacobson, "Augmentation Mammaplasty II: Further Surgical and Psychiatric Evaluation," *PRS* 27:3 (March 1961), 279–296.

24. Silas A. Braley, "The Use of Silicones in Plastic Surgery: A Retrospective View," *PRS* 51:3 (March 1973), 280–288.

25. Kurt Wagner, *How to Win in the Youth Game: The Magic of Plastic Surgery* (Englewood Cliffs, N.J.: Prentice Hall, 1972), 126; Deborah Larned, "A Shot—or Two or Three—in the Breast," *Ms.,* September 1977, 55; Paul Bernstein, "Newest Wrinkles in Cosmetic Surgery," *LA Magazine,* January 1979, 141; *New York Times,* January 18, 1992, 1.

26. *Chicago Daily News,* May 14, 1964, section 3, 25. See also *Harper's Bazaar,* October 1964, which warned women about this new and experimental practice.

27. Simona Morini, *Body Sculpture: Plastic Surgery from Head to Toe* (New York: Delacorte, 1972), 119–141; James O. Stallings, *A New You: How Plastic Surgery Can Change Your Life* (New York: Mason/Charter, 1977), 43. Numerous critics have called into question the efficacy—both intended and actual—of Dow Corning's affidavit program. Participants were plastic surgeons Franklin L. Ashley (University of California at Los Angeles), Ralph Blocksma (Grand Rapids, Mich.), Reed O. Dingman (University of Michigan), Milton T. Edgerton (University of Virginia), Dicran Goulian, Joseph E. Murray, and Thomas D. Rees (New York), and dermatologist Norman Orentreich (New York).

28. *San Francisco Chronicle,* November 15, 1965, 1, 15; November 16, 1.

29. Ibid.; see also "Illegal, Immoral and Dangerous," *Science News,* February 17, 1968, 173.

30. "Abreast of the Times," *JAMA* 195:10 (March 7, 1966), 863; Franklin L. Ashley, Silas Braley, Thomas D. Rees, Dicran Goulian, and Donald L. Ballantyne Jr., "Present Status of Silicone Fluid in Soft Tissue Augmentation," *PRS* 39:4 (April 1967), 411–415; Khoo Boo-Chai, "The Complications of Augmentation Mammaplasty by Silicone Injection," *British Journal of Plastic Surgery* 22:3 (July 1969), 281; C. Hal Chaplin, "Loss of Both Breasts from Injections of Silicone (with Additive)," *PRS* 44:5 (November 1969), 447. No national statistics on complications are available, but one San Diego physician told a reporter that 20 percent of the approximately four hundred complications he saw between 1967 and 1974 required amputation. See Larned, "A Shot."

31. "Illegal, Immoral and Dangerous." Records showed that the recipient of the illegal shipment was Harvey Kagan, one of silicone's pioneers. See Larned, "A Shot." M. E. Nelson responded to this article for Dow Corning, criticizing the attribution to Dow Corning of responsibility for the distribution of silicone. According to Nelson, fourteen U.S. manufacturers produced industrial-grade silicone; as for medical, "we have always enforced rigorous controls to prevent unauthorized use of this material" (*Ms.,* January 1978, 4). Dow Corning has conceded that it should have made more of an effort to ensure that its product was not being used in humans; see *San Francisco Chronicle,* January 20, 1971, 4.

32. Silas Braley, "Letter to the Editor," *PRS* 45:3 (March 1970), 288; *San Francisco Chronicle,* August 6, 1974, 16; February 10, 1975, 34; January 30, 1976, 14; Al Reinert, "Doctor Jack Makes His Rounds," *Esquire,* May 1975, 114; see also Donald T. Moynihan and Shirley Hartman, *Skin Deep: The Making of a Plastic Surgeon* (Boston: Little, Brown, 1979), 102–103. According to *Ms.,* the problem in Las Vegas was so bad that in April 1975 Nevada enacted emergency legislation making it a felony; California made it a misdemeanor in 1976. See Larned, "A Shot."

33. According to C. Hal Chaplin, vegetable and mineral oils, including castor oil, were used as additives in order to provoke a "moderate fibrous tissue response" that would prevent silicone migration. Silas Braley, in 1970, reported that of three cases where tissue samples were sent to the Dow Corning laboratory for analysis, the substance in question was not silicone at all but a "linear hydrocarbon, most likely paraffin." One of the women had received injections in New York in 1964; the other two in Fukuoka, Japan, between 1965 and 1970. In Toni Kosover, "Fill Her Up," *W,* November 3, 1972, 20, dermatologist Michael Kalman of New York's Orentreich group is quoted as attributing problems to Japanese doctors who added peanut, sesame, and olive oil. According to Moynihan, the use of "industrial grade raw silicone . . . a cheap commercial material that sells for about fifteen dollars a gallon and is manufactured as a base for floor waxes, polishes, electrical insulation, and water-repellent sprays" was responsible for Tijuana Silicone Rot. John Conley, *Face-Lift Operation* (Springfield, Ill.: Charles C. Thomas, 1968), 92. Despite the publicity, women continued to see silicone as an easy option. See, for example, "For Women Only," *San Francisco Chronicle,* December 14, 1971, 21, in which a woman wrote to ask why silicone injections, which sounded so easy, were illegal.

34. "The Silicone Injection Story Updated," *Harper's Bazaar* 100 (May 1967), 148; Simona Morini, "A New Aid to Plastic Surgery: Silicone," *Vogue,* March 15, 1971, 84; Kosover, "Fill Her Up"; *Newsweek,* December 11, 1972. A few articles were more cautious; see, for example, William and Ellen Hartley, "How We're Saving Bodies and Psyches with Silicones," *Science Digest,* August 1974, 25.

35. Larned, "A Shot"; Reinert, "Doctor Jack."

36. Larned, "A Shot." A March 1979 article in *FDA Consumer* reported: "Despite its popularity, most liquid silicone surgery practices are condemned both by FDA and the American Medical Association. While surgery per se is outside FDA's jurisdiction . . . sterile liquid silicone is considered a medical device, and is subject to regulation by FDA under the Medical Device Amendments of 1976." In the spring of 1978, FDA approved a new Dow Corning test program that, on a limited, nonprofit basis, would enable doctors to experiment with liquid silicone as a solution for severe disfigurements that could not be corrected in any other way. "New Face Lift Not All Smiles," *FDA Consumer,* March 1979, 15.

37. Schalk, "History," 89; Braley, "Use of Silicones," 285–286; *New York Times,* November 13, 1988, IV 9:1.

38. Permeation by breast tissue was a significant problem with the polyurethane-covered implants that were developed in an effort to solve the contracture problem, a topic that is covered later in this chapter.

39. Schalk, "History," 89; Braley, "Use of Silicones," 285–286; see Ralph Blocksma and Silas Braley, "Implantation Materials," 3–148, in *Plastic Surgery,* ed. W. Grabb and J. Smith (Boston: Little, Brown, 1965).

40. *Time,* March 27, 1964, 48; T. R. Broadbent and Robert M. Woolf, "Augmentation Mammaplasty," *PRS* 40:6 (December 1964), 517–523; Colette Perras, "Plastic Reconstruction of the Small Breast," *Journal of the American Women's Medical Association* 20:10 (October 1965), 951–952.

41. *Time,* March 27, 1964, 48; "Yes, You Can Have a Bigger Bosom!" *Cosmopolitan,* January 1970, 66.

42. Morini, *Body Sculpture,* 74; see also Simona Morini, "Breast Sculpture," *Vogue,* January 15, 1971, 82–85. Arthur Frank and Stuart Frank, "Health," *Mademoiselle,* November 1975, 74; Barbara Lynn, "Taking Shape," *Cosmopolitan,* June 1977, 136; "Bosom Surgery: The Latest News," *Cosmopolitan,* June 1978, 188; Maxine Abrams, "Cosmo's Update on Plastic Surgery," *Cosmopolitan,* December 1981, 212; "Beauty and Health Report," *Glamour,* January 1985, 182. Over the years, popular magazines have presented a range of opinions on cosmetic breast augmentation, often offering alternative viewpoints in back-to-back issues (for example, an article one month touting the benefits and an article the next month profiling a case that went wrong). In general, coverage was positive until the late 1980s and in some cases the early 1990s, when stories about risks and problems, often sparked by one of the widely publicized court cases or by FDA action, began to appear.

43. Rose Kushner, a dedicated advocate for breast cancer patients, marshaled convincing evidence that the practice of immediate mastectomy following a "frozen section" biopsy had developed for the surgeon's convenience rather than for any compelling medical necessity. See "Before Breast Surgery: What Every Woman Should Know," *Family Circle,* May 1976, 64. More recently, debate has

arisen surrounding the issue of immediate reconstruction. Surgeons have insisted that immediate reconstruction endangers patients' health and gives them no time to mourn their loss, while women often argue the procedure's benefits. Connie Boyd, a plastic surgical nurse, in 1989 advocated more attention to patients' emotional needs and argued that immediate reconstruction is one of the ways in which medical caregivers can meet women's needs. See "Meeting the Psychological Needs of the Breast Reconstruction Patient," *Plastic Surgical Nursing* 9:3 (Fall 1989), 129.

44. "Rebuilding the Breast," *Time*, April 14, 1975, 76; Gilbert Cant and Toby Cohen, "The Operation Women Never Dreamed Would Be Possible," *Good Housekeeping*, September 1975, 56.

45. Betty Rollin, "First, You Cry," *Family Circle*, September 1976, 118–122; "Gazette," *Ms.*, February 1978, 22.

46. Margaret Markham and Toby Cohen, "The Miracle of a New Breast," *Harper's Bazaar*, September 1976, 148; "In Her Own Words," *People*, September 11, 1978, 69; "For Mastectomy Patients," *McCalls*, May 1980, 61; Abby Avin Belson, "Breast Reconstruction," *Ms.* August 1983, 96 (silicone bleed is the only side effect not mentioned; it was known to occur in 1983 but its health effects were not known); "To Be Whole Again," *Life*, May 1987, 78. See also Thomas D. Cronin, Joseph Upton, and James McDonough, "Reconstruction of the Breast after Mastectomy," *PRS* 59:1 (January 1977), 1–14.

47. Jack Star, "How Silastic Transformed Breast Surgery," *Look*, July 27, 1971, 12.

48. On subcutaneous mastectomy, see Bromley S. Freeman, "Whither Subcutaneous Mastectomy?" and Daniel L. Weiner, "On Subcutaneous Mastectomy," *PRS* 49:6 (June 1972), 654–655; Morini, *Body Sculpture*, 105; Moynihan and Hartman, *Skin Deep*, 106; C. Lawrence Slade, "Subcutaneous Mastectomy: Acute Complications and Long-Term Follow-Up" and Jack Fischer, "Discussion," *PRS* 73:1 (January 1984), 84–90; Letters to the Editor (four), *PRS* 74:1 (July 1984), 151–153.

49. John E. Hoopes, Milton T. Edgerton, and William Shelley, "Organic Synthetics for Augmentation Mammaplasty: Their Relation to Breast Cancer," *PRS* 39:3 (March 1967), 263; Tibor de Cholnoky, "Augmentation Mammaplasty: Survey of Complications in 10,941 Patients by 265 Surgeons," *PRS* 45:6 (June 1970), 573.

50. John Goin was quoted in *Medical Economics*, February 21, 1977; Marjorie Nashner and Mimi White, "Beauty and the Breast: A 60% Complication Rate for an Operation You Don't Need," *Ms.*, September 1977, 53.

51. Nashner and White, "Beauty and the Breast"; Letters, *Ms.*, January 1978, 4.

52. Letters, *Ms.*, January 1978, 4.

53. Gregory P. Hetter, "Satisfactions and Dissatisfactions of Patients with Augmentation Mammaplasty," *PRS* 64:2 (August 1979), 151–155; Norman S. Levine and Robert T. Buchanan, "Decreased Swimming Speed Following Augmentation Mammaplasty," *PRS* 71:2 (February 1983), 255–256.

54. Madalyn Eisenberg, "The Biggest Mistake a Woman Can Make," *Good Housekeeping*, March 1980, 82.

55. John A. Brossman and Ruth Winter, "Breast Augmentation Surgery," *Glamour*, November 1981, 255; Melva Weber, "Breast Augmentation," *Vogue*,

October 1984, 678; Melva Weber, "Breast Reshapers," *Vogue*, July 1986, 201; "How Safe Are Breast Implants?" *Good Housekeeping*, April 1989, 237.

56. Harriet LaBarre, *Plastic Surgery: Beauty You Can Buy* (New York: Holt, Rinehart and Winston, 1970), 88–93; Wagner, *How to Win in the Youth Game*, 70–80; see also Richard B. Aronsohn and Richard A. Epstein, *The Miracle of Cosmetic Plastic Surgery* (Los Angeles: Sherbourne Press, 1970), 279, and Sylvia Rosenthal, *Cosmetic Surgery: A Consumer's Guide* (Philadelphia and New York: Tree Communications/J. B. Lippincott, 1977), 200.

57. James L. Baker Jr., Roger J. Barkels, and William M. Douglas, "Closed Compression Technique for Rupturing a Contracted Capsule around a Breast Implant," *PRS* 58:2 (August 1976), 137–141; Gerald D. Nelson, "Complications from the Treatment of Fibrous Capsular Contracture of the Breast," *PRS* 68:6 (December 1981), 969–970; see also *PRS* 69:5 (May 1982), which carried three articles and five commentaries on capsular contracture, 794–814; and Abrams, "Cosmo's Update on Plastic Surgery."

58. B. R. Burckhardt, Letter to the Editor, *PRS* 73:2 (February 1984), 329–330. The definitive article on the Même is Regush, "Toxic Breasts"; see also Sybil Niden Goldrich, "Restoration Drama," *Ms.*, June 1988, 20–22, which played a significant role in sparking the recent controversy, and Blakeslee, "The True Story," which details the early history of the polyurethane-covered implant. For an example of how the Même was discussed in the popular press, see Joan L. Lippert, "A Better Breast Implant," *Health*, April 1983, 21–22.

59. Eugene Courtiss and Robert M. Goldwyn, "Breast Sensation before and after Plastic Surgery," *PRS* 58:1 (July 1976), 1–13; Hetter, "Satisfactions and Dissatisfactions," 151–155; see also "How Safe?"

60. Garry S. Brody, "Fact and Fiction about Breast Implant Bleed," *PRS* 60:4 (October 1977), 615–616.

61. Thomas J. Sergott, Joseph P. Limoli, Curtis M. Baldwin, and Donald R. Lamb, "Human Adjuvant Disease, Possible Autoimmune Disease after Silicone Implantation: A Review of the Literature, Case Studies, and Speculation for the Future," *PRS* 78:1 (July 1986), 104–110.

62. "Silicone Breast Implants on Trial," *Science News*, December 10, 1988, 380; "Breast Implants: A Safer Method," *Newsweek*, September 25, 1989, 52; Bruce W. Van Natta, J. Bradley Thurston, and Thomas S. Moore, "Silicone Breast Implants—Is There Cause for Concern?" *Indiana Medicine* 83:3 (March 1990), 184–185.

63. Garry S. Brody, "Humpty Dumpty on Capsular Contracture and Complications," *PRS* 73:4 (April 1984), 658–659.

64. Courtiss and Goldwyn, "Breast Sensation," 1–13; "How Safe?"

65. *New York Times*, January 29, 1992, C1; Regush, "Toxic Breasts."

66. LaBarre, *Beauty You Can Buy*, 79, 81–82, 85; Morini, "Breast Sculpture." See also Susan Seliger, "What Price Beauty?" *Washingtonian*, April 1979, 159; Harriet LaBarre, "Making More (Or Less) of Your Bosom," *Ladies Home Journal*, May 1972, 87; Rosenthal, *Cosmetic Surgery*, 207; Phyllis Lehman, "Your Choice: Breast Reshaping," *Vogue*, July 1979, 178.

67. John R. Lewis Jr., "The Augmentation Mammaplasty," *PRS* 35:1 (January 1965), 51; Hugh A. Johnson, "Silastic Breast Implants: Coping with Complications,"

PRS 44:6 (December 1969), 588–591; see also Aronsohn and Epstein, *The Miracle,* 274, 283–285.

68. Paule Regnault, Thomas J. Baker, Matthew C. Gleason, Howard L. Gordon, A. Richard Grossman, John R. Lewis Jr., W. Reid Waters, John E. Williams, "Clinical Trial and Evaluation of a Proposed New Inflatable Mammary Prosthesis," *PRS* 50:3 (September 1972), 220; James L. Baker Jr., Irving S. Kohn, and Edmund S. Bartlett, "Psychosexual Dynamics of Patients Undergoing Mammary Augmentation," *PRS* 53:6 (June 1974), 652–659; Reinert, "Dr. Jack."

69. Reinert, "Doctor Jack"; A. Richard Grossman, "Psychological and Psychosexual Aspects of Augmentation Mammaplasty," *Clinics in Plastic Surgery* 3:2 (April 1976), 167–170.

70. Josephine Lowman, "Why Grow Old?" *Oakland Tribune*, May 1, 1953, 38:4; *San Francisco Chronicle*, July 31, 1954, 9; November 5, 1957, 5. On postwar fashions in breasts, see Bailey, *From Front Porch to Back Seat*, 73–74.

71. Susan S. Lichtendorf, "Are Your Breasts Too Small, Too Large?" *Harper's Bazaar*, September 1976, 145; "New Bodies for Sale," *Newsweek*, May 27, 1985, 64–69; on East v. West, Lawrence Reed quoted in Laura Green, "The Brave New World of Cosmetic Surgery," *Cosmopolitan*, July 1986, 208–212. On changing seasons: Patricia Morrisroe, "Forever Young," *New York Magazine*, June 9, 1986, 42–49, quotes Steven Herman ("When May rolls around, I see a lot of women who want nicer breasts"); William E. Geist, "About New York," *New York Times*, December 11, 1985, II 3:1, quotes Elliot Jacobs on holiday parties.

72. Thomas D. Rees, Cary L. Guy, Richard J. Coburn in *PRS* 52:6 (December 1973), 609; Green, "Brave New World," 208–212; "Sizing Up Breast Implants," *Health*, August 1987, 23. The literature on shape and size is substantial; only a few examples are given here. Medical: see John E. Williams, "Experiences with a Large Series of Silastic Breast Implants," *PRS* 49:3 (March 1972), 253–258; Garry S. Brody, "Breast Implant Size Selection and Patient Satisfaction," *PRS* 68:4 (October 1981), 611–613; Sherman G. Souther and Morgan L. Lucid, Letter, *PRS* 69:6 (June 1982), 1025. Popular: "Breasts," *Glamour*, November 1981, 252, gives ideal geometric measurements. "The More the Mariel," *People*, November 21, 1983, 41, cited Hemingway's augmentation as an example of the lengths to which stars will go to fit a role's physical requirements. Hemingway, who played Playmate Dorothy Stratton in *Star 80*, denied that her implants were tied to the part, saying, "Since making this movie, I feel I've become a real woman, and I like it." Holly Brubach, "Beauty and the Breast," *Vogue*, July 1986, 204, quotes Norma Kamali. Joanne Kaufman, "Whose Breasts Are They, Anyway?" *Mademoiselle*, August 1987, quotes Steven Herman ("The full-breasted European look is definitely in"); Eileen Ford ("Surgery would be very ill-advised. . . . Models are youngsters. They just love that kind of thing"); Jule Campbell, model selector for *Sports Illustrated*'s swimsuit issue ("The girls want to be noticed, and if having large breasts is what it takes, they'll get them"); and Frances Grill, founder and president of Click Models ("I do think it's tough on women. . . . It's hard to feel beautiful unless you fall into the 'right' category that's popular at the moment"). Breast augmentation increased all over the world in the 1970s and 1980s (see the *San Francisco Chronicle*, November 29, 1974, 7, on British women), but nowhere except perhaps Brazil compared with the United States.

73. Lois Banner, *American Beauty* (Chicago: University of Chicago Press, 1983), 86–87, 94, 96; Nancy F. Cott, *The Grounding of Modern Feminism* (New Haven: Yale University Press, 1987), 12–13; Miriam Schneir, ed., *Feminism in Our Time: The Essential Writings, World War II to the Present* (New York: Vintage, 1994), 125; Susan Douglas, *Where the Girls Are: Growing Up Female with the Mass Media* (New York: Times Books, 1994), 139–140, 157–161.

74. "Cheers for Cher," *Ms.*, July 1988, 53.

75. Douglas, *Where the Girls Are,* 246; Barbara Kerbel, "Getting a New Face on Plastic Surgery," *Houston Chronicle,* September 29, 1996, C6.

76. Karen Offen, "Defining Feminism: A Comparative Historical Approach," *Signs* 14:1 (1988), 119–157; Susan Ware, *Still Missing: Amelia Earhart and the Search for Modern Feminism* (New York: W. W. Norton, 1993), esp. 117–143.

77. Robert H. Shipley, John M. O'Donnell, and Karl F. Bader, "Personality Characteristics of Women Seeking Breast Augmentation," *PRS* 60:3 (September 1977), 369–376.

78. Goldrich, "Restoration Drama"; Kendall H. Moore and Sally Thompson's 1979 *The Surgical Beauty Racket* was highly critical of the FDA's attitude. "Plastic Surgery: Prostheses Need More Regulation," *Science Digest,* August 1979, 78–81, took up the gauntlet: "Special interest groups control the FDA. The truth is: the specialty of plastic surgery has brought pressure to bear upon the FDA and has thus far managed to evade any restrictions whatsoever on breast, cheek or nose implant materials. The complications from these materials have simply been swept under the rug." But most periodicals ignored it. In 1982, Paul Tilton and Louise Fenner, "The Body Doesn't Always Take Kindly to Breast Implants," *FDA Consumer,* April 1982, 4–7, reviewed the history and side effects of breast augmentation (hemmorhage, infection, capsular contracture, silicone bleed, rupture and leakage requiring replacement, and cancer) but concluded that "Each woman must decide for herself whether it is worth the risk to try to provide what Mother Nature didn't." In 1986 the FDA noted: "Implants should not be confused with liquid silicone injections, which FDA banned due to the risk of cancer and other life-threatening complications. There is no evidence that silicone gel implants have these problems." See "Breast Reconstruction," *FDA Consumer,* May 1986, 11.

79. Goldrich, "Restoration Drama."

80. *New York Times,* November 10, 1988, I 18:1; November 24, 1988, II 16:5; "Silicone Breast Implants on Trial," *Science News,* December 10, 1988, 380.

81. "FDA to Require Safety Data on Breast Implants," *FDA Consumer,* March 1989, 2.

82. Cynthia Marks, "The New Breast Implant Scare," *Mademoiselle,* February 1989, 124–125; Robin Marantz Henig, "Are Breast Implants Too Risky?" *Vogue,* July 1989, 111–112.

83. Bruce W. Van Natta, J. Bradley Thurston, and Thomas S. Moore, "Silicone Breast Implants—Is There Cause for Concern?" *Indiana Medicine* 83:3 (March 1990), 184–185.

84. Hoehn quoted in Hait, "History of the ASPRS," 97A.

85. See "Breast Reconstruction," *FDA Consumer,* May 1986, 11. In 1987, Eugene Courtiss, then chairman of the American Board of Plastic Surgery, warned

that autologous fat transfer "may seem like a woman's dream come true, but that dream is likely to turn into a nightmare." See "Women Warned of Dangers of Fat Recycling Technique," *Jet*, July 6, 1987, 29; see also Jacqueline Rivkin, "Plastic Surgeons Nix Breast Fix," *American Health*, May 1988, 13; "Spare Parts Breast Surgery," *Health*, August 1988, 20; "Breast Implants: A Safer Method," *Newsweek*, September 25, 1989, 52; *New York Times*, August 23, 1990, B 9:4. In 1988 two surgeons reported seeing several women who had received "cadaver fat allografts" in the Soviet Union in the mid-1970s; although these women had experienced few problems, the surgeons did not advocate this method. See Pamela B. Rosen and Norman E. Hugo, "Augmentation Mammaplasty by Cadaver Fat Allografts," *PRS* 82:3 (September 1988), 525–526. On the latest possibility—the "engineered tissue" described as a "grow your own" alternative—see Steve Sakson in *Knoxville News-Sentinel*, September 19, 1995, C1. "Database: Body Work," *U.S. News and World Report*, October 17, 1994, 15; "The Long and the Short of it: Answers from 1,000 Men," *Glamour*, January 1995, 138.

EPILOGUE   ***The Eye of the Beholder***

1. Norma Lee Browning, "New Mecca for Face-Lifts," *Saturday Evening Post*, November 1978, 68–69, 102–103; Warren Hoge, "Doctor Vanity: The Jet Set's Man in Rio," *New York Times Magazine*, June 8, 1980, 42–46, 52–62, 66–70; Alessandra Stanley, "Lifting the Spirit (and Face) in Russia," *New York Times*, June 6, 1995, A6.

2. M.S.W. to American Board of Plastic Surgery, August 13, 1961 (NAPS, ABPS #302).

3. For an early perspective on body contouring, see Max Thorek, "Possibilities in Reconstruction of the Human Form," *New York Medical Journal and Medical Recorder* 116:2245 (November 15, 1922), 572–575, and Max Thorek, "The Possibilities of Surgical Esthetic Remodeling of the Human Form," *Tri State Medical Journal* 3:10 (July 1931), 621–622.

4. For a quick trip through liposuction's emergence in the United States, see B. Teimourian and J. B. Fisher, "Suction Currettage to Remove Excess Fat for Body Contouring," *PRS* 68:1 (July 1981), 50–58; *New York Times*, November 22, 1982, II 12:2 and July 3, 1989, I 12:2; Robert M. Goldwyn, "The Advent of Liposuction," *PRS* 72:5 (November 1983), 705; Carson M. Lewis, "Early History of Lipoplasty in the United States," *Aesthetic Plastic Surgery* 14 (1990), 123–126; and Yves-Gerard Illouz, ed., *Liposuction: The Franco-American Experience* (Beverly Hills, Calif.: Medical Aesthetics, 1985), 36–38, 54–55, 72–73. For a sampling of the enormous popular literature, see P. Harrison, "Fat by the Pocketful," *McLeans*, September 13, 1982, 53; K. Feld, "A Vacuum Cleaner for Fat," *Washingtonian*, February 1983, 15; N.E. Hugo, "Saddle-Bag Surgery," *Health*, April 1983, 8; "Fat Vacuuming—A New Fad?" *Science Digest*, October 1983, 79; W. A. Nolen, "Fat Vacuuming: How Safe Is It?" *McCalls*, January 1984, 45–46; L. Vaughn, "All about Fat Removal Operations," *Prevention*, May 1984, 75–80; R. Blaun, "Vacuum Leaner," *New York*, December 3, 1984, 128, 130; S. M. Sims, "Fat Vacuum," *Vogue*, August 1985, 144, 146; M. Gentle and M. Siegel, "The Operation That Did . . . ," *Good Housekeeping*, September 1985, 54–61;

"Good-Bye Thunder Thighs," *Dance Magazine,* May 1987, 114–115; R. B. Pearce, "Miracle Cure for Saddlebags," *Women's Sports and Fitness,* July 1987, 38–39; "Fat Loss," *Consumers Research Magazine,* September 1987, 2; R. M. Henig, "The High Cost of Thinness," *New York Times Magazine,* February 28, 1988, 41–42 and "Liposuction," *Vogue,* October 1989, 292–296; S. Montgomery, "Vacuuming the Fat Away," *Working Woman,* May 1988, 132–134; P. Boyer, "The Lowdown on Liposuction," *Prevention,* August 1988, 42–43, 127; L. Ashland, "Liposuction: Fat Loss or Fiasco?" *Harper's Bazaar,* August 1988, 144–145; J. O. Stallings, "A Plastic Surgery Cure for Cellulite," *USA Today,* November 1988, 68–69; S. Asken, "The Importance of Accurate Reporting on Liposuction Surgery to the Public," *Journal of Dermatologic Surgery and Oncology* 16:3 (March 1990), 228–230.

On calf implants, see Adrien E. Aiache, "Calf Implantation," *PRS* 83:3 (March 1989), 488–493, and Elisabeth Rosenthal, "Cosmetic Surgeons Seek New Frontiers," *New York Times,* September 24, 1991, B5:1.

5. Giora G. Angres, "Eye-Liner Implants: A New Cosmetic Procedure," *PRS* 73:5 (May 1984), 833–836; "Read This First," *U.S. News and World Report,* October 14, 1996, 79.

6. *San Francisco Chronicle,* February 21, 1994, D7; Kathleen Doheny, "Plastic Surgery Lite," *Mirabella,* May/June 1997, 68–70.

7. Walter R. Siemian and M. Reza Samiian, "Malar Augmentation Using Autogenous Composite Conchal Cartilage and Temporalis Fascia," *PRS* 82:3 (September 1988), 395–401.

8. Linton A. Whitaker and Michael Pertshuk, "Facial Skeletal Contouring for Aesthetic Purposes," *PRS* 69:2 (February 1982), 245–253.

9. Judy Shapiro, "New Faces for Down's Kids," *McLeans,* December 27, 1982, 38; Maya Pines, "Plastic Surgery for Down's Children," *Psychology Today,* September 1983, 85, 88; Carol Turkington, "Changing the Look of Mental Retardation," *Psychology Today,* September 1987, 45–46; Deborah C. May, "Plastic Surgery for Children with Down Syndrome: Normalization or Extremism?" *Mental Retardation* 26:1 (February 1988), 17–19; Shlomo Katz and Shlomo Kravetz, "Facial Plastic Surgery for Persons with Down Syndrome: Research Findings and Their Professional and Social Implications" and Barbara Dodd and Judi Leahy, "Commentaries," *American Journal on Mental Retardation* 94:2 (1989), 101–111.

10. Rosenthal, "Cosmetic Surgeons Seek New Frontiers." Significantly, while 55 percent of men agreed that they would encourage their partners to have breast implants if the process were "painless, safe, and free," only 33 percent would have pectoral implants themselves under the same conditions. "The Long and the Short of It: Answers from 1,000 Men," *Glamour,* January 1995, 136, 139.

11. I first learned about penile enhancement when a friend brought me an advertisement clipped during a weekend trip to Los Angeles that advised interested parties to call 1–800-U-DISTINCT; this number is no longer in service. See Claudia Morain, "Men Who Think Bigger Is Better," *San Francisco Chronicle,* October 3, 1994, E7; Reynolds Holding, "Physician Sued over Penis Surgery," *San Francisco Chronicle,* April 24, 1995, A9–11; David Perlman, "Few Penis Enlargements Necessary, Doctors Say," *San Francisco Chronicle,* April 27, 1995, A7; Lisa Bannon,

"How a Risky Surgery Became a Profit Center in Los Angeles," *Wall Street Journal*, June 6, 1996 (interactive edition; thanks to Keith Wailoo for forwarding this). As used for faces, the technique, known as autologous fat transplantation, is described in Bernice Kanner, "Postponing the Knife," *Mirabella*, September 1993, 124–126, 131.

12. On explanation, see 1993 and 1994 issues of *Plastic and Reconstructive Surgery*.

13. On the FTC episode, see Frederick J. McCoy, "Report on the Activities of the ASPRS," *PRS* 59:3 (March 1977), 315–317; Peter Randall, "Federal Trade Commission vs. Reliance upon Board Certification in a Specialty," *PRS* 63:4 (April 1979), 453–456; Mark Gorney, "F.T.C., Woodstock, and Plastic Surgery," *PRS* 65:2 (February 1980), 245; Mark Gorney, "The Morning After," *PRS* 66:5 (November 1980), 751–752; Francis X. Paletta, "History of the American Society of Plastic and Reconstructive Surgeons, Inc., 1931–1981: Its Growth, Change, Unity," *PRS* 68:3 (September 1981), 314–317; Norman E. Hugo, "Five-Year History of the American Society of Plastic and Reconstructive Surgeons, 1979–1983," *PRS* 75:4 (April 1985), 596–602; Claire G. Fox and William P. Graham III, "The American Board of Plastic Surgery, 1937–1987," *PRS* 82:1 (July 1988), 182–183; Pam Hait, "History of the ASPRS," *PRS* 94:4 (September 1994), 72A–74A.

14. The debate on advertising may be followed through George V. Webster, "Whatever Happened to Ethics?" *PRS* 60:1 (July 1977), 100; Eugene H. Courtiss, "Our Past and Present Challenges," *PRS* 62:5 (November 1978), 671–675; Gilbert P. Gradinger, "The Roles and Goals of the American Society for Aesthetic Plastic Surgery," *PRS* 65:1 (January 1980), 72–73; Bernard L. Kaye, "Questions, Ruminations, and Illuminations: The State of the Society," *PRS* 68:5 (November 1981), 776–778; Leonard R. Rubin, "Advertising and PR Agents," *PRS* 69:1 (January 1982), 117–118; Arthur G. Ship, "To Advertise or Not to Advertise," *PRS* 74:1 (July 1984), 123; Robert M. Goldwyn, "Plastic Surgeons on the Make," *PRS* 75:2 (February 1985), 251–252; Robert Singer, "Advertising by Plastic Surgeons," *PRS* 80:5 (November 1987), 752; Carl Manstein, "Yellow Pages and False Credentials in Plastic Surgery," *PRS* 80:6 (December 1987), 870; Carl Manstein, "Marketing and Advertising: Different or the Same?" *PRS* 82:1 (July 1988), 202; Mark Gorney, "Who Is Responsible?" *PRS* 84:5 (November 1989), 801. Mark Holoweiko, "Is This the World Record for Malpractice Claims?" *Medical Economics* (April 17, 1989), 192–211, chronicles the case of Richard Dombroff's Personal Best clinics as a direct result, as does Laura Fraser's "The Cosmetic Surgery Hoax," *Glamour*, February 1990, 184–185, 220–224.

15. Hait, "History of the ASPRS," 69A, 86A.

16. Elizabeth Kaye, "The Case for a Polyester Face," *Savvy*, January 1986, 42–45; Holoweiko, "World Record for Malpractice Claims?"

17. Ibid.

18. *New York Times*, May 29, 1972, 22:1.

19. For examples of previous experiments with fat, see H. O. Bames, "Breast Malformations and a New Approach to the Problem of the Small Breast," *PRS* 5:6 (June 1950), 499; H. O. Bames, "Augmentation Mammaplasty by Lipo-Transplant," *PRS* 11:5 (May 1953), 404; Herbert Conway and James Smith, "Breast Plastic Surgery:

Reduction Mammaplasty, Mastopexy, Augmentation Mammaplasty and Mammary Construction," *PRS* 21:1 (January 1958), 8–14.

20. Susan Gerhardt, "The Beauty Morph," *San Francisco Bay Guardian,* February 2, 1994, 29–30; Sylvia Rubin, "Her Face Is a Work of Art," *San Francisco Chronicle,* February 4, 1994, C1, C16.

21. Gertrude Atherton, *Black Oxen* (New York: Boni and Liverwright, 1923), 142; *San Francisco Chronicle,* February 21, 1994, D7.

Illustration Credits

The author thanks the following individuals and organizations for permission to reproduce illustrations appearing on the indicated pages.

219   Archive Photos/Scott Harrison

222   *Hygeia,* American Medical Association, copyright 1931

248   *San Francisco Chronicle*

252   First published as "Dr. Jack Makes His Rounds, by Pierre Houles," in *Esquire Magazine,* May 1975. Reprinted courtesy of *Esquire Magazine* and the Hearst Corporation.

276   Archive Photos

291   Pamela Gentile

293   Cosmetic Surgery International

297   Dhome/SIPA

298   AP/Wide World Photos

299   REUTERS Joe Skipper/Archive Photos

Index

Page numbers for entries occurring in figure captions are followed by an *f*; note numbers are preceded by an *n*.

Haiken, Elizabeth.

    Venus envy: a history of cosmetic surgery / Elizabeth Haiken.

       p.   cm.

    Includes bibliographical references and index.

    ISBN 0-8018-5763-5 (cloth: alk. paper)

    1. Surgery, Plastic—Social aspects—United States.   2. Surgery, Plastic—United States—History.   3. Beauty, Personal—Social aspects—United States. 4. Surgery, Plastic—United States—Public opinion.   5. Public opinion—United States.   6. Beauty, Personal—United States—Public opinion.   I. Title.

    RD119.H35   1997

    617.9'5—dc21   97-19823

                                                       CIP